The Handbook of Microcomputer Applications in Communication Disorders

CONTRIBUTORS

Michael R. Chial, PhD
Department of Audiology and
  Speech Sciences
Michigan State University
East Lansing, MI 48823

Carol Cohen, MS
Schneier Communication Unit
Cerebral Palsy Center
Syracuse, NY 13104

Alan G. Galsky, PhD
Director, Office for
  Research and Sponsored Programs
Associate Dean, The Graduate School
Bradley University
Peoria, IL 61606

Stephen B. Hood, PhD
Professor and Chair, Department of
  Speech Language Pathology and
  Audiology
Bowling Green State University
Bowling Green, OH 43402

Elaine Z. Lasky, PhD
Professor, Department of Speech
  Pathology and Audiology
Cleveland State University
Cleveland, OH 44102

Robert B. Mahaffey, PhD
Director, Division of Speech and
  Hearing Sciences
University of North Carolina
Chapel Hill, NC 27514

Leland R. Miller, PhD
Professor and Chair, Department of
  Computer Sciences
Bowling Green State University
Bowling Green, OH 43402

James M. Mullendore, PhD
Dean, College of Health Sciences
Bradley University
Peoria, IL 61606

Gary E. Rushakoff, PhD
Speech & Hearing Clinic
New Mexico State University
Las Cruces, NM 88003

Arthur H. Schwartz, PhD
Director, Division of Speech and
  Hearing Sciences
Bradley University
Peoria, IL 61606

William M. Shearer, PhD
Professor, Department of Communicative
  Disorders
Northern Illinois University
De Kalb, IL 60115

Walter R. Wilkins, MS
Health Sciences Librarian
Bradley University
Peoria, IL 61606

Kent J. Wilson, PhD
Chief, Speech Pathology
Veteran's Administration Medical Center
Tucson, AZ 85749

The Handbook of Microcomputer Applications in Communication Disorders

Arthur H. Schwartz, Editor

Bradley University

Peoria, Illinois

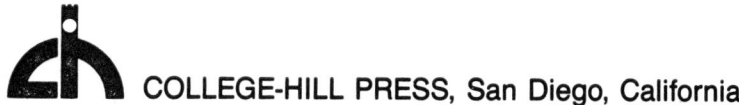
COLLEGE-HILL PRESS, San Diego, California

College-Hill Press, Inc.
4284 41st Street
San Diego, California 92105

© 1984 by College-Hill Press

All rights, including that of translation, reserved. No part of this publication may be reproduced, stored in a retrieval system, or transmitted in any form or by any means, electronic, mechanical, recording, or otherwise, without the prior written permission of the publisher.

Library of Congress Cataloging in Publication Data
Main entry under title:

The Handbook of microcomputer applications in communication disorders.

    Bibliography: p.
    Includes index.
    1. Communicative disorders—Data processing—Handbooks, manuals, etc. 2. Microcomputers—Handbooks, manuals, etc. I. Schwartz, Arthur H., 1942-
RC423.H326   1984   362.1'96855'02854   84-12716

ISBN 0-933014-13-9

Printed in the United States of America.

*I would like to dedicate this book
to my wife
Judi Schwartz
for putting up with the latest in
a series of causes and crusades.*

TABLE OF CONTENTS

CONTRIBUTORS	....	ii
DEDICATION	....	v
LIST OF FIGURES	....	xi
LIST OF TABLES	....	xii
PREFACE	....	xiii

SECTION I   **PREVIEW OR REVIEW**

Chapter 1   **Introduction to Microcomputers for Specialists in Communication Disorders**
Elaine Z. Lasky

Overview of Microcomputers and Applications for Speech-Language Pathologists and Audiologists ...	1
Essential Introductory Concepts	2
Administrative Applications	5
Clinical Applications	7
Instructional Applications........................	8
Trends: Microcomputer Technology, Accessibility, and Professional Issues	12

Chapter 2   **Implementing Microcomputer Applications**
Carol G. Cohen

Phases of Microcomputer Implementation	17
Implementing Microcomputers in Different Environments.................................	25
Before Implementing: Some Final Comments	31

SECTION II   **BASES FOR DECISIONS**

Chapter 3   **Funding Sources for Microcomputers**
Alan G. Galsky

Proposal Types	35
Considerations...................................	37
Information of Funding Opportunities..............	38
Proposal Generation	40

	Internal Proposal	44
	Funding Sources	45
Chapter 4	**Informational Resources, Systems, and Services** *Walter R. Wilkins*	
	Libraries	53
	Agencies and Associations	60
	Online Data Bases	62
	Consultants	67
	Users' Groups and Computer Clubs	70
	Dealers	72
	Training Sources	75
Chapter 5	**Evaluating Microcomputer Hardware** *Michael R. Chial*	
	Computers and Other Information Processors	79
	Evaluating Hardware Systems	81
	A General Architecture for Microcomputers	86
	Central Processing Units (CPUs)	86
	Communication Buses	92
	Memory Systems	93
	General Purpose Peripherals	99
	Interfaces	108
	Special Purpose Devices	111
	Implications for Communication Disorders	119
	The Marketplace and the Costs of Programs	120
Chapter 6	**Evaluating Microcomputer Software** *Arthur H. Schwartz*	
	Features of Microcomputer Software	126
	Steps in Software Evaluation	127
	Criteria for Software Selection	131
	Additional Software Considerations	140
	System Considerations	143
SECTION III	**MICROCOMPUTER APPLICATIONS**	
Chapter 7	**Clinical Applications in Communication Disorders** *Gary E. Rushakoff*	
	Rationale	147
	Historical Developments	149
	Hardware Needs	155
	Existing Clinical Applications	158
	Generating Clinical Reports	165
	Software Availability	166

	Limitations of Current Clinical Applications: Needs for Future Applications	167
	Clinician Microcomputer Education	168
Chapter 8	**Research Applications in Communication Disorders** *Robert B. Mahaffey*	
	A Research Framework	174
	Microcomputer Impacts on Research Directions	176
	Strategies for Research Applications	180
	Administrative Applications in Research	190
Chapter 9	**Academic and Instructional Applications for Microcomputers** *William M. Shearer*	
	The Microcomputer as Instructor Concept	193
	Applying Microcomputer Instruction	197
	A Microcomputer Instructional Program	202
	Instructional Languages for CAI	208
Chapter 10	**Administrative Applications for Microcomputers** *Stephen B. Hood and Leland R. Miller*	
	Administrative Functions: An Overview	219
	Mainframe Development of the Program............	221
	Custom Software Applications.....................	222
	Packaged Software Applications	233
SECTION IV	**A BROADER PERSPECTIVE**	
Chapter 11	**Issues and Controversies in the Use of Microcomputers** *Kent J. Wilson*	
	Computer Literacy	247
	Cyberphobia	248
	Issues in Selecting Software	250
	Controversies in Software Development	252
	Piracy	254
Chapter 12	**Microcomputer Applications: A Perspective in the Development of the Profession** *James M. Mullendore*	
	Reflections on the State of the Art	259
	Microcomputers in Perspective.....................	262
	Impact of the Microcomputer on the Profession	267

SECTION V	**MICROCOMPUTER TERMINOLOGY**	
Chapter 13	Glossary of Microcomputer Terms .... *Michael R. Chial*	275
Author Index	....	311
Subject Index	....	317

LIST OF FIGURES

Figure 3-1 Model of reverse pyramid structure for proposal preparation
Figure 4-1 Steps in systematic searching for information in a library
Figure 5-1 Generic architecture of a microcomputer
Figure 6-1 Five steps in the evaluation of applications software for microcomputers
Figure 6-2 Six factors to consider in evaluating microcomputer software
Figure 7-1 Garrett's automatic speech correction system
Figure 7-2 The /s/ meter as a dedicated device, circa 1964, and microcomputer version with speech recognition unit attached
Figure 7-3 Touch screen as an alternative to keyboard entry
Figure 7-4 Phonological Process Summary from Linquest 3 (from Palin & Mordecai, 1982; reprinted with permission)
Figure 7-5 Blissymbolics Bliss Drill (from Wertz, Kehrberg, & Wertz, 1982; reprinted with permission)
Figure 7-6 Lesson summary from First Words (from Fox & Wilson, 1982; reprinted with permission)
Figure 7-7 Lesson presentation from First Word (from Wilson & Fox, 1982; reprinted with permission)
Figure 8-1 Microcomputer and dedicated hardware that can be utilized for research applications (courtesy RC Electronics)
Figure 9-1 Diagram of computer-assisted instruction
Figure 9-2 CAI program listing for anatomy of the ear
Figure 9-3 CAI template outline

LIST OF TABLES

Table 1-1	Advantages of computer-assisted instruction
Table 2-1	Areas of consideration in the adoption of microcomputers in communication disorders
Table 2-2	Phases in the adoption of microcomputers
Table 2-3	Questions for consideration in deciding the need for microcomputers
Table 2-4	Personnel factors to consider when planning for microcomputers
Table 2-5	Final considerations
Table 3-1	Summary of proposal types
Table 3-2	Sections of a typical proposal
Table 3-3	Proposal checklist
Table 5-1	Comparison of selected features of five common central processing units (CPUs)
Table 6-1	Features of microcomputer software written in different levels of programming languages
Table 10-1	Student demographic and clinical data
Table 10-2	Clinical experience summary: Speech–language pathology
Table 10-3	Clinical experience summary: Audiology
Table 10-4	Client demographic data
Table 10-5	Billing invoice
Table 10-6	Clinic census data
Table 10-7	Selected examples of procedure codes and file maintenance
Table 10-8	Entering session data
Table 10-9	Spreadsheet example of five expense categories from three income sources
Table 10-10	Spreadsheet example of four clock hour categories for five student clinicians
Table 10-11	Equipment inventory–maintenance checks
Table 10-12	Employee personnel form
Table 10-13	Year and budget review: Total expenses
Table 10-14	Budget category summary for June
Table 10-15	Specific budget category summary for part-time student employment
Table 10-16	Specific budget category summary for part-time student employment
Table 10-17	Examples of printed output

PREFACE

Currently we are being bombarded with information about microcomputers. Newspapers, magazines, specialty periodicals, professional journals, specialty books, and advertising on radio and television allege that there is a revolution being created. Challenged by demands from employers, clients, funding agencies, and professional associations, we are legitimately asking if microcomputers can help us perform our roles. It is paradoxical that computers, which represent the most sophisticated technology, are publicized as easy to learn and use by nearly anyone for almost everything. The plethora of information about microcomputers seems awesome. Is this a legitimate or a media revolution? Are microcomputers a genuine technological improvement or merely a 1980s version of the CB fad? Are they as easy to use as claimed? Can they enable us to function more efficiently and productively? Will they put us out of jobs? Are the programs available for microcomputers nothing more than gimmicks? These and a host of other issues are immediately raised whenever an individual begins to give some thought to purchasing a microcomputer system.

HOW THE HANDBOOK CAME ABOUT

My own experience may be a typical example of the road traveled from confused observer to, however clumsy, a user of microcomputers. After reading brochures, talking to other users, and observing the performance of microcomputers, I proceeded to purchase one and obtain more intensive experience at trying to use it. As my proficiency developed, I found myself asking questions about specific applications that were pertinent to my area of specialization. Perhaps other specialists go through the same stages of progression. Without some accessible body of information, finding answers to these questions is difficult.

Information on microcomputer systems that seems pertinent to communication sciences and disorders has been scattered in a variety of places, most of which are not our own professional periodicals. Given a seeming void of information, I sensed a need for a centralized reference, no matter how quickly dated that reference might become. Out of this came the *Handbook of Microcomputer Applications*. Throughout my wanderings in the literature, a core of specialists who have been active in the use of microcomputers emerged. Communications with them revealed a similar concern for the lack of reference material on the topic as well as an interest and commitment to preparing a reference that reflected the state of the art in their area of expertise.

The handbook was prepared with the assumption that it would serve as the prototype reference for applications of microcomputers in communication sciences and disorders. It is logical to assume that topics, now treated as individual chapters or sections, will become monographs or books themselves as the information and knowledge based on that topic expands. Already there seems to be a nucleus of activity in specific areas that could justify a special book.

INTENDED AUDIENCE

This handbook was organized to address as broad an audience as possible. Attention has been given to trying to accommodate different levels of sophistication in microcomputer usage as well as diverse professional applications and environments. For individuals unfamiliar with microcomputers and beginning to wonder if these systems are legitimate, there is information in this book to orient them toward microcomputer functions and implementations. Similarly, the person with experience and proficiency using microcomputers will find several chapters relevant. Between these two levels (where most of us are at this time) is the thrust of this handbook. The handbook will be helpful for students, clinicians, and other specialists who have some knowledge and experience in using microcomputers and now want to find out how to exploit the technology.

HANDBOOK ORGANIZATION

The handbook is organized into five sections. Section 1 (Preview and Review) consists of two chapters that survey critical concepts regarding microcomputers. In Chapter 1, Lasky describes the components of microcomputer systems, their applications, and their uses. In a sense, this is an introductory chapter that surveys the entire content of the handbook. The focus of her chapter should enable the reader to answer the question, "What can microcomputers do?" Cohen's chapter on "Implementing Microcomputer Applications" suggests factors to be considered when installing a microcomputer system in different settings. Synthesizing information from a variety of sources, she presents a model for implementing microcomputer systems that will save time, effort, and false starts in selecting a microcomputer.

The second section (Bases for Decisions) organizes information and procedures to assist a specialist in making an intelligent and sensible decision about microcomputer systems. Four of the most commonly asked questions are (1) "How can I go about getting the funds to acquire a system?" (2) "Where can I find information about microcomputers, their components, and their applications?" (3) "What kind of equipment and instrumentation is needed to use a microcomputer?" (4) "What do I need to know about software to make the most intelligent use of the system?"

In his chapter on "Funding Sources for Microcomputers," Galsky (chap. 3) suggests possible sources for obtaining funds to purchase microcomputer systems. He reviews more commonly accessible sources and offers recommendations on preparing proposals for submission. For individuals unfamiliar with proposal writing, this chapter will provide a framework for developing and justifying microcomputer adoptions. In conjunction with Wilkins's chapter on informational resources, Galsky sets forth possible funding agencies (federal, state, local, and private) that might support the purchase of this technology. Besides funding sources, Wilkins ("Informational Resources and Services" —chap. 4) enumerates resources that can be consulted by specialists wanting to obtain information. Many of these resources are not commonly known. While many readers may be familiar with books, journals, and literature search services in university libraries, it is questionable whether the scope of resources available in state, local, or specialty libraries are widely known.

Once possible funding sources and strategies have been identified and information on systems has been located, the reader will need to know more about hardware and software. Frequently perceived as incomprehensibly technical, hardware is often the most intimidating aspect of microcomputers. Possibly because of the lack of explicit information about the applications of the hardware, it is frequently confusing to a novice trying to make decisions about which components are more appropriate. Working from his base as a communication sciences and disorders specialist, Chial provides a comprehensive and comprehensible explanation of the hardware and how it can be utilized by communication sciences and disorders specialists. Much of the literature on microcomputer systems presumes that software could be selected and then hardware should be obtained to operate the software. This premise needs to be questioned in the area of communication sciences and disorders. Many of the functions to be performed by microcomputer systems are software-driven, yet they are entirely contingent on the appropriate functioning of special input or output devices. The rule of "software before hardware" may not be applicable in communication sciences and disorders. For special application purposes, hardware has to be considered prior to the selection of software. It was for this reason that the chapter on hardware evaluation was deliberately placed ahead of the chapter on software evaluation. Following Chial's excellent survey of hardware, Schwartz (chap. 6) develops an approach to the selection of software. Much of the software currently available is overpriced, incomplete, poorly written, and simply does not perform the functions advertised. Given the high costs of software in communication sciences and disorders, it seems appropriate to be slightly cynical and highly skeptical when evaluating software. Despite the proliferation of pseudo-objective checklists and rating scales for microcomputer system software, most of these are superficial or only tangentially applicable to communication sciences. Schwartz defines principles and practices that can be followed in evaluating microcomputer software. These can be differentiated into two areas: *steps* involved in evaluating microcomputer software, and *principles* in the selection of microcomputer software. Concurrently with Chial's chapter, Schwartz imparts guidelines for software evaluation that assist users in making critical evaluations in order to utilize the system productively.

Section 3, intended as the core of the handbook, consists of four chapters focusing on current and future applications. In the preparation of this section, an assumption was made that there are four broad, overlapping areas of applications for microcomputers: clinical, administrative, instructional, and research. Depending upon the level of sophistication of the user, the setting, and the need, both commercially and specially adapted systems should be applied. In the time since the book was conceived, the interest in microcomputer applications in communication disorders has literally exploded to the point that any of the four topics within this section will, within a short time, have sufficient information available to justify elaborated monographs or textbooks.

Chapter 7 ("Clinical Applications") furnishes information about microcomputer systems used in the assessment and management of speech–language and hearing impairments in children and adults. While not intended to endorse specific products or programs, Rushakoff's chapter highlights some of the currently available software and hardware used in the clinical management of communication disorders. Mahaffey's chapter ("Research Applications") is not a chapter on statistical design nor special research instrumentation. Rather, he offers an approach for using microcomputers in research. Mahaffey concentrates on the impact that microcomputers can have on enabling specialists to ask questions, find new ways to study events, bridge the gap between clinician and researcher, and introduce some of the strategies that can be utilized in modifying existing technology to work with microcomputers. As the field of artificial intelligence expands and expert systems software becomes available, there will be programs that will guide the microcomputer user to ask answerable questions and set up designs. Given the portability of microcomputer systems and the availability of such expert systems software, it is possible that in the future, any practitioner will be capable of asking viable questions and conducting systematic and rigorous studies of aspects of communicative behavior using microcomputers.

"Instructional Applications" (chap. 9) by Shearer presents concepts that are of relevance to academicians and clinicians in settings where microcomputers could be used to develop computer-assisted instruction (CAI). Reviewing some of the appropriate and inappropriate applications of CAI, he proceeds to illustrate how some of the common software languages can be used to develop innovative and effective instruction to augment existing methods. Shearer explores strategies for developing computer-assisted instruction and explains the advantages and limitations of this format. Existing instructional programs in communication sciences and disorders are discussed and implications for the future development of this powerful pedagogical tool are presented.

Throughout the three chapters on applications, administrative uses for microcomputers are mentioned. However, in their chapter, Hood and Miller (chap. 10—"Administrative Applications") carefully examine the uses of microcomputers for monitoring and evaluating record keeping, financial matters, report writing, and information retrieval. Probably more than any other area, applications are the most advanced due to the availability of general-purpose software that can be adapted for administrative purposes. Hood and Miller explain a custom program developed on a minicomputer and discuss how microcomputer programs now perform segments of that program. Using microcomputers for administrative functions provides ease of accessibility, flexibility for formatting information, and saves time and effort. The information they discuss is of particular relevance to students, academicians, clinicians, or administrators who are faced with a deluge of paperwork and limited time to manage it.

The fourth section (Broader Perspectives) steps back and takes a view of some of the issues, controversies, and considerations in the applications of microcomputers. In our enthusiasm to adopt this new technology, it is possible that we may overapply this tool. Could there be a backlash against microcomputers similar to the one against teaching machines in the 1960s? Are microcomputers good for everything? Both chapters within this section explore the issues and questions and try to place microcomputers within a perspective in our field. Wilson (chap. 11) examines issues facing practitioners using microcomputers. How much knowledge and programming skill is necessary to use microcomputers? Of particular relevance is Wilson's discussion of legal aspects of microcomputers. He provides a succinct overview of the legal aspects of software usage, differentiating between legitimate archival copying and piracy. His discussion should enable practitioners to understand some of the problems faced by both users and developers regarding microcomputer software. As a capstone to the handbook, Mullendore (chap. 12) looks at the application of microcomputers from the perspective of over 35 years as a practicing clinician, researcher, academician, and administrator. In such a context, microcomputers could be regarded as a logical evolution in the application of technology to the management of communication disorders rather than the revolution touted by magazines and other media. Indeed, Mullendore raises vexing questions regarding the effect of microcomputers on services delivered, individuals providing services, and the justification for existing approaches. It is fitting to end a handbook that is designed to provide the direction for microcomputer applications with such a chapter that urges a balancing of euphoria with an appreciation of our heritage and the challenges that are to be met in the future.

The last section of the handbook consists of a single chapter containing over 400 definitions of terms that readers are likely to encounter. In chap. 13, Chial defines, many times with the addition of perspective and humor, the technical terminology used by microcomputer specialists. Earlier, Wilson (chap. 11) discussed the intimidating effect of "computerese" on novice users. Chial's chapter, with definitions that have been translated to apply to communication sciences and disorders, assists in demystifying many of the terms so glibly tossed about in the media and by microcomputer salespeople, yet so seldom defined. Using this glossary as a reference, specialists should have the information needed to answer questions regarding aspects of microcomputer applications.

ACKNOWLEDGMENTS

I express my gratitude to the students, faculty, and professional staff in the College of Health Sciences at Bradley University for their assistance in the preparation of this handbook. I owe my appreciation to Rosalie Hagaman for her encouragement and willingness to take the time to make telephone calls, run copies, or help with the numerous tasks associated with the production of this handbook. Cathy Carrara, Liz Foreman, Karen Koczot, and Anne Wickert are commended for their interest and assistance in the tedious preparation of the indexes. In addition, I thank Pat Knight for her willingness to type long manuscripts with little lead time. Finally, a note of thanks is offered to Karl Martin of Wallace Micromart, who has shown the utmost patience in answering a myriad of my naive questions. He willingly provided his time, knowledge, and help to answer questions and teach me how to get software to perform. This is the kind of service that most dealers advertise but relatively few provide.

A special note of appreciation is offered my brother, Jim Schwartz, Bill Berdine, Jim Nation, and Bill Scott for their unwavering faith and support before and during this endeavor. Without their encouragement and my wife's patience and tolerance, this handbook could neither have been initiated nor completed.

Finally, I acknowledge each of the contributors of this volume. Their willingness to commit to paper what exists in the minds of a smaller group of specialists who have seen the potential of this technology and forged ahead to develop a body of knowledge will make the journey easier and faster for those who follow. The fact that this project was completed with such harmony is a reflection of both the importance of the topic and of the caliber of people involved. It indeed has been a privilege to learn from them.

From a selfish point of view, this handbook was undertaken so that I could learn more about things that I did not know. As a result, not only have I learned much of what I sought, but I have made new friends and colleagues. Needless to say I have found that, although I have answered some of my questions and learned a great deal, I now have more questions. Indeed, as the prototypical reader of this handbook, I have learned enough not just to understand and appreciate what is being done with microcomputers, but to begin to comprehend the power and flexibility of this tool to help me work smarter.

A. H. Schwartz
Peoria, Illinois
April 2, 1984

SECTION I
PREVIEW OR REVIEW

Chapter 1

Introduction to Microcomputers for Specialists in Communication Disorders

Elaine Z. Lasky

OVERVIEW OF MICROCOMPUTERS AND APPLICATIONS FOR SPEECH-LANGUAGE PATHOLOGISTS AND AUDIOLOGISTS

By whatever criterion is selected as a measurement, an explosion can be observed in microcomputer technology and its applications. Articles relating to the effects of microcomputers appear routinely in virtually every type of periodical. Most people have recognized the increasing involvement of the microcomputer in their lives through their pay checks, utility bills, supermarket transactions, and files regarding aspects of medical, educational, work, and credit records. Many of the recent microcomputer applications, however, could not have been imagined even a few years ago by those not working with computers. Microcomputers can allow an individual to sketch a landscape or draw a house plan, diagnose an illness, play and write music, teach and play games even with small children, write and modify personal and business letters and papers, keep track of telephone numbers and addresses, recipes, or items in any storage unit, teach academic material, provide individualized instruction, analyze test results, and synthesize speech. For specialists in communication disorders, activities as diverse as maintaining client schedules, analyzing diagnostic test performance, generating progress or diagnostic reports, presenting language concepts, or providing varieties of communication devices for the severely impaired can be performed quickly and accurately. Applications for enhancing the communication, work, and recreation opportunities for the handicapped are just beginning to be explored.

The purpose of this chapter and the purpose of this book is to provide a reference regarding the nature, applications, and potential for microcomputers for speech-language and hearing. This chapter presents an overview of the components and functions of microcomputers for communication disorders. Topics discussed include: What does a speech-language pathologist or audiologist need to know? How much does a user need to know? Is it necessary to be computer-literate to make decisions about costs and possible ways to implement the technology? An introduction of some of the administrative functions that can be easily facilitated via a microcomputer is presented here and expanded by Hood and Miller (see chap. 10). Administrative applications include functions such as: record keeping for clients, students, and staff; billing; generating letters, reports, or individualized educational programs (IEPs); passing and protecting

©College-Hill Press, Inc. All rights, including that of translation, reserved. No part of this publication may be reproduced without the written permission of the publisher.

stored data. A survey of some instructional applications is presented here and amplified by Shearer (see chap. 9). Clinical functions introduced include assessment and diagnostic procedures that may be administered or analyzed by microcomputer. Intervention and teaching applications are highlighted, from those that are directed to the client with mild disorders to those developed for clients with severe impairments to those for the student in training in communication disorders. This is enlarged by Rushakoff (see chap. 7). Attention is drawn to considerations relating to updating skills and continuing education for the professional in the field. The last section of this chapter summarizes some of the trends in microcomputer technology and the effect on professional issues.

ESSENTIAL INTRODUCTORY CONCEPTS

Skills needed

Do clinicians, researchers, or academicians have to know how a microcomputer works to know *how to put it to work?* Not necessarily! It is not necessary to know how a television, video or audio tape recorder, or microwave oven works in order to use it. Professionals do need to know enough so that they are not intimidated by microcomputers. They must learn enough about components and operations to make informed decisions about the usefulness of various hardware devices and software that are available. Enough information needs to be known to begin to ask some questions, gain information and evaluate that information, and be able to run a program from a disk. If an individual or group needs to make decisions regarding purchasing specific types of equipment or programs, then specific information must be obtained and studied. If a specialist wants to adapt or modify any of the software programs to meet the individualized needs of selected clients or to handle specific office procedures, then the level of information and skills needed is further raised. If the user wants to prepare materials—develop programs—then, again, a higher level of knowledge is required. There are various levels of knowledge necessary to interact with a microcomputer depending on the intentions of the user. One should not assume that it is necessary to learn to program a microcomputer to *begin* to use some of the materials available.

The first six chapters of this handbook examine topics to enable communication-disorders specialists to make decisions related to the acquisition and implementation of microcomputer systems for different purposes in a variety of settings. An overview is presented in this chapter; the topics are covered in greater depth in the succeeding chapters.

Hardware

Hardware involves all equipment including the wires, cables, and plugs connecting the components. The *central processing unit* (CPU) is the microprocessor that controls, stores information, and performs all the computation and logic functions. To communicate with the CPU, input devices are needed. With a keyboard the user can enter information one character (symbol or letter) at a time. A joystick, a lever-like device, can be used to enter or input information and is frequently used to select an item or move an object on the monitor screen, as in a game. Control knobs, paddles, light pens, and various other devices have been developed as simpler input devices (see Chial, chap. 5). Other input devices include pads or tablets on which the user can draw or select a response from a display on the monitor. Some microcomputers can be equipped to recognize voice input while others have a touch-sensitive screen. Various input adaptations are available to make access possible by the very young or the handicapped. Specific adaptive devices are discussed in fuller detail by Rushakoff (see chap. 7 on clinical applications.)

Audiotape cassette players can be used to input previously stored information. Similarly, a disk drive can read or enter stored information into the CPU from the magnetic (record) disk or floppy disk.

Once that information has been entered into the CPU, devices are needed for the output. The *monitor* is a screen specifically developed for microcomputer display, although a television screen may be used. The monitor is an output device that provides an ongoing visual display of the information entered (e.g., the user's typing or drawing from the keyboard), the CPU's calculations, or segments of the information stored on the floppy disk (e.g., programs, data). A printer is also an output device. The CPU can direct information displayed on the monitor, stored in memory, or stored on a disk to be printed on paper by the printer. Other output devices of specific interest in communication disorders include tone generators, music synthesizers, speech synthesizers, *X-Y* plotters, and signal generators. A MOdulator/DEModulator or *MODEM* provides a link for one microcomputer to communicate with another via standard telephone receivers and telephone lines.

Although taking considerable space in memory, much-improved speech synthesizers allow speech reproduction that does not have a "computer accent." (See for example, Stolker, 1983.) The use of an audiocassette player for reproducing speech can certainly produce high-quality speech, although a problem arises with accessing the playback. With an audiotape cassette, the tape must be wound forward or back to search sequentially for the desired speech signal. If data are stored on a disk or in memory, a random access approach is significantly easier and more rapid than the mechanical access necessary with the audio tape. Newer, improved speech synthesizers offer outstanding potential for generating quality speech stimuli for programs for remediation.

Software

Software comprises the sets of instructions necessary to govern activities of the microcomputer. Packaged software programs are available that instruct the microcomputer to do a variety of tasks. Most of these programs are *interactive*, that is, the user must respond by entering data at certain times. The responses of the CPU are dependent upon the program and the information entered by the user. Programs designed for remediation may present an item that requires the client to select a picture or a word. Following the response, the microcomputer indicates whether the response was correct or incorrect. If correct, another item can be presented; if incorrect, a clue may be supplied or an explanation presented. When the client completes all the items, the number correct and number incorrect may be tallied and displayed.

Many software programs start out with a menu, or table of contents, listing the options of activities within the total package. The desired option can be selected by pressing a specified key. Often the first section of the menu is a tutorial program that teaches the user how to use the rest of the program. A combination of instructions, diagrams, or graphs appear on the monitor to guide the user. This information is similar to the programmed texts of the 1960s. Branching routines, depending on the type and frequency of the user's errors, may be available to assist the user in mastering the program content.

A few software constraints need to be identified. One: different brands of microcomputers do not use the same language. Special languages have been developed for different purposes, users, or hardware. BASIC (Beginner's All-purpose Symbolic Instruction Code) is a software language that is not difficult to learn and yet has some sophisticated capabilities. COBOL (COmmon Business-Oriented Language) was developed for business applications; FORTRAN (FORmula TRANslations) and ALGOL (ALGOrhythmic Language) were originally developed for science and math applications. Some other languages used for microcomputer software include FORTH, Pascal, and LOGO. Programs currently available for use on microcomputers by those in communication disorders are frequently written in BASIC.

Two: Not all computers use the same dialect of a particular language. Many of the microprocessors can run on software programmed in BASIC, but the software written in BASIC for one system generally cannot be read by a different system. Similarly, the operating system for one microcomputer is not identical to the operating system for a different computer (see Schwartz, chap. 6). The operating system provides the instructions necessary to perform all operations to use the microcomputer. Whatever software is purchased must be compatible with the operating system of the user's microcomputer. Most software, then, is device specific at this time.

Some brands of microcomputers are considered to be clones of other microcomputers. Software programs written for one microcomputer will operate on any clones of that microcomputer. Many software programs are written specifically for a particular microcomputer while others have modifications for different computers. These are so advertised and listed, but it is necessary to carefully examine the ads and the labels.

Three: Some software is called "user friendly." This characteristic refers to routines in the package that guide the user in learning the program's features and operations, provide further assistance if requested by the user, and confirm the user's intentions before executing certain functions (e.g., clear memory, write new data over previously stored data).

These and other software considerations are discussed in depth by Schwartz (chap. 6). Information on software features is important for making decisions about purchasing selected hardware.

Gaining information

Initial attempts to obtain information by scanning through catalogues and listings of hardware and software, talking to salespersons at computer stores, or reading through microcomputer publications can be frustrating, confusing, and intimidating. The technical jargon bombarding users is abstract and requires some familiarity. The number of new concepts is large; some concepts are defined by other equally unfamiliar terms; and the terminology may not make much sense until a user has some direct opportunity to operate and interact with a microcomputer. While current manuals are *much* improved over earlier versions, the information in the manual is more comprehensible and valuable after some experience in using the program or the system.

An additional problem related to the state of the art is that salespersons in local microcomputer shops may or may not be knowledgeable about hardware, software, or applications for speech–language and audiology. The advice of more than one person should be sought; publications should be read, other users need to be consulted, and user groups should be investigated (see Wilkins, chap. 4).

Speech pathologists and audiologists may eventually wonder whether it is necessary to learn one or more of the languages to prepare programs for a microcomputer. This depends on individual and organizational needs and interests. Understanding the concept of programming through writing and designing programs may take time and effort. Some initial experience with simple programs can enable the specialist to internalize the task and/or acquire some skills in adapting a program for applications specific to a particular setting or client.

Introductory workshops can be very helpful, but they will *NOT* take the place of the direct involvement of sitting down in front of a microcomputer, turning it on, loading a program, and working through it. This can be simple or more difficult depending on what is selected as the initial program. Newer programs seem to be becoming easier to learn to use.

Microcomputer fairs or exhibits provide an opportunity to sample available hardware and software. The software emphasis may not be specifically applicable for use in communication disorders and hardware designed for the handicapped may not be shown unless the fair is sponsored by organizations with persons serving the handicapped (e.g., special education, American Speech, Language, and Hearing Association). Some local microcomputer stores provide opportunities to sample hardware and software; many have classes to teach introductory skills. At this time, one national chain provides up to 30 hours of free hands-on instruction for individuals who have a letter indicating their involvement with some aspect of education.

Wilkins (see chap. 4) describes a variety of resources to be consulted, including Special Education Regional Resource Centers (SERRC), colleges, and continuing education centers for information on microcomputer classes or sessions requiring various levels of proficiency. SERRCs and consortiums of schools may serve as libraries for users to borrow complete programs or disks containing sample segments of programs to try. Some centers also have a copy service for reproducing programs that are within the public domain.

Another source for surveying the market is the plethora of publications in bookstores and computer stores. Magazines are published with specialized emphases such as business, education, hobbyist, and game. Ads and reviews of hardware and software are informative and demonstrate clearly the range of equipment and programs on the market. Prices vividly portray the competitive nature of the market. Discounts on popular programs are listed. Spinoffs with slight modifications in name and program appear at fractions of the original cost. Consulting firms offer services to help adapt programs for specialized needs. The reviews and articles do not obviate the need to become sufficiently informed to make decisions, but they do offer information and creative approaches to solving problems that specialists will find helpful. A recent issue of *Consumer Reports* (Sept., 1983) elaborated advantages and disadvantages of purchasing through mail-order discount suppliers. Respondents to their questionnaire and reports from consumer affairs offices sampled generally reported satisfaction with either retail or mail-order suppliers.

For the novice, there is much to explore. There are, however, many resources available to support this effort.

ADMINISTRATIVE APPLICATIONS

What are the kinds of administrative applications that may be considered? How helpful are they? Are they expensive? Are they necessary? Do they help in professional decision making? This section introduces this topic with a few examples and a few cautions. Hood and Miller (chap. 10) provide extensive details about administrative applications of microcomputers.

The professional records in communication disorders may be divided into those necessary for maintaining clinical information and those necessary for maintaining academic and training information regarding student classes and clinical practice. Clinical applications are reviewed first.

For any client, records must be kept of quantitative data for billing purposes, for monitoring procedures administered and progress made, and for generating reports. These data are kept in various formats.

How much time is currently used in documenting, recording, and retrieving these records for individual clients? What kinds of reports need to be sent? To whom? Can records be maintained with less time and greater ease by using microcomputerized procedures?

Many administrative questions asked by speech–language pathologists or audiologists are business functions and are similar to those related to automating individual files in medical offices, dental offices, and hospital settings. Software programs are available to adapt and set up specialized client files. Data can be entered for filing, for storage, for billing, and for subsequent report generation. Numerous software packages have been developed to handle the financial operations (accounting/spreadsheet procedures) necessary to run a clinic.

Other data-processing procedures can be adapted for special application. Project Special (Oltman, 1983) is one model of a microcomputer-based information management system related to special education needs. The amount of time professional staff must spend in performing clerical tasks is reduced so that planning and direct intervention time with clients can be increased. The project was developed by the Educational Testing Service, school districts of Mercer County, New Jersey, and the New Jersey Department of Education. Maintaining pupil records is one component of the group of programs in the system. Special filing procedures add, delete, modify, and display information, including identifying information (e.g., name, address, date of birth), due process information (e.g., referral, classification, and conference information), evaluation data (e.g., tests administered, scores, comments, messages), and program information (e.g., school, class, related services). Measures are included to protect privacy and limit access to files.

A report-generation and transmission program extracts information from these records and generates the reports necessary for local, county, and state departments. A special option termed "Ad Hoc Inquiry" gives professional staff options to compose other reports as needed. The mailing label program generates address labels to facilitate mailing of reports to parents. One program can generate letters to parents or progress reports to other professionals.

Catalogues of microcomputer software offer programs that are adaptable for communication specialists. Programs can be adapted to set up files so that the data can be entered, updated, merged, or deleted into appropriate files on a continuing basis.

Obtaining input from professional colleagues and support staff is critical when selecting any microcomputer system or procedure (see Cohen, chap. 2). If those who must use the procedure or system do not see it as an advantage, full use will not be made of it. Any applied technology must make less work for professional and support staff.

Cost factors must be considered when using microcomputers for administrative purposes. The base price of a microcomputer may comprise less than half of the total cost. Acquisitions of add-ons or peripherals such as speech synthesizers, printers, graphics tablets, or MODEMs to serve important applications must be anticipated. Costs of the software and operating supplies should be tallied. In addition, the time and expense of training staff has to be calculated. Most of these costs are not ongoing, but rather are start-up costs that save in the long term—if the system is needed, used, and properly implemented.

Administrative functions to maintain academic and professional training records for students may be set up relatively easily and inexpensively using commercially available software. Setting up a microprocessor within a college department and, when greater memory is needed, hooking into the university's minicomputer or mainframe computer is usually feasible. Most computer centers within universities are willing to provide technical assistance if the user attempts to become somewhat conversant with the task, materials, and equipment at hand.

Among the earliest administrative applications of computers to communication disorders were those set up by departments to maintain records regarding students' clinical experiences. Files are set up and automatically updated as new data on student hours are entered. A listing can be readily obtained that documents clinical experiences including number or units of client-contact hours, type of disorders, type of activity (e.g., diagnostic, therapy) site or location of the activity, and supervisor. Performance evaluation information can be added in various formats from checklist ratings to longer comments. Hood and Miller (chap. 10) describe how one such system developed on a minicomputer can be adapted for a microcomputer.

Decision making for clinics, hospitals, or universities requires the examination and analysis of selected aspects of an operation. Specialized programs can be developed or adapted to facilitate this task. Hixson (1983), for example, proposes using a personal computer and several packaged statistical analysis programs to make projections regarding marketing of hearing aids. Information can be analyzed that is critical for effective budgeting and planning. She argues that, although helpful, it is not essential that an administrator be able to program a computer, only that the administrator be able to enter the requested data—data, for example, reflecting number of unit sales, styles, and demographic information related to purchasers.

Administration of any facility requires handling, storing, and using data in a myriad of ways. Microprocessors can facilitate many of these functions.

CLINICAL APPLICATIONS

Client assessment

The great speed, accuracy, and patience of a microcomputer become useful in a variety of clinical tasks. The analysis of diagnostic instruments and the preparation of diagnostic reports are especially suitable clinical applications. In this section a few such applications are reviewed.

Sonies and Larkins (1982) reported on a computerized assessment system developed by the speech pathology service of the National Institutes of Health (NIH), Clinical Center, Department of Rehabilitation Medicine, to report information more efficiently, retrieve data for purposes of accountability, and disseminate information with greater facility. While this system uses a mainframe computer, it can be adapted for use with a microprocessor. A master evaluation matrix is used into which is fed the type of evaluation performed, objective findings, and subjective comments. Data are stored in a patient's file and can be readily updated. A standard reporting format is established so that systematic record-keeping facilitates the generation of clinical reports. The procedure expedites reporting to referral agencies or other professionals, reduces clinician time spent on writing and proofreading the report, and provides data to determine quality of patient care and cost effectiveness.

Harlan (1983) developed software to accept, store, retrieve, and report case history information and audiologic test results for adult clients. Other programs function similarly so data can be entered in response to requests regarding case history data and test results for children referred for speech–language pathology evaluation. The program automatically compares an individual's performance to stored normative data. Performance on a test can be reported and printed out in various formats such as percentiles or thresholds.

Katz (1983) found it helpful to explain a client's hearing loss and present remedial actions available by using a graphic display on the video monitor. He reported improvement in service *and* time-saving advantages in simulating hearing aid fitting options by comparing manufacturers' specifications of various hearing aids in combination with various types of ear molds. These data are then compared to a patient's hearing loss via a computer program. Relative to a clinician's making these comparisons manually, the microcomputer makes these analyses easier, faster, and with less chance of error.

Software is available from several publishers that allows the user to enter raw scores from subtests of specific tests, such as the Wechsler Intelligence Scale for Children (R) or The Woodcock–Johnson Psychoeducational Battery. The client's performance is analyzed to evaluate strengths and weaknesses in relation to variables such as normative data, scores on other tests, chronological age, and grade level. An individualized report is generated that describes and analyzes performance and suggests specific intervention strategies. Certainly the human diagnostician could produce the report; the computerized analysis, however, is faster, easier to obtain, and cheaper in professional hours. The program considers many aspects of the client's performance and frees the diagnostician from hours of repetitious paper work—providing the program was prepared properly.

Several software packages are commercially available that generate individual educational programs (IEPs). Interactive in nature, the program requests identifying information, test scores, meeting dates, and professionals involved. A printed output can be prepared that includes listings of components required by law, identification data, results of testing, meetings, and previous reports indicating intra-individual differences in performance and current levels of functioning. Options to select goals and objectives in specified academic and/or developmental ability areas and a bank of hundreds of possible short-term and long-term instructional objectives are available. Objectives can be selected by the clinician to reflect students' strengths and/or weaknesses.

A potentially useful clinical development is adaptive testing for persons with speech-language and/or hearing problems. Adaptive testing tailors a test or procedure to the individual (Wainer, 1983). The procedure utilizes a method of determining the level of difficulty of items and the microcomputer quickly selects those items most closely matching the client's ability (Wainer, 1983). The client's time and energy are not wasted with many items that are too easy nor does he become frustrated with items that are too hard. This procedure can be valuable in a number of areas with clients with communication disorders, especially those with problems of attention or those easily upset and frustrated (e.g., those with aphasia, learning disabilities, or mental retardation). A large supply of prepared questions or activities at selected levels of difficulty can be coded and stored. After the client's initial responses, the program evaluates the level of difficulty of correct and incorrect responses plus the response time and hones in and presents items at the client's level of performance at that time. Voice-synthesized items or videotaped segments can be utilized to vary the session and evaluate different response modes. These testing procedures use the microprocessor's capability to perform tedious statistical analysis rapidly and accurately.

INSTRUCTIONAL APPLICATIONS

Applications for instruction cover a spectrum from synthesizing speech sounds for nonvocal persons to producing braille to teaching academic coursework. Microcomputers have been used in a variety of ways to enhance learning. Computer-assisted instruction (CAI) provides tutorial drill, simulation, or problem-solving approaches to intervention that may be designed specifically for a normal or impaired learner. Early use of CAI did not catch on or even begin to approach expectations. Nickerson (1982) argues that carefully designed CAI programs used under appropriate conditions offer certain advantages over traditional educational or remedial approaches of comparable cost.

What can CAI offer?

The learning situation can be adapted to specific needs of the individual. Interactive software can be utilized to keep a client actively involved at his or her optimum level of challenge. The response mode can be altered if a keyboard is not usable by handicapped children or adults.

Activities can be self-paced. Software can be prepared and modified to allow the subject to set the rate at which stimuli are presented and responses are required. This is of particular importance for the communicatively impaired. Throughout the literature, reference is made to the poor performance of speech- and language-impaired individuals with rapidly presented

Table 1-1 Advantages of Computer-Assisted Instruction (CAI)

1. The learning situation can be readily *adapted* to the specific needs of the individual learner.
2. Activities can be *self-paced*.
3. *Branching* tasks can be added.
4. Immediate *feedback* is provided.
5. The computer is infinitely *patient*.
6. *Interaction* with the computer is highly motivating.
7. Engaged *time-on-task* is increased.
8. *Stimuli* can be increasingly varied.
9. Use of *examples* and analogies can be increased.
10. Fine motor *control* and eye–hand control can be developed through a number of computerized activities.

---

items. Controlling the rate of presentation has been shown to facilitate performance. Programs can allow clinician or learner control of the pace.

Branching tasks can be developed as needed. If a client demonstrates mastery over a task, she or he progresses to the next appropriate level of difficulty. If performance is inadequate, more items, a lower level item, or special supplementary instruction needs to be provided. If a lack of understanding in any aspect of the task is indicated, the learner can select a branch for additional work in the necessary area.

Immediate feedback can be provided. Whether it is the answer to a question or the initial attempts at solving a problem, the learner is shown immediately if the response is correct or incorrect. There is general agreement as to the value of knowing immediately if a response is correct and of being guided through a process and corrected if performance is in error.

Care must be taken, however, in determining what is reinforcing and what is not. Some severely and profoundly impaired persons reportedly enjoyed the supposedly negative acoustic feedback associated with Pacman being eaten. The clients liked the sounds of losing and did not grasp the negative implication.

The microcomputer can be infinitely patient. Learners can review and move along at their own rate. No verbal or nonverbal punitive statements need be encountered by the learner. The professional needs to monitor this, however, since there have been reports of software that flashes, "Dummy!" if the user makes more than a few errors.

Motivation has been a major aspect of the newer instructional software. The almost addictive quality of computer games for some children has been detailed in the popular media and has led to civil ordinances prohibiting use of computer video games during selected hours. Educational software is relatively new and, for some children and adults, it, too, is almost addictive. The color, sound, and movement on the monitor attracts, excites, and maintains a client's interest.

McCorkell (1983) discussed uses of the microcomputer with developmentally disabled adults in teaching living skills. Some persons found the interaction with the program so highly satisfying and motivating that there was difficulty in getting students away from the microcomputer when it was time to quit. Papert (1980) and Weir, Russell, and Valente (1982) cite examples of motivated interaction and progress with children of all ages and abilities. Particularly dramatic was the progress made by children with autism, cerebral palsy, and learning disabilities in using the LOGO language.

Engaged time-on-task is reported to be the critical aspect of learning. Nickerson (1982) has suggested that the longer the learning activity maintains a student's interest, the greater the learning—both as related to the learning of the task itself *AND* as it affects learning to *ATTEND*. It is not as much *time* on task but, rather, *engaged* time—time that is spent actively interacting with the task, that is important. The more actively engaged the learner is, the more that is learned (Walk, 1978). The deeper the level of processing (i.e., no superficial or trivial responses required), the more learned and remembered (Jacoby & Craik, 1979). Effective microcomputer programs engage the learner frequently, actively, and deeply, and hold promise for increasing skills, information, and concepts.

Stimuli can be increasingly varied. Stimuli that are most meaningful and motivating for the student should be used. With the newer software packages developed to generate high-quality, more realistic graphics, more varied stimuli can be used. Videotape segments, improved speech synthesizers, and improved music synthesizers can provide new dimensions to augment instructional microcomputer programs.

Simulation of examples and analogies is possible with CAI. More examples that are meaningful and familiar can be used as stimuli in the preparation of any procedure. As a consequence, the maintenance and generalization of the learning is more likely.

Fine motor control and eye-hand control can be developed through a number of computerized activities. Programs have been prepared that teach eye-hand coordination through control of a joystick (Heyer et al., 1983). Even severely retarded adults have been able to work through a variety of movements leading to mastery of selected skills. Controlling the joystick and recognizing the relationship between movement of the joystick and movement of an object on the monitor was the first step.

All of the above advantages of using CAI are possible. A major problem at this time appears to be the limited amount of high-quality educational software especially for nonreaders and those who will not become readers. There are no standards regarding quality of educational software. Increasing numbers of programs are being produced for the special child, however, and many programs can be adapted to suit the needs and skill level of the impaired child. Schwartz (chap. 6) delves into this topic more deeply and presents criteria by which the user can select software.

What kinds of CAI programs have been developed?

Tutorial

Instructional packages have been categorized according to the major goal of the program. Some present new information to the learner using a *tutorial* approach. Examples of this tutorial method are those programs that teach a programming language, typing, or present a new concept. Programs are currently available to teach shape discrimination and letter recognition, basic concepts (Lasky et al., 1983), numbers, addition, and to plot numbers on a grid and graph (Raleigh, 1983). First-year algebra can be taught with available software, as can logic, grammar, and aspects of history. Other programs present tutorial approaches to flying an airplane or sailing. Tutorial programs could be prepared to teach college students audiometric testing, how to perform and interpret a language sample, sections of anatomy and physiology, hearing and speech science, and research methods. A tutorial program for a language-delayed client may teach selected concepts or introduce adjectives or pronouns. A few programs directed at preschool children are tutorials for teaching letters of the alphabet or concepts related to numbers and counting skills.

Drill and practice

Drill and practice programs provide exactly that: drill and practice with activities such as comprehension of vocabulary or comprehension or production of syntactical constructions. Drill and practice or tutorial programs can be directed to the college student in communication disorders or training or to the client. Computer Users in Speech and Hearing (CUSH), an ad hoc committee of the American Speech, Language, and Hearing Association, distributes a list of programs prepared to provide both tutoring and drill and practice for language-delayed children or for children or adults who have sustained brain damage. Undoubtedly more and more materials will become available. Extreme care must be taken, however, in evaluating the quality, costs, and usability of software (see Mullendore, chap. 12). Some of the drill and practice routines can provide little more than expensive electronic workbooks. High-quality interactive drill and practice routines require creativity and sophistication from the developer.

Simulation

Taber (1983) describes several uses of simulations: to substitute for an activity when necessary equipment is unobtainable; to substitute for experience; to provide exposure to a situation but collapse the time scale and eliminate the danger. One such simulation program called *Oregon* was developed, evaluated, and revised over a period of years through a statewide effort in Minnesota to effectively implement computers into the schools. *Oregon* simulates a trip by wagon cross-country and includes all of the adversities one might encounter on such a trip.

Programming the microcomputer

Some writers have argued that a user should be able to take control rather than being controlled by the microcomputer (e.g., Moursund, 1981; Papert, 1980). Learning to program a computer can be an activity that enables the learner to develop problem-solving strategies, specific cognitive skills, and acquire the programming language itself.

Papert (1980) argues that in many applications, microcomputers are being used to program the child. Rather, he sees the child as the programmer of the computer. He has designed a programming language, LOGO, as a natural way of thinking, communicating, and learning by using a computer. To think, and to think about thinking, Papert developed an object to think with: a turtle. Programming is introduced as the child exercises control and commands the turtle to move. The interaction of the movement of the object on the screen with commands entered by the child introduces the child to concepts about microcomputers and concepts about space and spatial relations. The LOGO language contains a powerful set of graphics and increasingly sophisticated programming capabilities. It has been used with young children and adolescents of various ages and abilities; it has been used with learning disabled children, physically disabled children, autistic children, and dyslexic children (Weir et al., 1982).

For some disabled students, LOGO and the microcomputer is a first experience in which they can tackle problems and initiate solutions; they can try out a solution, comprehend and respond to direct feedback, and decide what to do next (Weir et al., 1980). Spatial and mathematical concepts can be learned through manipulation of shape, length, angle, size, position, and number. A language such as LOGO not only has educational implications, but also has vital vocational implications for the handicapped and the nonhandicapped that society has not yet considered in great depth.

Among the tasks a microcomputer can do for a language-learning disabled child or a physically handicapped child is to allow access for gaining and expressing information. The mildly disabled person can begin to write without the problem of trying to correctly print or write a letter in the right location on the paper, dropping pencils and erasers, or tearing the paper. Only a key or alternate input device need be activated.

Severely disabled individuals have often been almost totally dependent on others to interpret or produce messages. Their role has been passive and dependent. Through adapting input devices in any one of many ways, from placing a hard cover over the keyboard and adding large, spaced input buttons to obtaining input from an action potential of a muscle, the microcomputer shifts initiative and control to the user. It allows a direct interaction with the environment. The Trace Center has been actively involved with developing hardware and software to facilitate communication and learning for the severely handicapped (Vanderheiden, 1983).

Using microcomputer technology coupled with any combination of methodological approaches, the communications specialist can create needed intervention schemes and provide services not previously available. REMATE is one example of a creative technological approach to communication problem solving (Vaughn, 1982). REMATE (Remote Machine Assisted Treatment and Evaluation) utilizes telephone communication as an outreach health care delivery system. Supplementary treatment, evaluation, and rehabilitation services are developed on and stored by computer-managed programs. Services are made available, accessible, and cost effective nationwide through telephone communication of drills in speaking, listening, reading, and writing. The related evaluation, records, reports, scheduling, and paperwork associated with any system are automated in REMATE. Clinicians prepare the materials, analyze responses, and interact with patients through a variety of telephone and computer-assisted devices.

TRENDS: MICROCOMPUTER TECHNOLOGY, ACCESSIBILITY, AND PROFESSIONAL ISSUES

What has occurred in the past 20 years has been remarkable; what is likely to occur in the next 20 years is virtually unpredictable. Some trends in the characteristics and operations of microcomputers have been identified and projected. Trends that have affected and will increasingly affect microcomputer usability include decreasing size of the components, decreasing costs of these components, increasing reliability of the equipment, and increasing demands and applications. Each of these is reviewed briefly.

Decreasing component size

The first large electronic computer, Electronic Numeric Integrator and Calculator (ENIAC), built in 1946, used 18,000 bulky vacuum tubes, 70,000 resistors, 10,000 capacitors, 6,000 switches, and was housed in a 30 by 50 foot room. Currently, a more powerful computer than ENIAC is possible using a silicon chip of less than one-quarter inch in size. This chip is a microprocessor and contains thousands of microscopic transistors and the connections among them (integrated circuits). By 1981, the equivalent of 750,000 vacuum tubes could be etched onto a microchip (Shane, 1982). The number of elements that can be placed on a microchip has increased approximately 10 times every 5 years since 1960 (Nickerson, 1982). With computers designing and modeling the circuitry and with increasing technology, the limits are undefined.

Decreasing component costs

Costs of components have dropped dramatically from the hundreds of thousands of dollars necessary for a system in the 1960s. Costs now range from $100 to $3,000 to $5,000 or more depending on what is purchased, where it is purchased, and what accessories or peripheral components are desired.

Increasing reliability

While the cost of production of a logic gate has decreased from more than $10.00 to less than $0.10 during the decades from 1960 to 1980, the reliability of the logic gate has increased about 100,000 times (Nickerson, 1982). The reliability of some of the earlier equipment was certainly questionable. Since some of the equipment seemed to fail randomly, but very frequently, many users were observed to develop chains of lucky gestures that seemed to function as starters similar to a "sequence of secondary symptoms." Today's microprocessors outperform the early large mainframe computers and many of the minicomputers that began appearing in research and business applications in the late 1960s and early 1970s.

Increasing demands and applications

In the mid-1960s, working with large, mainframe computers, large organizations developed specialized departments that were physically and administratively separate. Only a few small businesses were involved in early time-sharing projects developed to obtain affordable computer time and services. Fewer schools, clinics, or university training programs provided more than very limited opportunities for most students to gain any computer experience.

Less than 20 years later, in April, 1982, IBM predicted that in the near future, 75% of the work force will need some computer skills to do their jobs. The number of electronic circuits per capita in the United States, estimated to have been about 3 in 1965, was estimated to be about 10,000 in 1980, and is expected to be about 2,000,000 in 1990 (Nickerson, 1982). Computers are a vital part of industry, banks, hospitals, retail stores, transportation systems, and countless other areas. By 1990, at least 80% of all schools will use microcomputers to assist in instruction and/or for administrative purposes. Some universities require entering freshmen to purchase or have access to a microprocessor. Some hotels have installed terminals in rooms so guests can "log-on" with proper identification to check stock quotations, order flowers, receive or send electronic messages to other computers back at their homes or offices or hook into a network to check the electronic newsletter or play electronic games with others, and hold conferences with other professionals, perhaps in several distant cities.

Implications of these trends for specialists in communication disorders

Concerns for any professional, and certainly for those who have clinical, teaching, research and/or administrative roles in speech–language pathology and audiology, relate to how specialists can become knowledgeable and proficient in using microcomputers and how will this impact the profession. As specialists become more aware of the value of the microcomputer and demonstrate a need and desire for more information, resources will be developed. Workshops can be organized to provide specific information at introductory or advanced levels. Books about microcomputers are becoming increasingly abundant; many are well written, thorough, and provide examples illustrating points made. Microcomputer stores offer short courses with hands-on experience. Community adult education programs and universities offer introductory and advanced courses.

To gain competence in using and interacting with the microcomputer, it is essential, however, to practice in conjunction with the instruction manuals and software documentation. The new user should not be intimidated or frustrated by confusion or trepidation in beginning the experience. Entering the world of microcomputer interaction requires some risk taking, concentrated attention, thinking, struggling, and problem solving. While many will find this challenge fun, the user should be informed that: (a) the task is not simple or trivial, but one that requires some discipline; (b) the information cannot be acquired passively (to be a user it is necessary to decide to become *actively involved*); and (c) there is a need to set aside time to practice, keep to it, and do it.

With a good bit of repetition, the jargon becomes familiar and comprehensible. A gradual immersion into the demonstration materials at stores, libraries, computer consortiums, resource centers, and commercial exhibits allows users to sample the wide range of programs available—and the range is wide in terms of quality, topics, and approaches. Documentation for usable programs is printed in each issue, usually in BASIC, for one brand of computer, followed by adaptations in the code to make it compatible with other units; adaptations may be made for use by the specialist in communication disorders.

For advanced users, information sources are varied. The reviews of software and hardware, questions and answers, and issues raised by magazines directed to the hobbyist or educator can be valuable resources. Documentation for usable programs are printed in each issue, usually in BASIC, for one brand of computer followed by adaptations in the code to be compatible with other units; adaptations may be made for use by the specialist in communication disorders.

Users' groups composed of people with a common interest can be supportive, informative, and stimulating. Local groups may attract owners of one brand of microcomputer, persons interested in special education applications, or others with similar interests. Regional or national groups are developing to serve varied interests.

The committee on Personal Computers and the Handicapped (COPH-2) serves disabled persons, their families, friends, and the professionals involved. (For more information, write: COPH-2, 2030 Irving Park Road, Chicago, IL, 60618.) The committee on Educational Technology of the American Speech Language and Hearing Association publishes a newsletter and a software registry.

Professional groups are organizing activities and raising issues specifically for users of microcomputer technology. One valuable activity is the electronic forum or conference via a telephone, MODEM, and computer hookup that enables professional groups or transdisciplinary teams to exchange views (see Wilkins, chap. 4). Another expedient activity is electronic mail in which messages, information, and ideas are exchanged rapidly from one computer to another and printed out if hard copy is desired. Electronic mail can be sent to a teletypewriter, deafnet, or to a mechanical hand which can finger spell into the palm of a deaf-blind user (Programs for the Handicapped, Department of Education, May–June, 1982). Computerized data bases provide bibliographic listing for defined topics, thus saving search time and facilitating assessing.

Issues

Some issues will need to be considered, those that are related to use of microcomputers in many areas and those specific to specialists in communication sciences. Developing and instituting safeguards to protect privacy of clients and security of files is of general concern. Preventing piracy and protecting copyright of software packages are likely to be critical concerns for many areas; the solutions may be complex.

What effects will computer technology have on development of language comprehension and production in the young? What will be the effects on their learning to read? To write? What effect will computer technology have on those with communication disorders? What variables need to be controlled in designing computer programs for special target groups? These are some of the issues that professionals in communication disorders need to examine.

CONCLUSION

The potential value of the microcomputer for the field of communication disorders is significant. A myriad of applications currently available can assist the clinician, the researcher, the teacher, and the administrator. The specialist in communication disorders has both the opportunity and the responsibility to gain the information to utilize this microcomputer technology. This chapter presents an introduction to microcomputer technology and to some of the applications for the communicatively impaired child and adult, for the student in training, and for the active members of the profession. Subsequent chapters in this volume delve into various topics relevant to gaining the requisite information.

REFERENCE NOTES

Oltman, P. (1983). Project Special: A microcomputer-based management information system for special education. Paper presented at National Convention, Council for Exceptional Children, Detroit, MI.

Sonies, B. C., & Larkins, P. G. (1982). Diagnostic reporting simplified: Use of a computerized system. Paper presented at the Annual Convention of the American Speech Language and Hearing Association, Toronto, Canada.

Harlan, D. (1983). *Adult audiology case history and audiologic diagnostic test summary.* Colorado Springs, CO: Apropos Systems.

McCorkell, W. (1983). Impact of instruction for disabled adults in independent living skills. Paper presented at Council for Exceptional Children, Detroit, MI.

REFERENCES

Consumer Reports. Computers. (Sept. 1983). pp. 446–461.

Heyer, J., Lasky, E., Fontana, Woznak, D., Yutzy, M. (1983). *Maze days.* Cleveland, OH: The Learning Place.

Hixson, J. (1983). Information management: What to do with the computer in your office. *Hearing Instruments, 36,* 6.

Jacoby, L., & Craik, F. (1979). Effects of elaboration of processing at encoding and retrieval: Trace distinctiveness and recovery of initial context. In L. Cermak & F. Craik (Eds.), *Levels of processing in human memory.* Hillsdale, NJ: Lawrence Erlbaum Association.

Katz, K. R. (1983). Computers...Every office needs one! *Hearing Instruments, 34,* 7.

Lasky, E., Woznak, D., Yutzy, M., & Heyer, J. (1983). *Learning concepts.* Cleveland, OH: The Learning Place.

Moursund, D. (1981). *Introduction to computers in education for elementary and middle school teachers.* Eugene, OR: International Council for Computers in Education.

Nickerson, R. S. (1982). *Three uses of computers in education.* Report #5178. Bolt, Beranek & Newman.

Papert, S. (1980). *Mindstorms: Children, computers, and powerful ideas.* New York: Basic Books.

Raleigh, C. P. (1983). Give your child a headstart. *Personal software, 1:*1, 36–51.

Shane, H. G. (1982). The silicon age and education. *Phi Delta Kappa, 63:*5, 303–308.

Stolker, B. (1983). CompuCorder speech storage and output device. *Creative Computing, 9:*7, 22–24; 28–30.

Taber, F. (1983). *Microcomputers in special education.* Reston, VA: Council for Exceptional Children.

Vanderheiden, G. (1983). *Rehabilitation resource book: Telecommunication and environment control devices.* Baltimore: University Park Press.

Vaughn, G. (1982). *Exchange of information programs. Telecommunicology; remate: Communication outreach; EC-H-CO: Ecology of human communication.* Birmingham, AL: Veterans Administration Medical Center.

Wainer, H. (1983). On item response theory and computerized adaptive tests. *The Journal of College Admissions,* 28.

Walk, R. D. (1978). Perceptual learning. In E. C. Carterette and M. P. Friedman (Eds.), *Handbook of perception, V. IX Perceptual processing,* (pp. 257–297). New York: Academic Press.

Weir, S., Russell, S., & Valente, J. (Sept. 1982). LOGO: An approach to educating disabled children. *BYTE Publications,* 350–360.

Chapter 2

Implementing Microcomputer Applications

Carol G. Cohen

Microcomputers can save time and energy, eliminate tedious paperwork, increase productivity, and stimulate creativity if utilized appropriately. Because of the flexibility with which microcomputers can gather, manipulate, and send information this tool offers a broad scope of applications in the field of communication disorders. As Plummer (1984) noted:

> "Last year the major question was 'Which microcomputer do we need to buy?' This year the question being asked is 'How many of them do we need?'"

Increasingly, individuals, departments, and entire organizations have converted from more traditional approaches of client and information management to a microcomputer-assisted or managed format. Further, as evidenced by the number of special workshops and shortcourses, significant numbers of clinicians, researchers, and administrators are clamoring for comprehensible information about microcomputer systems and their applications in order to decide if they offer a more efficient and productive way of doing things (Asha, 1983).

Four of the basic reasons for considering the adoption of microcomputers are that: (1) tasks can be performed more accurately and completely; (2) operations can be done faster; (3) more tasks can be done at once; and (4) the tasks can be done in a cost-effective manner. Without positive responses to these queries, it would be difficult to justify the implementation of microcomputers in any setting regardless of application and intention.

Table 2-1 identifies questions associated with the four criteria to contemplate. Increased accuracy, augmented speed, greater flexibility, and reduced costs should be the direct result of microcomputer utilization. Increased motivation, stimulation, development of new solutions to old problems, and the creation of new programs are indirect benefits of microcomputers.

PHASES OF MICROCOMPUTER IMPLEMENTATION

Determining whether microcomputers are warranted can be complex, confusing, and occasionally intimidating. Assimilating microcomputers into any setting can be regarded as a succession of phases with successful — or unsuccessful — implementation (or rejection).

©College-Hill Press, Inc. All rights, including that of translation, reserved. No part of this publication may be reproduced without the written permission of the publisher.

Table 2-1 Areas of consideration in the adoption of microcomputers in communication disorders

Area		Questions
Accuracy	1.	Will a microcomputer help do the task correctly?
	2.	Will it do all aspects of the task completely?
	3.	Can it make the task simpler?
Speed	1.	Can it do the task faster than current procedures?
	2.	Can it handle more information than the present system?
	3.	Will it save time?
Flexibility	1.	Will it process information to meet our needs?
	2.	Can it be expanded as needs expand?
	3.	Will it accept additional functions?
Costs	1.	Will it cost less than current approaches once the system is operational?
	2.	Can existing personnel be trained to use it?
	3.	Is the expense of training personnel worth the savings?
	4.	Are maintenance costs less than current procedures?

Understanding these phases, particularly the early ones concerned with determining needs, can enhance the probability of making good decisions. The process of examining and implementing microcomputer hardware and software can be divided into seven phases as depicted in Table 2-2. Specific activities for each of the phases are identified.

Phase I: Planning and preparation

Whether a microcomputer is being considered for use by an individual, a small organization, or for a unit within a larger institution, some individual(s) need to be responsible for determining the need and applications and obtaining information on various products or services. The larger the organization, the more people affected by these changes and the greater the need for input from personnel at all levels (Schaffert, McDowell, & Levine, 1982). While the number of individuals involved in a school, hospital, or university may be larger, the phases involved in the implementation of microcomputers and the issues addressed at each stage are similar.

To plan adequately for the acquisition and acceptance of a microcomputer, an individual or group of personnel representing a variety of disciplines should coordinate activities surrounding the acquisition of microcomputer systems. For the purposes of this chapter, the term "planning person/committee" will be used to refer to that individual or group guiding and directing the microcomputer implementation process. A planning person/committee develops an atmosphere of support and validity for the process and secures staff input for the decision-making process (Naiman, 1982). In larger organizations, the composition of a planning committee could include delegates from administration, clinicians, parents, business office staff, and personnel from other relevant disciplines.

The planning person/committee should gather and evaluate information to make recommendations to responsible individuals who will make decisions about systems acquisition and implementation. This person/committee will ultimately be responsible for demonstrating the need and applications for the system as well as the components needed. It is on the basis of planning recommendations that decisions on the purchase of hardware and software are made.

Table 2-2 Phases in the adoption of microcomputers

Phase	Task		Activities
I	Planning & preparation	a.	Designate responsible individual(s) to gather information.
		b.	Determine staff interest and support.
II	Task analysis	a.	Identify current tasks (1) Volume (2) Speed (3) Accuracy (4) Costs
		b.	List current procedures.
III	Needs analysis	a.	Specify performance criteria for tasks and procedures.
		b.	Identify current tasks that take too long, cost too much, have high error rates, or are too large to handle with staff and procedures.
		c.	Determine discrepancies between current procedures and needs.
		d.	Project needs for 1, 3, and 5 years.
IV	Systems investigation	a.	Consult resources on microcomputer systems.
		b.	Investigate and observe hardware and software operation.
		c.	Determine costs and sources of financial support.
V	Staff preparation	a.	Develop procedures for staff training and supervision.
		b.	Work out policies for access and operation.
VI	System installation	a.	Establish timetable for installation of system.
VII	Operations evaluation	a.	Develop review of system operation.
		b.	Assess support mechanisms.
		c.	Reassess tasks, procedures, and operations.
		d.	Develop plans for future uses.

A review of organizational goals and a determination of how the objectives and policies coincide with microcomputer usage should be one of the first tasks addressed by the planning person/committee. Asking some direct questions about needs, attitudes, and uses is justified during the initial phase of planning for microcomputer implementation. Poirot and Heidt (1982) prepared a questionaire for educators that may be adapted to suit the needs of speech-language pathologists and audiologists interested in polling how staff members feel about the need to use microcomputers.

The extent to which the question/interview process is conducted is dependent on the size of the organization. For small clinics or agencies, information can be gathered informally. However, for large organizations considering microcomputers in several areas, a questionnaire can be developed or modified that explores pertinent information about needs, tasks, attitudes, and interests. Surveys of staff/faculty can determine tasks needing improvement, staff attitudes

Table 2-3 Questions for consideration in deciding the need for microcomputers[a]

Topic	Question
Improvement	Will this really improve things or is it a gadget?
Utilization	Will the personnel in the facility use it or be intimidated and alienated?
Availability	Is the software available to do the task needed?
Costs	Can the microcomputer pay for itself?
Tasks	What are the specific tasks that will be done on the microcomputer?
Support	Will there be a resource person?

[a]From Punch, Levitt, Mahaffey, and Wilson (1983).

and skills, and individuals with some existing skills that could be used to ease the transition period.

Phase II: Task analysis

The planning person/committee's next act, after surveying staff attitudes, is to analyze current procedures, that is, engage in a task analysis (Naiman, 1982). Identifying and listing various clinical, administrative, and instructional tasks and reviewing the manner in which activities are executed is fundamental to the process of evaluating current procedures. Many of the same procedures described by Mager (1973) in analyzing performance, developing goals, and preparing objectives can be adapted to analyzing functions.

"Tasks" are defined as those activities which are completed on a day-to-day basis. The planning person/committee needs to ask three generic questions about current tasks:
1. What are the current tasks being performed?
2. What are the staff and material requirements?
3. What are the time considerations for managing the task?

A delineation of specific tasks includes all activities such as file contents and management, intake records, budget records, letter and report writing, daily therapy logs, inventory recording, attendance, scheduling, individual education plans (IEPs), mailings, appointment confirmations, and maintaining accounts payable and receivable. Each task presently performed needs to be identified as explicitly as possible and the procedures involved in completing the task need to be specified.

Phase III: Needs analysis

The function of the needs analysis phase is to evaluate all current tasks to determine whether the tasks completed meet standards and to identify any procedures that do not achieve the desired results. Both current and future applications have to be considered. One of the best ways to do this is to list the desired outcome for each task, then determine if current procedures achieve that outcome. Simultaneously, the adequacy of existing procedures to do the task accurately and efficiently with current resources has to be evaluated. In those instances where there are errors in task performance, delays in preparation, difficulties managing the volume of material, or personnel who cannot handle the demands, an alteration in procedures is warranted. Whenever there is a discrepancy between the desired product and the actual product, a need for modification exists.

Determining needs represents a continuation of Phase II. Those tasks which need increased accuracy, volume, or faster processing lend themselves to technological assistance. Needs which require human judgment, perspective, and intuition are not amenable to being performed by microcomputers. The software in microcomputer systems performs certain functions. In many cases those functions coincide with needs for improved task performance (Cohen, 1983b). For example, where necessary information on clients cannot be obtained quickly or accurately using a manual filing system, there is a need for a faster, more accurate, or more flexible procedure to do the task. As discussed by Hood and Miller (see chap. 10) microcomputer data base management programs are specifically designed to organize large volumes of information quickly. As many organizations preparing accreditation reports find, when staff have to cease their regular activities to gather information manually, valuable time and effort are taken from other activities. This is one of the first signs that "there has to be a better way." In such instances, computerization is now possible with microcomputer systems and should be seriously considered. When staff insist that they can no longer maintain records accurately and completely, when it requires an inordinate amount of time to retrieve information, or when there is no longer adequate space to contain paper records, computerization is a feasible alternative.

During Phase III it is also the planning person/committee's role to estimate future requirements. The person/group will then need to specify, as objectively as possible, criteria for performance of these tasks. If the task and performance characteristics are consistent with microcomputer functions, consideration for switching is justified.

Several important considerations are recommended when considering revision of existing procedures and products:
  (1) each function being conducted;
  (2) how microcomputers can meet these needs;
  (3) future growth in terms of increased activities; additional services, or changing facility policies;
  (4) the time and effort to make any change;
  (5) how the staff will react to the changes and technology to make the change;
  (6) the effect revisions will have on the present level of internal control;
  (7) who will operate system and where it will be installed;
  (8) the need to resolve people-based problems must be handled differently from task-based problems.

Phase IV: Systems investigation

Once tasks and needs are identified, information on technology to perform those tasks must be obtained and evaluated. There are over 100 brands of microcomputers available and several have many different models within their line. In addition, there are over 10,000 software programs for microcomputers. Not all software programs will accomplish the tasks required by a specific agency, not all microcomputers can be used with all software, and special hardware devices for clinical and research applications require some study. The topic of hardware and software evaluation is introduced in this chapter only as part of the overall process of implementation. In separate chapters, Chial (see chap. 5) and Schwartz (see chap. 6) provide detailed discussion of features of hardware and software, as well as the implications of these features for speech-language pathologists and audiologists. The reader is refered to these chapters for a thorough examination of each topic.

Material requirements invoke visions of a plethora of hardware unfamiliar to most personnel. The amount of hardware and software necessary will be a direct reflection of the specific tasks to be accomplished. The microcomputer and its peripherals (accessory equipment such as printers) are precision equipment that will not function properly in rooms that are dusty, hot, or poorly ventilated (Datapro, 1982). Most systems can be used with a standard 110V AC receptacle. Other instrumentation such as audiometers, electronic aids, and office equipment may have to be moved to other circuits, since their operation could cause fluctuations in electricity that can "crash" (undesired termination) a program. Since electricity "builds up" in rooms that are not humid, a relatively static-free environment is helpful to ensure proper functioning. Often an antistatic carpet or spray solution can prevent the buildup of electrical charges and potential loss of data.

Consideration needs to be given to current and future costs, both direct and indirect, as well as acquisition and upkeep. Obviously, adequate funding is necessary to acquire microcomputer systems. Galsky (see chap. 3) has identified potential sources and strategies for obtaining funding. It has been this author's experience that organizations do not fully anticipate actual expenditures when implementing microcomputer systems. Software needs must be examined in relation to the tasks and needs of the professionals and clients affected prior to any hardware consideration. Individuals and agencies repeatedly purchase hardware and then discover they have inadequate software resources and/or find themselves without the financial means to acquire support programs to operate the newly purchased technology. Do not spend all the budgeted money at once. Save some for ongoing enhancement of the equipment, education of staff, and for additional software. It may become feasible to add a hard disk or a letter-quality printer. For treatment of clients with communication disorders, a speech synthesizer may be a valuable acquisition. Allocating a software budget of at least one third the price of the hardware is recommended (see chap. 6). The initial outlay of funds represents only the beginning of costs to the organization or individual. It has been estimated that in the first year of operation, an additional 30-50% of the initial cost of hardware will be spent on software, staff, materials, supplies, and maintenance. This must be examined and anticipated when developing a funding plan for microcomputer implementation.

Elsewhere, Wilkins (see chap. 4) enumerates sources of information that can be used when investigating microcomputers. Within his chapter, he describes the use of consultants. Consultants act as facilitators of dialogue and can assist when staff members need to express concerns and anxieties to administrators and funding officials (Bar, 1983). Consultative services provide overviews of issues and factors to consider when determining the need to introduce technological adaptations and/or assist with product decisions.

Consultants who can provide accurate information and anecdotal accounts significantly assist the decision-making and ultimately the implementation process. It may be advisable to seek consultation from other specialists who have expertise with microcomputers and an understanding of speech-language and hearing disorders. Another approach often employed involves the participation of a consultant outside of the field of communication disorders. A business consultant can analyze administrative needs and offer objective recommendations on apparatus and vendors. Typically, these individuals are knowledgeable though costly.

Phase V: Staff preparation

A point Mullendore discusses elsewhere in this volume (chap. 12) is that specialists in communication disorders have historically shown an interest in and ability to adapt technology into their professional repertoires. The immediate benefits of microcomputer systems are improved information management and planning and a reduction in paperwork (Norwood,

1983). However, some professionals express apprehension about computerization, often for reasons such as fear that the microcomputer will not do the task accurately or efficiently, that they will not be able to learn to operate the equipment, or that they will be replaced by the microcomputer.

Staff must be reassured that microcomputers will not usurp their responsibilities, but rather will enhance their effectiveness. Lay-offs, or even the misperception that technological advances can reduce staff, can have a devastating morale effect (Datapro, 1982). Employees need to be oriented to the computer and as many as possible should be trained to use the system. Staff preparation includes all activities beginning with surveying staff needs and attitudes through the training and supervision of staff on the use of the system.

Rogers and Shoemaker (1971) identified five factors that affect the rate of adoption of any innovation: (1) the relative advantage over traditional tools; (2) complexity; (3) trialability; (4) observability; and (5) compatibility. The degree of staff training and participation that will be required, in addition to their typical routine, must be critically and pragmatically analyzed. Phase V is critical to the ultimate level of adoption. Without adequately trained staff, systems will not be used to their maximum potential and in some cases will remain idle (Taber, 1983). Improperly educated personnel will eschew interaction with the microcomputer or react negatively when offered the opportunity to interact. Individuals who do not possess the necessary information and skills could, if urged to operate the microcomputer, inadvertently cause the hardware to jam or the software to crash.

Guidelines for usage and access need to be devoloped. Ideally, it is the agency's responsibility to provide incentives and opportunities to obtain training. Staff education can be accomplished in a variety of ways, including in-house instruction during working hours or after hours, or off-site tutelage. Education can be offered on a regular basis or at periodic intervals. In any regard, microcomputer training must be ongoing so that the staff acquires a full appreciation for the many applications and approaches to treatment and client management with microcomputers. Further, it is incumbent on personnel to keep abreast of new advances in hardware and software technology. An introductory orientation to the hardware is usually provided by the vendor at the staff's convenience. This session usually addresses only rudimentary operation and maintenance.

Phase VI: System installation

In a sense, the installation of a system is an extension of Phases IV and V. Once hardware and software systems have been identified that meet the individual/organizational requirements for task performance and steps have been made for staff training and supervision, actual set up of the system is appropriate. One more personnel-related issue needs to be considered as part of the installation phase — the designation of an individual responsible for all activities directly or indirectly related to the microcomputer. Taber (1983) recommends designating one person to coordinate microcomputer implementation. Logically, this individual would be an active participant in the first three phases of implementation. Preferably, this person should have an interest in working with microcomputers, be able to work well with other staff, and have some competency in using microcomputers. Of these three factors, interest and compatability with other staff are the most important. Table 2-4 identifies nine tasks that a coordinator can do to facilitate the installation of a system.

Naiman (1982) has recommended that, prior to installation of a system, a timetable for the physical set up of the system(s) be developed. This agenda would incorporate the estimated time of arrival and a time allotment for actual installation including unexpected electrical and environmental modifications. Prior to receiving the system, the location of the microcomputer

Table 2-4 Personnel factors to consider when planning for microcomputers

1.	Who will be in overall charge of the equipment?
2.	Who will see that all equipment users are properly trained?
3.	Who will make decisions about maintenance and repair?
4.	Who will investigate sources of software and evaluate programs?
5.	Who will schedule use of the microcomputer?
6.	Who will make arrangements for ongoing inservicing?
7.	Who will involve parents and community?
8.	Who will keep abreast of new technological developments and research?
9.	Who will be responsible for arranging periodic review of operations?

needs to be designated. In addition to space for the hardware and its peripherals, some working area for materials and space for storage of manuals and supplies should be provided.

In negotiations for the system, consideration should be given to making the purchase contingent on having the vendor set up all of the equipment in the facility. If this is not feasible, then the system should be assembled and tested at the vendor's location and the responsible staff member shown how to reassemble the system. Dealer installation of special cards, devices, or other devices will simplify on-site installation.

Most software for microcomputer requires little if any modification prior to usage. Elsewhere, Schwartz (see chap. 6) describes the types of preparation for software that may be needed. One additional factor to consider in preparing for installation pertains to access to software and its documentation. Because of the costs involved, care must be taken to ensure that programs are not damaged or lost. Many software programs come with duplicate copies or permit the purchase of backup copies Wilson (see chap. 10) explains some of the distinctions between legitimate copying and illegal piracy of software. If permissible, arrangements should be made to obtain backup copies of software and documentation. The original disks and manuals can then be stored and the copies placed in general use. In the case of damaged or misplaced software, the originals can be used while arrangements are made to obtain replacements from the manufacturer.

Phase VII: Operations evaluation

For at least 3 months following installation of the microcomputer, constant monitoring and evaluation of operations needs to be done. A parallel (the original manual procedures) operation should be maintained to avoid loss of information in the case of system problems (Schwartz, chap. 6). A written log of staff comments, suggestions, and reactions concerning system operation is most helpful in evaluating performance.

Once an operation has been computerized, procedures must be reevaluated periodically to assess adequacy, efficiency, and cost effectiveness (Schaffert, et al., 1982). Systems which are inflexible or difficult to maintain may not accommodate all the tasks and requirements previously enumerated. A system must also be able to accommodate future needs of an agency, its staff, and its clients. Microcomputer system expansions and modifications will depend upon current utilization and perspicacious planning. If additional units or expansion of a single system is planned, some means to document needs should be developed for presentations to appropriate administrative offices.

Final considerations

If careful planning and systematic implementation are conducted, the probability of successful implementation and use of microcomputers is enhanced. There are, however, some other items that need to be considered during the seven phases of implementation discussed above. Newer, more powerful, and less expensive systems are being marketed regularly. Waiting for better prices or more powerful systems may be a dubious strategy. The time lost while waiting for the "right" system could be used to make operations more effective. The delay in waiting for the "ideal" system will be endless since new and better technology is always "around the corner."

For a system to be cost justified, it needs to be used for approximately 2 years. Therefore, in planning, it is wise to give consideration to tasks and procedures that will be used for at least that period of time. Hardware and software should be evaluated from the perspective that the system selected will be used for this period of time. It will take time and effort to convert records, modify procedures, train staff, and incorporate the system into daily operation. Constantly changing hardware or software can be more expensive than retaining manual procedures. Other considerations, mostly nontechnical in nature, are described in Table 2-5. Some if not all, of these need to be taken into account when incorporating microcomputers into different settings for clinical, instructional, administrative, or research applications.

IMPLEMENTING MICROCOMPUTERS IN DIFFERENT ENVIRONMENTS

Introduction

As Lasky (chap. 1) has indicated, microcomputers have applications in diverse settings and for a variety of purposes. Some of these uses are generic and cross settings while others are specific to particular types of organizations. Elsewhere in this volume, several authors have provided in-depth information on uses of microcomputers for different functions. The following section applies Phases II and III (Task Analysis and Needs Analysis) to the application of microcomputers in different settings. The focus, therefore, will be on tasks and needs in the different types of environments in which communication disorders specialists function.

In a 1983 ASHA survey, Punch indicated that a majority of members work in public school settings (41.3%), followed by nongovernmental health services (17.7%); third are "other" settings and finally, college and university settings account for 11.0%. Only a small percentage of ASHA members are in private practice (5.7%).

The justification for employing an environmental approach for microcomputer use in daily routine should be apparent. While there are common characteristics of microcomputer technology that make it applicable to all sections of the profession, there exist individual differences in environments or site of service. The features of technology that make it attractive to communication disorders specialists are universal and indigenous to many systems: motivational quality, individualized instruction, adaptation to the needs of special children and adults, reliability, cost effectiveness, and the ability to increase accuracy and efficiency of managers (Stallard, 1982).

Applications of microcomputers in the schools

Speech-language pathologists employed in school settings can successfully use microcomputers clinically (see Rushakoff, chap. 7), administratively (see Hood & Miller, chap.

Table 2-5 Final considerations

1.	There is a distinction between needs and uses. Tasks determine needs. People determine use. Staff must believe that microcomputers can help them do a task better.
2.	Staff members do not have to be programmers to use microcomputers.
3.	Planning is essential. Hasty unilateral mistakes are time consuming and difficult to rectify.
4.	Microcomputers can improve efficiency of operation but not human judgment underlying organizations.
5.	Microcomputers augment—not supplant—personnel performance.
6.	A supportive environment—regardless of setting or application—may be more important than system of hardware and software.
7.	Build networks and encourage collaborative efforts to share information, resources, and evaluations.

10) for inservice instruction (see Shearer, chap. 9) or for research purposes (see Mahaffey, chap. 8). Typically, microcomputers are acquired by a school district for use in a particular school rather than for a specific individual. Often, one site is designated as the "microcomputer" school. When a decision has been reached (traditionally by school administrators with meager input from professional or administrative staff) to implement microcomputer technology, a location that is most convenient for intended users has to be identified. There are two important roles that the communication specialist can provide in the schools. First, he/she can function as an active lobbyist for the acquisition of a microcomputer. Suggest to the school principal or district administrators charged with the computer adoption process that a steering committee be formulated. A comprehensive utilization proposal explaining how the system would be used to provide services is necessary. Justify that the speech-language pathologist be an integral member of that committee. Second, document applications that other school personnel could use. The provision of examples of successful implementation in the field of communication disorders services and treatment would enhance the credibility of a request for microcomputers. Demonstrations, for administrators and teachers, of the systems' ease of use and relevance in an educational setting should be arranged.

Administrative and managerial applications

Historically, clinicians have struggled with the large amount of client information that needs to be stored and managed for both clinical and administrative matters. The demands made for record keeping are herculean. Files require constant updating of test results, progress notes, and parent contacts. Often these tasks are a serious burden on professional staff, diverting their attention from service delivery (Bennett, 1982). Hood and Miller (chap. 10) explain how data base management software allows clinicians to efficiently locate, manipulate, and report data about services, including types and numbers of clients served and locations of services.

Access to student records for information needed for state and federal audits can be complicated, time consuming, and labor intensive. Considerable time and effort may be spared by converting manual record keeping to a data base program. Any clinician having more than 15 IEPs to generate could save time by using one of the commercially available IEP software packages or by developing one using a data base software program.

The generation of diagnostic, progress, or summary reports is tedious and repetitious. Word processing software programs can alleviate the drudgery of repetitive writing. Consisting of a group of subprograms, word processing software simplifies the updating or revision of reports. Electronic preparation, storage, retrieval, editing, and printing using word processing programs assists the school clinician when writing reports, developing letters to parents, organizing therapy logs, and preparing activity reports.

Delivery of services

Rushakoff (chap. 7) describes many of the assessment and intervention applications for microcomputer systems. Clinicians processing large volumes of information in short periods of time, as in the case of annual speech and hearing screenings, could save time and effort by using vertical applications software (see Schwartz, chap. 6) for analyzing and reporting performance. In many districts, the reporting of screening results for articulation and language performance follows a similar format for each student. The CUSH Software Registry lists specific packages in these areas (Fitch, 1983a). The time saved in writing individual screening reports can be used for starting clients in follow-up diagnostics or therapy sooner. Additional clients could be treated without compromising the therapist's effectiveness.

The assessment of children with special needs provides information for making decisions about service eligibility, diagnosis, classification, educational programming and therapeutic objectives, scheduling, placement, and progress review (Bennett, 1982). It is increasingly common to find assessment programs (software) containing information analysis and reporting options (Fitch, 1983b; Rushakoff & Toossi, 1983; Yorkston & Beukelman, 1983) which have unique and timesaving features to assist the teacher/therapist maintain individual records on many students simultaneously.

Certain aspects of instruction and treatment can be enhanced by microcomputers. While the microcomputer is a tool that has the capability of delivering some aspects of treatment it is not designed to supplant a clinician (Hofmeister, 1982). It can facilitate treatment by eliminating much of the repetition of certain of redundant intervention, and supply the clinician with time and means to develop new, exciting, and highly motivating forms of stimulation (Naiman, 1982). Shearer (see chap. 9) comments on the types of instructional applications that clinicians may utilize to supplement therapy.

A recent national survey (Ahl, 1983) indicated that the attitudes of school personnel toward microcomputers are generally enthusiastic and positive. However, in response to the questions on microcomputer availability, 32.6% of the teachers who responded to the survey indicated that at least one computer was available in their school. It was estimated that in the spring of 1982 there were approximately 131,000 computers in the 25,350 polled schools nationally. This study indicated that microcomputers are more likely to be found in secondary schools. It is probable that school clinicians will have to share computers, particularly at the elementary level, since the greatest proportion of speech-impaired students are of elementary school age (Asha, 1981). Limited access to computers is presently a serious dilemma faced by public school clinicians. While more and more schools are acquiring microcomputers it does not appear that the number of microcomputers available for use exclusively by speech-language clinicians is improving drastically.

Special applications

Teleconferencing, an aspect of telecommunications, offers potential for increased effectiveness and better communication among school clinicians. Telecommunications is defined as the transmission of information over distances (Hedberg, 1984). Teleconferencing is a strategy often employed by business and industry to save time and money spent in travel when it is necessary to bring people together without heed to geographic proximity. The use of microcomputer communications can solve problems in two ways: (1) detecting problems before they become serious by predicting future trends and projecting alternative solutions, and (2) discovering hitherto unknown problems to be solved by these kinds of systems, problems typically very complex, protracted, and not straightforward (Cross, 1982).

Teleconferencing could be a functional tool in a school setting for staff conferencing, case review and presentation, and remote data base access. There are a number of information systems or brokers (see Wilkins, chap. 4) which can log-on to networks of educational, special educational, and clinically oriented information bases. Vast amounts of data may be accessed by means of a telephone MODEM easily, efficiently, and in a cost-effective manner.

In summary, the primary tasks and needs of the speech–language pathologist in the school setting would seem to be for the management and reporting of information on direct services. Within the realm of the school-based clinician, it is important to realize that often the situation will not be one of determining need per se, but determining how the speech–language professionals in the school and/or district will utilize the technology that has been purchased by the administrators of the district.

Applications for microcomputers in private practice

Efficient, cost-effective records management is perhaps the most pressing need for private practitioners. The support services typically found in school, hospital, or clinical settings often do not exist for individuals in private practice. Commercially available software programs can be utilized for administrative activities, thereby enabling the practitioner to spend more time directly with patients or developing the practice.

Administrative applications

Data base management. Efficient organization of information allows the private practitioner rapid access to data about a client. There are several easy-to-use, yet powerful, data management programs that are especially adaptable for professional environments. Client scheduling and tracking systems are available that are flexible and sophisticated (Bolton, 1982). Such programs are often designed to interface with mass storage devices such as hard disks, thereby giving the private practice greater range in data base management and scheduling.

Word processing. Word processing is an indispensible tool for private practitioners. The work load of a single private-based clinician may not be significant enough, relative to the practice size, to justify the costs of a full time secretary. With word processing software and a suitable printer the communication disorders specialist can use the microcomputer to handle most of the correspondence. As Hood and Miller (chap. 10) explain, reports do not have to be completely retyped to insert an additional or customized paragraph.

Financial planning and management. For the private practitioner, managing of financial matters including expenses, income, projections, and tax-related records can be costly. Using financial software on the microcomputer provides an inexpensive way to monitor expenditures, salaries, accounts payable/receivable, tax returns, and a myriad of other financial planning tasks. The expenses saved — time and cost — can justify, in many instances, the implementation of a microcomputer.

Delivery of services

The utility of microcomputer-assisted direct client service warrents consideration. Many private practitioners travel to private homes or contract with private facilities such as nursing and residential care centers to offer therapeutic intervention for hospitalized and convalescent patients. With the advent of portable self-contained units it may become more feasible for practitioners to augment traditional methodologies and strategies with some computerized instruction and treatment (Morris, 1983). It also goes without saying that if the practice is based in one location the microcomputer(s) might be employed in some aspects of direct clinical service (see chap. 7).

One area of application to consider is the computerization of therapy prescriptions. Adherence to many third party guidelines regarding types of services and eligibility criteria can be complex and involved. This aspect of direct client service might lend itself extremely well to automation. A data base might be organized to comply with funding requirements and third party payment schedules. This might be an important subsection of the data base management system and would prove infinitely useful to many private practice professionals.

Applications for microcomputers in academic settings

Microcomputers are valuable tools for professionals providing preservice or inservice education. For clinicians in nonuniversity settings, microcomputers offer a means to use and develop innovative and effective materials for staff, education, or community education. For university faculty, microcomputer-assisted instruction (see Shearer, chap. 9) offers an opportunity to develop and refine skills, simulate processes, provide individual tutorials, and aid in the problem solving of clinical situations.

Instructional applications

Relatively few institutions have or utilize computer-assisted instruction (CAI) for students in speech-language pathology and audiology. However, interest in the development of CAI for such purposes is evolving at a few locations. Subject areas that involve discrete and voluminous information, such as anatomy and physiology, instrumentation, or test scoring, are particularly appropriate for CAI. Similarly, topics that require extensive drill and practice to reach proficiency, such as masking or phonetic analysis, are cost-effective instructional aids once materials are developed. Shearer (chap. 9) surveys the instructional applications of microcomputers for the development of tutorials for specific subjects, demonstration of assessment or intervention procedures, or simulation of events.

Research applications

Research in academic institutions is an integral part of most instructional positions. The microcomputer is ideally suited to process numbers at great speeds (Moursund, 1981). The microcomputer can be the researcher's most devoted ally, analyzing the vast amounts of data and information collected. Further, the microcomputer may be utilized to evaluate, store, and report facts gathered in the investigatory process.

There is, unfortunately, an impression that research is conducted primarily in laboratories and clinics that are specially staffed or equipped for research. This is an artificial dichotomy that may be obscured through the use of microcomputers, according to Mahaffey (see chap. 8). The portability of microcomputers, the scope of hardware and software that are supported and used, and the ease of client/clinician operation make this instrument accessible to any practitioner in any setting who is asking questions and seeking information about communicative disorders. With microcomputers, it is possible that any clinician can be a clinician scientist: asking pertinent questions, systematically investigating events, and quantifying performance.

Software development

Colleges and universities have been instrumental in the development and dissemination of microcomputer software for assessment and treatment of communication disorders (Fitch, 1983a). Programs which allow for the monitoring and tracking of students' clinical hours (Rushakoff & Toossi, 1983), student data base management (Fitch, 1983a), and diagnosis of dysarthria (Yorkston & Beukelman, 1983), to name but a few, are representative of the burgeoning interest in the creation of software by academically based speech-language pathologists.

Applications for microcomputers in clinical and hospital settings

Administrative applications
The functions to be performed in hospital and clinical settings include client file maintenance, writing of reports, letters, and therapy logs, budget preparation and monitoring, and maintenance of ledgers for accounts payable and receivable. More specific setting-oriented applications include appointment scheduling, inventory, staffings, telecommunications, and remote data base access. Given escalating costs, increasing volumes of information to be processed, and personnel costs such organizations need to find effective ways of doing these tasks. Considerable time and energy can be conserved by implementing microcomputers in a cost-effective manner.

Clinical applications
In organizations serving orthopedically, cognitively, or neurologically impaired patients, the microcomputer may prove to be a workable aide to the clinician as well as a means of expressive communication for the nonspeaking client. Software, called authoring programs, for developing other programs is available to enable clinicians to create their own lessons and actually write programs according to a particular client's needs without knowledge of computer programming.

Special clinical applications for microcomputer systems is an area receiving increasing attention. Many speech-language pathologists treating severely communicatively impaired individuals have found that computer systems facilitate the treatment process and often provide nonspeaking, physically disabled individuals with the only meaningful way of interacting with and controlling their environments (Cohen & De Ruyter, 1982). Low-cost computing technology promises unprecedented opportunities for the disabled person (Luttner, 1981). These factors deserve consideration when determining the need to implement microcomputers in a clinical-hospital setting.

The use of speech synthesis and speech or voice recognition systems can add an ingredient to therapy that traditional methodologies are incapable of approximating. Synthesized speech, either digitized or text-to-speech, allows for the production of unlimited utterances and can provide the client with vocal output. Voice recognition offers the communicatively impaired user technology capable of responding to virtually any consistent vocalization; these productions do not have to be intelligible utterances. Perhaps the most exciting and innovative application potential is programming the system to accept an unintelligible client's vocalizations as if such utterances were indeed recognizable words. Many impaired persons are also nonreaders due to mental retardation, visual involvement, and/or perceptual difficulties. Many can utilize computers despite the lack of reading skills through the implementation of graphics. Software that incorporates graphics, such as the "Talking Blissapple" (Trace Research and Development, 1982) and "Magic Cymbals" (Schneier Communication Unit & Carlson, 1984), provides nonorthographic communication systems applicable for a variety of children and adults (Cohen & De Ruyter, 1982).

Augmentative communication
Clinicians working in settings with orthopedically or neurologically impaired patients need to explore electronic technologies as a source of communication. The use of microcomputers as augmentative aids has been limited, to some extent, to stationary types of systems (Vanderheiden, 1981). Microcomputer-based communication systems for individuals who are nonspeaking and/or nonwriting have included applications such as writing and filing systems, telephone control and telecommunications incorporating speech synthesis, and graphics software for expressive language. Nonportable devices have not solved the conversational needs of individuals with severe communication impairments (Vanderheiden, 1981). In a clinical setting,

the microcomputer offers the clinician an exemplary means by which to evaluate and select the most appropriate augmentative communication approach. Through software and special accessing devices the microcomputer can facilitate the evaluation of communicative prerequisites (Cohen, 1983a). These potential applications should certainly be a consideration when determining the need to implement microcomputers in a setting serving severely involved populations. The new generation of portable computers when interfaced with voiced output makes it possible to have a portable, accessible, microcomputer-based prosthesis and conversational communication aid all in one.

Special control interfaces increase the information-transfer rate between disabled individuals and the devices they are trying to control (Vanderheiden, 1981). The physically disabled person, regardless of the level of disability, can access a microcomputer through special interfaces such as single switch mechanisms, keyguards, emulators, and special software and firmware. Therefore, when determining the need to implement microcomputers for severely physically handicapped persons, the cost of interfaces and accessing systems must be considered along with overall cost and training for staff. Dedicated (microprocessor-based) communication aids that are more portable in nature, such as the *VOIS* systems and Express III, have addressed the needs of the nonspeaking population more completely than have microcomputers.

BEFORE IMPLEMENTING: SOME FINAL COMMENTS

Although there are many tasks a microcomputer can perform diligently and accurately, it is not the anodyne for all clinical, administrative, or instructional needs. The thrust of this chapter is on the time and effort that the microcomputer can save in processing large amounts of information (clinical, administrative, or research) quickly and efficiently. Some perspective is needed, however, since the microcomputer will execute all properly given directions regardless of the accuracy of the information or the appropriateness of the task.

The microcomputer is ideally suited for certain tasks. It will not solve broad or poorly defined problems. Furthermore, rather than creating organization from chaos, a microcomputer will amplify the pitfalls of inadequate or inaccurate manual procedures. It is doubtful, given the state of artificial intelligence in computers today, that microcomputers can replace the judgment and experience of clinicians in the diagnosis and management of communication problems. Lastly, microcomputer systems are fallible. Equipment and circuits are not perfect. Software, both the programs and the supporting documentation, may have errors. Practitioners implementing microcomputer systems must remember that the microcomputer is a tool that enhances user effectiveness rather than replaces the individual.

In conclusion, it is not a trivial task to revitalize outmoded or unproductive manual procedures with technologically based functions. The process requires considerable time, energy, and tenacity. Many factors should be investigated, individuals consulted, systems evaluated, and needs and tasks analyzed. The information presented in both this chapter and the previous chapter is designed to provide information about how microcomputers can be implemented into a variety of settings and organizations for different applications.

REFERENCE NOTES

Apple Computer Company (1981). *Apple pilot (program and manuals)*. Cupertino, CA: Author.
Asha (1984, June). *Final report of the Asha task force on information services*. Rockville, MD: American Speech Language Hearing Association. Unpublished paper.
Bar, A. (1983, August). *Personal communication.* New York, NY: Mount Sinai Hospital.
Burke, R. L. (1982). *CAI sourcebook*. Englewood Cliffs, NJ: Prentice-Hall.

Cohen, C. (1983a). *Microcomputer systems: management, application, and treatment.* Shortcourse presented at the 1983 Director's Conference (American Speech-Language-Hearing Association), San Antonio, TX.

Cohen, C. (1983b). *The use of software in augmentative communication evaluation and treatment.* Seminar presented at the Minnesota State Speech and Hearing Association Annual Convention Minneapolis, MN.

Fitch, J., Ed. (1983a). *Software registry.* Computer Users in Speech and Hearing (CUSH). University of South Alabama, Mobile, AL.

Fitch, J. (1983b). *Computer managed articulation treatment.* Gulfport, MS: Communicology Associates.

Governmental Affairs Review (1981, July). "Do you have an average caseload?" *Asha, 23;* 79.

Lutus, P. (1982). *Applewriter IIe operating manual.* Cupertino, CA: Apple Computer Company.

Plummer, H. (1984). *Future encounters.* Presented at the 1984 American Speech and Hearing Foundation Conference, Las Vegas, NV.

Punch, J., Levitt, H., Mahaffey, R., & Wilson, M. (1983). *Computer technology: The revolution has started without us.* Miniseminar presented at the Annual Convention of the American Speech-Language-Hearing Association, Cincinnati, OH.

Rushakoff, G. & Toossi, M. (1983). *Therapy data collector.* Las Cruces, NM: New Mexico State University.

Schneier Communication Unit, & Carlson, F. (1984). *Magic cymbals.* Syracuse, NY: Cerebral Palsy Center.

Schwartz, A. H. (1984). *Introduction to administrative applications for microcomputers.* Miniseminar presented at the 1984 American Speech-Language-Hearing Foundation. Las Vegas, NV.

Trace Research and Development Center (1982). *Talking blissapple.* Madison, WI.

REFERENCES

Ahl, D. (1983). School uses of microcomputers. *Creative computing, 9:2,* 185-186.

Bennett, R. (1982). Application of microcomputer technology to special education. *Exceptional Children, 49:2,* 106-115.

Bolton, B. (1982, March-April). Solving administrative problems in the schools: Students scheduling and tracking for the microcomputer. *Educational Computer, 2:2,* 24-26.

Cohen, C., & De Ruyter, F. (1982). Technology for the communicatively impaired: A perspective for future clinicians. *Journal of National Student Speech, Language, and Hearing Association, 10:1,* 67-76.

Cross, T. (1982). Tele-conferencing: The new school tool. *Educational Computer, 2:6,* 25-28.

Datapro Research Corp. (1982). *Guidelines: Analyzing your business for the addition of a computer* (MC41 050 201). Delran, NJ: Author.

Hedberg, G. (1984). Personal computers. *Money Guide* (pp 78-87). New York, NY: Time Publishing Co.

Hofmeister, A. (1982). Microcomputers in perspective. *Exceptional Children, 49:2,* 115-123.

Luttner, S. (1981). Computers for the handicapped. *Apple, 2:1,* 26-29.

Mager, R. F. (1973). *Measuring instructional intent.* Belmont, CA: Fearon Publishers.

Morris, D. (1983, September). The portables are here. *Educational Computer, 3:5,* 13.

Moursund, D. (1981). *Introduction to computers in education for elementary and middle school teachers.* Eugene, OR: International Council for Computers in Education (ICCE).

Naiman, A. (1982). *Microcomputers in education: An introduction* (pp 5-10). Cambridge, MA: Northeast Regional Exchange.

Norwood, D. (1983). Here's a logical way to plan for microcomputers. *Illinois School Board Journal,* 22-24.

Poirot, J., & Heidt, M. (1982). Planning for educational computing: A questionnaire for educators. *Educational Learning,* 34-38.

Punch, J. (1983, January). Characteristics of ASHA members. *Asha, 25:1,* 31.

Rogers, E., & Shoemaker, F. (1971). *Communications of innovations.* New York: The Free Press.

Schaffert, T., McDowell, C., & Levine, S. (1982, Winter). Automated information systems for physicians. *Topics in Health Care Financing,* 1-13. Aspen Systems Corp.

Stallard, C. (1982). Computers and education for exceptional children: emerging applications. *Exceptional Children, 49:2,* 102-106.

Taber, F. (1983). *Microcomputers in special education.* Reston, VA: Council for Exceptional Children.
Vanderheiden, G. (1981). Computers can play a dual role for disabled individuals. *Byte, 7:9,* 136.
Yorkston, K., & Beukelman, D. (1983). Assessment of intelligibility of dysarthric speech. Tigard, OR: C. C. Publications.

SECTION II
BASES FOR DECISIONS

Chapter 3

Funding Sources for Microcomputers

Alan G. Galsky

This chapter is written as a guide for those organizations (and individuals) who have the talent, time, and energy to obtain microcomputers through the external funding process. Although this represents one alternative by which to obtain microcomputers, this route is time consuming, energy requiring, and often frustrating. It represents, however, a unique opportunity to obtain microcomputers for organizations that cannot readily afford to purchase them (or enjoy challenges).

Although in theory any agency or individual is eligible to seek external funding through the proposal process for a microcomputer, in practice those organizations with nonprofit status have the best opportunities for success. These include elementary and secondary schools, colleges and universities, hospitals and clinics, and a variety of other agencies. Each of these organizations will find varying degrees of success depending on the agency and type of proposal. These will be discussed later in the chapter.

If this brief description of the funding process is not discouraging and you are encouraged about the chances of obtaining funding, it is necessary to discuss the possible types of proposals.

PROPOSAL TYPES

Research proposal

Perhaps the most common type of proposal, at least in the minds of many, is the *research proposal*. This type of proposal can be written by almost any nonprofit organization or agency carrying out theoretical or applied research. The proposal often allows for the purchase of equipment necessary to conduct any facet of the research. The proposal could require a microcomputer for data analysis or the microcomputer could be the object of research such as "The Role of the Microcomputer in Analysis of ____ ." Since most microcomputers can be purchased for under $5,000, the addition of this item to the proposal will not drastically affect the budget.

The disadvantage of this type of proposal is that it is often difficult to justify the purchase of more than two microcomputers for research use per proposal. The advantage is that the

---

©College-Hill Press, Inc. All rights, including that of translation, reserved. No part of this publication may be reproduced without the written permission of the publisher.

Table 3-1. Summary of Proposal Types

Proposal type	Example of agency	Major advantage
Research	National Science Foundation National Institutes of Health Department of Education	Microcomputers can often be obtained as a small part of the total grant.
Curriculum	Department of Education National Science Foundation	Chance to obtain a large number of microcomputers.
Equipment	National Science Foundation National Institutes of Health	Proposal usually short, does not require much preparation.
Consortium or network proposal	National Science Foundation National Institutes of Health Department of Education	Chance of many organizations to work together; interinstitutional proposals are favored by many agencies.
Special projects or workshops	National Science Foundation National Institutes of Health Department of Education	No real advantage unless your organization is on the "cutting edge" of the field.
RFP or "Requests for Proposals"	National Institutes of Health Private foundations	Agency issuing RFP is interested in microcomputers.

microcomputer is often a small part of the total budget and proposal, and thus can be obtained as part of a larger scale project.

Curriculum proposal

Another type of proposal is the so-called *curriculum proposal*. This is usually available from several agencies depending on the particular year or what seems to be fashionable. This proposal is limited to organizations that have education programs in communication disorders. The key to a successful proposal in this area will be to convince the reviewers that the applicant has an innovative plan for curriculum change that involves the microcomputer in almost every aspect of the new curriculum and not as an afterthought.

For successful proposals, the harvest will be fruitful and it will allow the organization to obtain many microcomputers. For proposals that cannot convince the reviewers of the necessity to change the curriculum, the news will not be good. Both the curriculum and research proposal are often lengthy and require a good deal of time and thought to prepare.

Equipment proposal

Another type of proposal is the *equipment proposal*. This is rather self-explanatory and is offered as a separate program by a variety of agencies, including the National Science

Foundation and the National Institute of Health. The main road to success in this venture is to have an ongoing research or educational program in which there is a need for a microcomputer to improve the program or venture into new avenues using the existing program as a base. The advantages of equipment proposals are that they are usually short and do not require a lengthy preparation time, since the request is based on an already existing program. Although it will be difficult to obtain more than several computers per proposal by this process, this is an attractive mechanism for those organizations with sound research or educational programs.

Special projects

A fourth type of proposal involves funding for a special project or workshop. This type of proposal is most successful when the topic of the project or workshop is at the "cutting edge" of the field or is a matter of controversy. It will be advantageous if the project involves the leading experts in the field. Even then, it will be difficult to obtain equipment by this method. It is best to check the guidelines carefully before pursuing a project of this type to obtain microcomputers.

Consortium or network proposal

Another type of proposal can be best phrased as a *consortium* or *network* proposal. This proposal allows several (or many) institutions to join together to write a proposal dealing with an area or program of mutual interest in communication disorders. This would be an ideal situation for perhaps a hospital clinic, a university, a school system, or a series of universities or school systems. This proposal has many advantages including interinstitutional cooperation, a combination of working expertises, and the strength of numbers. This type of cooperative effort is usually favored by most agencies because more individuals can be served by a common grant. Although these proposals are often complicated and involved, each institution shares in the work.

It is possible from this type of proposal to obtain considerable numbers of microcomputers. This is presently the approach that must be taken in order to compete for the Apple Foundation awards (to be discussed later in this chapter).

Requests for proposals

The last type of proposal that will be discussed is the RFP or *Request for Proposals*. This differs greatly from the other proposals, in that the topic, format, and guidelines are not issued on a regular basis and are usually very specific in nature. These may be issued by government and/or private agencies. The advantage of such a proposal is that the rules are very clear—either the agency is looking for projects dealing with microcomputers or they are not. The other advantage is that the grant is a high priority of the agency. The disadvantage is that in many cases the time allotted for preparation is short and the awards are often few.

CONSIDERATIONS

Regardless of which of these proposals an organization is interested in, there is a variety of factors to consider even if, based on the guidelines, all factors appear favorable. Among these are:

1. What will be the cost to the organization (if the proposal is successful) in terms of purchasing additional software or hardware, or in the necessity of adding additional personnel? In other words, will it cost more than the grant is worth? In most cases the answer will be "no," but it is important to determine this prior to applying.
2. How urgently does the organization need this equipment? Since most proposals take 6 to 9 months to process, if the microcomputer is needed next month, the facts speak for themselves.
3. What are the requirements of the agency if the proposal is successful? These requirements could include ultimate ownership of the equipment, types of reports that are required by the agency, when these reports are due, and specific agreements concerning maintenance of the equipment.

If there is still enthusiasm about pursuing external support for obtaining microcomputers at this time, the next questions to be asking are, "How do I find out what is available?" "How can I keep up with the information?" The answer is that an institution or individual "must" subscribe to one or more of the many publications which are available.

INFORMATION ON FUNDING OPPORTUNITIES

The second part of this chapter discusses many of the major publications that list on a weekly or monthly basis the available funding opportunities.

The *Federal Grants and Contracts Weekly* is a weekly publication which is usually six to 10 pages in length and deals with federal programs. These programs are either new or have upcoming deadlines, or are about to issue guidelines.

The material is presented in short, easy-to-follow fashion and includes pertinent information such as the agency addresses, program officer, and deadline due date. Information is listed as "Grants Alert," "RFPs Available," "Sources Sought," and "Agency Profile." The publication is published by Capitol Publications, Inc., 1300 N. 17th St., Arlington, Va 22209. The 1983 yearly subscription price was $177. The publication is also available by electronic mail. The advantages of this publication are that it is available on a weekly basis and thus is extremely current. In addition, the general scope of the publication allows one to keep tract of the information available from many agencies. The disadvantage, which stems from one of its advantages, is the general nature of the publication. If an organization is a hospital-based clinic, much of the information is this publication may be of only indirect interest.

The *Medical Research and Funding Bulletin* is published three times each month and is available from the Science Support Center, P.O. Box 587, Bronxville, NY 10708. The annual 1983 subscription cost was $48. It contains short descriptions about current programs (from a variety of agencies) dealing with health-related issues. All pertinent information concerning these programs is contained in these descriptions. The information is listed under the following headings: "RFP," "More Upcoming Deadlines," and "Special Announcements." This publication contains information from federal agencies, private foundations, and industrial sources. Although not all the information directly relates to medical programs or speech and hearing programs, this publication is an obvious advantage to medical and medically related institutions.

The *Research Monitor* (*News* and *Profiles*) is published weekly by the National Information Service, 1754 Church St., NW, Washington, DC 20036. The 1983 subscription price was $450. Although possibly too expensive for an individual research office, it can be purchased by an institution's library. The *Research Monitor* is also available over electronic mail. This publication is different in many respects from the two previously described. It consists of two items, each of which can be purchased separately. The *Research Monitor—News* consists of articles describing federal agencies and programs. In addition, it contains information about pending legislation, budgets, and administrative policy. It also contains pertinent *Commerce Business Daily* excerpts and brief descriptions of articles from the *Federal Register*. The *Research Monitor—Profiles* is essentially a set of 9½ × 11 fact sheets, each containing a detailed description of an agency's program. Included on these fact sheets, in addition to the usual pertinent information, are sections dealing with the disciplines supported, types of awards, judging criteria, examples of research, program plans and objectives, and budget and award histories.

The advantages of this publication include the immense amount of factual material that it contains; the disadvantage, especially for small single-purpose institutions, is probably the price.

News Notes—The Grant Advisor is published monthly, except July, by Robert J. Toft, Box 3553, Arlington, VA 22203. The 1983 subscription price was $75 for 11 issues. This publication, which varies from eight to 12 pages in length, contains two- to three-paragraph descriptions of currently available programs from a variety of federal agencies as well as other nonprofit organizations. Each of the program descriptions contains subtitles such as "funding history," "eligibility," "overview," "priorities," and "requirements." In addition, at the end of the publication, there is a six- to eight-page detailed calendar of upcoming deadlines, listed alphabetically by agency, entitled "Deadline Memo."

The advantage of *The Grant Advisor* is that it provides the subscriber with up-to-date information about a variety of different programs and a detailed calendar of deadlines. The main disadvantage of the publication is that it is only published monthly.

The *NSF* (National Science Foundation) *Bulletin* is issued monthly, except July and August, by the Foundation's Public Information Branch. As its title indicates, the *Bulletin* contains information on current and new programs of the Foundation. In addition, the *Bulletin* contains a list of deadlines for upcoming NSF programs, news of meetings to be held at the Foundation, staff changes, and positions that are available at the Foundation. The *Bulletin* also contains a section that lists a variety of publications available from the Foundation (this section can be cut out and used as a request form for these publications). There is no charge for this publication and it can be obtained from the National Science Foundation, Public Information Branch, 1800 G St., NW, Washington, DC 20550.

Similar to the National Science Foundation, the National Institute of Health also issues a bulletin. This worthwhile publication, especially for those agencies with active clinical programs, is the *NIH Guide for Grants and Contracts*. The *Guide* is published at irregular intervals to announce scientific initiatives and to provide policy and administrative information. The *Guide* is published by the Guide and Contracts Distribution Center, National Institutes of Health, Room B3BN10, Building 31, Bethesda, MD 20205. As with the NSF publication, the price is right—there is no charge for the guide. The *Guide* usually contains between 20 and 40 pages and contains information on a variety of upcoming NIH programs. Each program description is between two and four pages and includes material on the background, general characteristics, mechanism of support, review criteria, and method of application dealing with the program. Programs are listed under the general titles "Notice," "Announcement," and "Request for Research Grant Applications."

Another worthwhile publication is the *Chronicle of Higher Education*. The *Chronicle* is published weekly except for the last 2 weeks in August and the last 2 weeks in December. The main editorial and business offices are located at 1333 New Hampshire Ave., NW, Washington, DC 20036. The subscription address is P.O. Box 1955, Marion, OH 43305. The 1983 subscription price was $41. The *Chronicle* contains news articles about *all* aspects of higher education. Of particular interest are the announcements of special programs being offered by a variety of agencies. Although it does not routinely list, as do the other publications, the funding programs available, it does provide a list of recent federal grant recipients as well as recipients of foundations and industrial awards. By reviewing the list one can obtain an idea of what "types of projects are being funded" and which agency (public, private, or industrial) is awarding microcomputers. In addition the *Chronicle* contains excellent articles on current and future trends in education and research, including the use of microcomputers.

PROPOSAL GENERATION

Once the decision has been made to pursue the proposal process and subscribe to one or more publications, the next question that should be asked is "How does one write a successful proposal?" Although there are no guarantees that any proposal will be successful, systematic preparation of a proposal increases the chance for success. The next part of this chapter deals with such issues.

Before one writes a proposal, in addition to considering some of the factors already mentioned, one should carefully examine the funding history and priorities of the donor agency. This information is usually available from the agency or can be obtained from one or more of the publications previously described. If these seem favorable, the next step is to obtain the proposal guidelines. These are available from the agency and in many cases are routinely sent to organizations. It is imperative to carefully read the guidelines prior to initiating the proposal. The guidelines contain information on the sections that the proposal should contain, the proposal deadline, the number of copies that are required, and the mailing address for the proposal. In addition, most guidelines contain the necessary application and budget form. Most guidelines also contain information on major points that should be addressed in the proposal as well as on criteria that are used in reviewing the proposal. This section should be read extremely carefully because proposals that do not follow guideline instructions are doomed to failure.

One final word of caution about the guidelines. Be sure to check whether the proposal due date refers to a postmark date or whether the proposal is due at the agency on that date.

Proposal contents

Abstract and title page

Most agencies provide within the guidelines a title or application face page. The information required on this page provides the agency with the facts it needs about the applicant's organization. These usually include the project title, name and address of project director, starting and termination date of the project, and total funds requested. In addition the page usually requires the signature of the individual authorized to sign for the institution as well as the project directors. Many Department of Education proposals also require the institution's federal identification number.

In addition to the title page, many of the guidelines also have an abstract page or require an abstract; the abstract should summarize the project, usually within a three-paragraph limit. Since the abstract is, in most cases, the reviewer's first introduction to the project, considerable care and thought should be put into its preparation.

Project description

In general, the project description consists of an introduction to the problem as well as pertinent background material relating to the problem. This information should be relevant, up to date, and immediately provoke the reviewer's interest. It should include material from a variety of literature sources.

The best way in which to view an introduction is in terms of a reverse pyramid (Figure 3-1). Start out with a broad description of the project and begin gradually to focus on what

Table 3-2. Sections of a Typical Proposal

General sections	Points to remember
Title page	Most often supplied by agency—supplies agency with the facts it needs to know about the applicant's organization.
Abstract	Most often supplied by the agency. Contains a short summary of the project and in most cases is the reviewer's first introduction to the project.
Project description	Contains introduction to the problem as well as pertinent background material relating to the problem and procedural methods.
Budget	May contain an itemized description of costs requested from agency, costs provided by institutions, as well as the applicant's indirect cost request.
Budget explanation	Contains detailed description of the budget.
Appendices	Contains supplemental materials such as letters of recommendation.

is being proposed. Be sure to include a statement on past work in the area, and clearly delineate what work is now proposed and the methods by which this work is to be accomplished. The project description should conclude with a list of specific project objectives. These should be listed (a, b, c, or 1, 2, 3) in an indented fashion. Many times funding decisions are influenced by whether the objectives are clearly stated, and, in the opinion of the reviewer, can be accomplished by the project staff in the time allocated.

If the project is one that lends itself to setting up a schedule or calendar of activities for the project, this should also be included at the end of the project description. This always impresses the reviewers, since it implies that the project has been planned and thought out. If the objectives to be accomplished can be listed next to a particular activity statement in the schedule, this will definitely add to the quality of the proposal.

EXAMPLE

Date	Activity	Objective met
October 12	Meet with staff	A
October 19	Bring in microcomputer consultant	B
October 26	Select patient sample	D

Budget

All proposals have a budget section. These can be extremely simple or complex, depending on the agency and the type of proposal being prepared. The budget may consist of three sections: direct costs, indirect costs, and cost sharing. Direct costs are those expenditures necessary to

Figure 3-1. Model of reverse pyramid structure for proposal preparation.

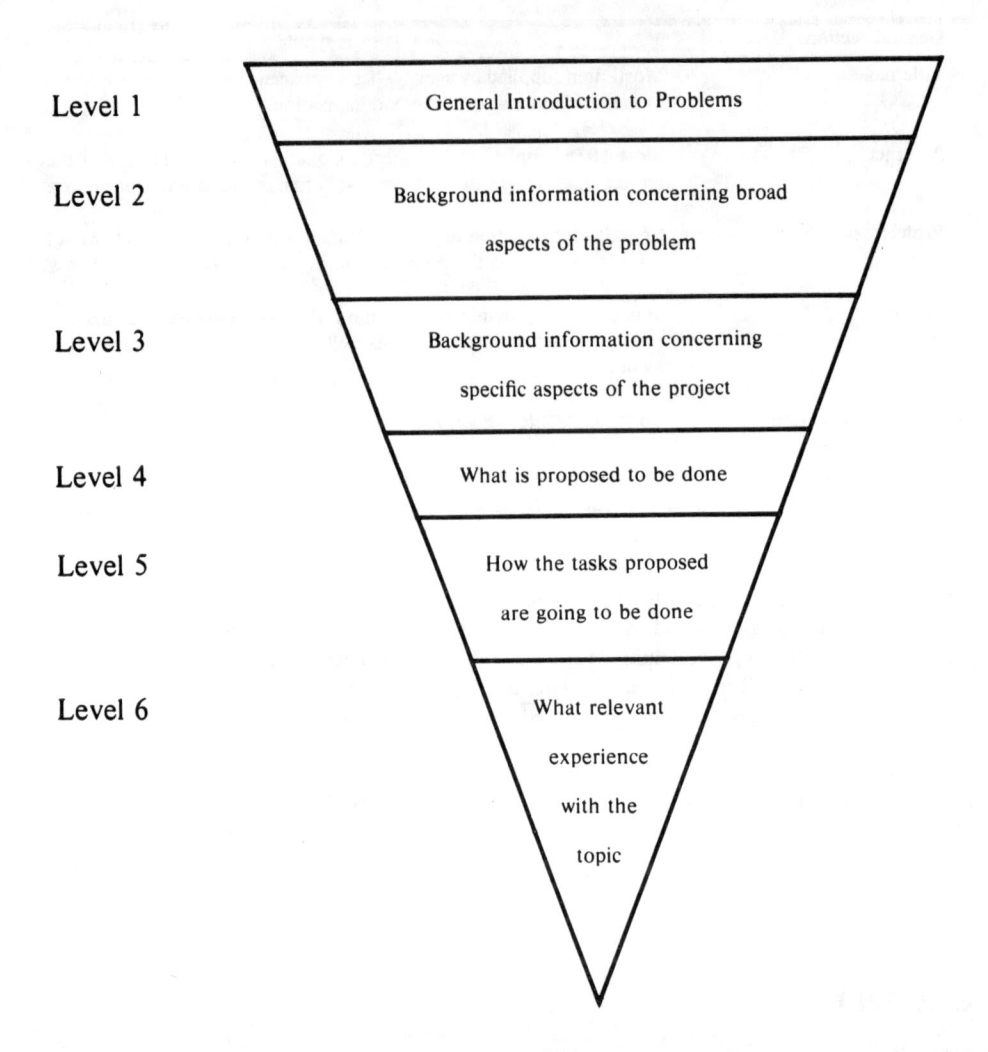

Level 1	General Introduction to Problems
Level 2	Background information concerning broad aspects of the problem
Level 3	Background information concerning specific aspects of the project
Level 4	What is proposed to be done
Level 5	How the tasks proposed are going to be done
Level 6	What relevant experience with the topic

carry out the project. They consist of such items as salaries, equipment, supplies, travel and publication costs, and costs for mailing and photocopying. Most equipment grants only allow direct costs for the purchase price of the equipment, and thus are easy to prepare. In fact, many of these have a maximum in terms of dollars or items of equipment. Indirect costs represent those expenditures necessary to support the project, including items such as building space, utilities, janitorial service, library facilities, and grant administration. Most nonprofit organizations have a percentage indirect cost rate that has been negotiated with a government agency, in most cases with Health and Human Services (HHS). The indirect cost rate is based either on a percentage of the total direct costs or on a percentage of total salary and wages. Many equipment proposals and private agencies do not allow indirect cost charges. Cost-sharing represents the percentage of the total cost of the project that must be contributed by the organization preparing the proposal. This is usually unique to a particular program. For example, most programs at NSF and NIH do not require cost sharing. Cost-sharing expenditures can usually be met by an actual dollar contribution or by contribution of faculty and secretarial time or space. In some cases, it may be necessary to waive some of the indirect costs in order to meet the cost-sharing requirements.

It should be noted, however, that many of the equipment proposals require a matching costs contribution by the applicant.

In many cases, especially if the budget is complex, it is helpful (and may be required by the agency) to provide a budget explanation. The budget explanation describes each item listed in the budget. For example, under salaries the applicant may have to provide information on how the salary requests were calculated; under travel the applicant may have to provide information on when, where, and for what purpose the travel is being requested; and certainly under equipment the applicant will be required to describe, in detail, the equipment requested. This will include the model, type, and manufacturer.

A well-prepared budget explanation will help the reviewers and agencies understand the budget and provide an indication that a good deal of planning went into the preparation of the proposal.

Appendices

It is helpful in most proposals to attach an appendix. The appendices usually contain information that is indirectly related to the proposal, such as letters of support for the project or complete resumés of the project staff. The appendices may, however, contain information directly related to the project, such as a detailed schedule of activities, which if placed within the proposal would exceed the proposal page limit.

Letters of support should be obtained from those individuals who are experts in the project area or would benefit directly if the proposal were funded. Examples of such individuals may include school and health administrators, leaders of organizational groups, and administrators of the applicant's organization. Although it is important to have a sufficient number of support letters, do not obtain them simply to fill up space.

For those proposals that are being submitted to federal agencies and involve several applicant organizations or will benefit a particular segment of the local population such as teachers or retarded students, it is helpful to obtain letters of support from US senators and representatives. Most Congressmen will be more than happy to issue such support letters. A letter to the representative requesting support should contain the following: the title and a brief description of the project, the name and address of the agency where the proposal was sent, and the grant number assigned to the proposal by the agency.

It is also helpful to include a cover letter with the proposal application. This letter should be addressed to the program director and read as follows:

> Enclosed you will find ____ copies of a proposal entitled "Microcomputers for Improving Articulation Therapy" which is being submitted by _____ . We would be happy to furnish additional information upon request.

Sincerely,

The review

Once the proposal has been sent to the agency, it is important to wait for a notification of proposal receipt from the agency. This usually comes in the form of a self-addressed postcard that was part of the application package. This should take between 2 and 4 weeks from the time the proposal was submitted. In many cases the card will contain a proposal number which was assigned by the agency. Any future correspondence between the applicant and the agency concerning the proposal should include the proposal number. It is strongly recommended that the agency be contacted if a notification of proposal receipt has not been received within 4 weeks. There is too much at stake to merely hope that the proposal has arrived.

Table 3-3. Proposal Check List

1.	Is the title page completely filled out including authorized signatures?
2.	Does the abstract adequately present a summary of the project?
3.	Do the budget figures adequately reflect the costs of the project; are there any math errors?
4.	Have you followed the agency's mailing instructions?
5.	Do you have a sufficient number of copies?
6.	Have you prepared a cover letter?

The proposal review process takes from 3 to 9 months, depending on the agency. In most cases at least 6 months can be expected to elapse before receiving the long-awaited news. There is probably no advantage to contacting the agency during this time period. However, it is certainly advisable to phone the agency if nothing has been heard after 6 months. In many cases, the agency might indicate if the proposal was successful once the reviews are completed.

Regardless of the proposal type and the agency, the review is almost always "peer review." This means that the proposal is reviewed by individuals who have some expertise in the field represented by the proposal. The review is either done by mail or reviewers are brought to a central location to review the proposals. In many cases, the reviewers are provided with specific review criteria as well as a score sheet. Almost all proposals are funded on a competitive basis, and it is not atypical to expect changes to be no better than 33%.

Finally, often after what always seems like a longer time than it is, the news from the agency arrives. If the proposal is successful, all the time and effort will have been worthwhile. One word of caution: be sure to carefully read the instructions on how to secure the grant. In some cases, they will require the signing and returning of several forms.

If the news is not favorable, there is bound to be initial disappointment. After this period, it is strongly advised that the applicant request the reviews from the agency. These reviews, in many cases, will be extremely valuable. They can tell what the reviewers did and did not like about the proposal, give an estimate of how close the proposal might have been to being funded, and most importantly, provide sufficient information to make an intelligent decision on whether to submit the proposal once again. It is sometimes helpful to discuss the reviews with the program director.

In concluding this part of the chapter, it is important to emphasize that throughout the proposal preparation stage one should *call the agency* if there are any questions.

INTERNAL PROPOSALS

Many times hospital or school clinicians find themselves forced to deal with the problems of convincing a supervisor, vice president, or chief executive officer of the necessity of obtaining a microcomputer for a particular unit or project. If there are no specific organizational forms or guidelines to follow, it would be helpful to approach this challenge in terms of preparing an *internal proposal*. This proposal should follow the same format as previously mentioned, but should have more of a "local flavor" than proposals submitted to external agencies. In other words, the proposal should not only emphasize why the microcomputer is important to the project, but should stress how this project would help other units within the organization, and how the microcomputer would be used after the project is completed. It should also emphasize, where appropriate, why these microcomputers will be cost effective in the long run. The proposal should be modified accordingly to eliminate those sections, such as indirect costs and cost sharing, which are specifically associated with external proposals. In many cases, the internal proposal need not be as lengthy as the proposal prepared for submission to an external agency.

These proposals, however, require the same thought and attention during their planning and preparation as do external proposals. This is particularly true since it is reviewed by individuals who are familiar with the organization and in many cases are responsible for governing the organization. A well-written internal proposal, therefore, will reflect most positively within the organization on the author's abilities.

FUNDING SOURCES

If the proposal process seems to be a reasonable alternative for a particular institution, it is helpful to investigate specific programs most likely to provide microcomputers as part of the proposal process. This is difficult to determine, since program guidelines and funding priorities change rapidly. Thus the further from the copyright date that one is reading this chapter, the more urgent it is to check on the current guidelines of the programs. The last section of this chapter deals with the agencies and their programs (as of 1983–1984) that are most likely to provide microcomputers through the funding process.

Tandy TRS-80 Educational Grants Program

The objectives of the Tandy Shack program are to (1) encourage and support the successful application of microcomputer technology in educational institutions in this country; (2) ensure a fair and objective evaluation of the relative merits of all such requests to the educational community before any commitments are made.

The program is administered by Tandy TRS-80 Educational Grants Program, Radio Shack Education Division, 1400 One Tandy Center, Fort Worth, TX 76102.

The program consists of four separate competitions each year. Each competition has a particular topic or category that is emphasized. The application and information concerning a particular topic that is emphasized during a funding cycle can be obtained by writing the aforementioned address.

The proposal consists of a cover sheet, abstract, and the body of the proposal. The proposal body should consist of an introduction, needs assessment, objectives, activities, proposal equipment lists section, and program evaluation section. The guidelines of this program limit the grants to Radio Shack-marketed TRS-80 hardware, courseware/software, and accessories only, with a maximum retail value of $15,000. Grants requesting equipment totaling less than $10,000, however, are encouraged. Service contracts cannot be included as part of the grant.

The proposals are reviewed by the Educational Grants Review Board. The Board consists of distinguished educators and meets quarterly throughout the year to rank the proposals for funding. The identity and names of the institution are removed from each proposal before being reviewed by the Board. The processing time is usually 2 months.

The advantages of the program are many. It is offered by the educational foundation of a well-known and respected microcomputer corporation, and thus the only priority of this program is the funding of microcomputers. The proposal, although not usually lengthy, requires one to give considerable thought to how the microcomputer is to be used in the project. In addition, the turn-around time is short compared to many other funding programs. The only disadvantage is that each competition is limited to proposals within a specific category.

All grants under the program will be made only to noncommercial educational institutions, or to individuals who are active as professionals in the field of education and who need assistance for noncommercial educational purposes and/or research.

The Apple Education Foundation

The Apple Education Foundation was established in 1979 to support the development of new methods of teaching and learning through the use of microcomputer technology. The primary goal of the foundation is to direct its resources to educational institutions for projects aimed at improving the quality of students' learning, and to improve teachers' ability to use microcomputers appropriately and effectively to enhance learning.

From 1977 to 1983, grants totaling nearly three quarters of a million dollars were awarded by the Foundation to more than 130 projects for the proposed development of quality, instructional courseware. Some of the projects that have been funded, which may be of particular interest to the reader, are
- *Communication for the Autistic Child;*
- *Computer Speech for Cerebral Palsy Children;*
- *Understanding the Handicapped Child;*
- *Synthesized Speech.*

This program was similar in many respects to the Tandy TRS-80 program until July 1983, at which time the guidelines were drastically changed. In response to a variety of reports concerning the declining status of American education, the Foundation wished to reaffirm its position that microcomputer technology, when used effectively and appropriately, offers a powerful tool for enhancing educational achievement. Thus, the Foundation will now support 2-year collaborative, school-based implementation and training projects that demonstrate the promise of microcomputer technology to develop active learning environments.

Priorities of the Foundation are
1. Models and simulation—particularly student-programmed simulation that teaches skills and procedures.
2. Microworlds—such as logic and logic-based microworlds.
3. Software that gives students intellectual tools such as word processing, image processing, and information retrieval and processing.
4. Tools providing access to activities that are otherwise inaccessible to many students.

The Foundation will provide equipment grants to cooperative projects of K–12 schools and colleges/universities that
1. Use microcomputers to create active learning environments;
2. Integrate students' uses of the computer into the development of systematic knowledge in major curricular areas, other than computer science and computer literacy;
3. Educate teachers to develop the knowledge and skills necessary to do the above successfully;
4. Demonstrate the improvement in the students' learning and gain in achievement resulting from the above efforts.

The successful applicants will be expected to produce one or more of the following products.
1. Collection of students' work—both on disc and hard copy;
2. Description of implementation and teacher-training models;

3. Curriculum materials focused upon integrating computer-based experiences into development of knowledge in language, mathematics, science, and so forth.

Applicants are requested to complete and submit a "concept paper" prior to any full proposal. Concept papers should be sent to: Teachers Can't Wait, Apple Education Foundation, 10201 N. De Anza Boulelvard, Cupertino, CA 95014.

The Foundation planned to award 12 grants for microcomputer equipment in 1984. Each grant consists of the following:
- 30 Apple IIe microcomputers;
- 60 Apple disk drives;
- 30 Apple monitor units IIe;
- 4 pages micromodem II and telecommunication software (donated by Hayer-Microcomputer Products, Inc.)

The advantages of this program are obvious. It allows for a university and local school district to collaborate on a project in which microcomputers will be used to enhance the educational/teaching process. This is a unique opportunity for a department or division of speech and hearing sciences to interact with their local school districts to enhance the use of the microcomputer in the "speech and language therapy" process. The prize—30 microcomputers and the appropriate software—is worth seeking. For further information on the Apple Foundation contact Barbara Bowen, PhD, Director, The Apple Foundation, 10201 N. De Anza Boulevard, Cupertino, CA 95014.

Other Government Agencies

Among the federal agencies, whose priorities and programs are subject to constant change, the agencies most likely to fund microcomputers for speech pathology-related projects are the National Institutes of Health, the Department of Education, and to a much smaller extent, the National Science Foundation.

NINCDS

The program at the National Institutes of Health that would be of interest to individuals in speech–language pathology is the National Institute of Neurological and Communicative Disorders and Stroke (NINCDS). The program has the following subdivisions:
a. Research Project Grants;
b. Program Project Grants;
c. Clinical Research Center Grants;
d. Cooperative Agreements;
e. Conference Grants;
f. Research and Development Contracts;
g. NINCDS Research Training and Development Programs;
h. National Research Service Awards;
i. Research Career Development;
j. Awards;
k. Teacher Investigator Development Awards.

Among the many missions of this program are studies of human communication, including speech and language, disorders of hearing and equilibrium, and disorders of speech and other central nervous system functions.

It is clear that one or more of the divisions within the program would be applicable to the types of proposals mentioned earlier in this chapter.

The director of the division is Dr. F. J. Brinley, Jr., Director, Convulsive Developmental and Neuromuscular Disorders Program, National Institute of Neurological and Communicative

Disorders and Stroke, National Institutes of Health, Federal Building—Room 812, Bethesda, MD 20205, (301) 496-6541.

Material for individual programs within the division can be obtained by writing or calling the following: Research Grants, Program Projects, and Centers, Director, Extramural Activities Program, NINCDS-NIH, Bethesda, MD 20205, (301) 496-9248; Research and Development Contracts, Contracting Officer, Extramural Activities Program, NINCDS-NIH, Bethesda, MD 20205, (301) 496-9203; or Training Grants and Awards, Deputy Director, Extramural Activities Program, NINCDS-NIH, Bethesda, MD 20205, (301) 496-4188.

Department of Education

Perhaps the most important program for communication disorders at the Department of Education involving the use of microcomputers in training is the "Training Personnel for the Education of the Handicapped Program." This program, which is offered by the Office of Special Education and Rehabilitative Services, has as its major purpose improving the quality and increasing the supply of special education and support personnel.

An applicant for a grant may propose a project period of up to 36 months. Generally, awards are made for periods ranging from 24 to 36 months. In 1984 the Secretary, because of a pressing national need to integrate services in education, health, and rehabilitation for handicapped adolescents and young adults, and because there is an extreme variability in the quality and level of services available for newborn and infant handicapped children, urged submission of applications which would prepare personnel to assist handicapped students in the transition from school to employment and community living, and to prepare personnel to provide services to newborn and infant handicapped children.

The Secretary also urged the submission of applications to prepare personnel to educate minority or underserved populations and provide training for members of groups that have been traditionally underrepresented. Within the program the following division will be of particular interest to the reader.

Handicapped—Preparation of special educators—New projects.

The priority of this division includes the preparation of speech-language pathologists and audiologists. The average grant for FY 1984 was expected to be $50,000. Applications submitted under this competition will provide for the preservice preparation of special education personnel. Projects should be designed to assist agencies and institutions in developing and maintaining quality training programs in order to alleviate the effects of identified shortages (national, state, local level) in the supply and distribution of certified special educators. Preservice activities may include training for the baccalaureate, masters, and specialists degrees—no doctoral or postdoctoral training activities are supported under this competition. Examples of training efforts which may be supported under this competition include (a) The preparation of instructional personnel to serve low-incidence populations, such as seriously emotionally disturbed, autistic, usually handicapped, deaf, and hard-of-hearing children and youth; (b) the preparations of other special education personnel including supervisors and administrators of special education programming and those who serve in diagnostic instructional capacities within the school setting; (c) the training of speech-language pathologists and audiologists; (d) the graduate training of minority students in speech-language pathology and audiology to serve handicapped preschool children.

Applications are reviewed according to the following criteria:
a. extent of need
b. participation
c. plan of operation
d. evaluation plan
e. evaluation design
f. quality of key personnel

g. adequacy of resources
h. contribution
i. budget and cost effectiveness.

Guidelines, information, and application forms can be obtained by writing Dr. Herman Sattler, Acting Director, Division of Personnel Preparation, Special Education Programs, US Department of Education, 400 Maryland Ave., SW, Donohue Building, Room 4805, Washington, DC 20202, (202) 245-9886.

FIPSE. Another program from the Department of Education that is worth considering in terms of possibly obtaining microcomputers is the Fund for the Improvement of Postsecondary Education (FIPSE) (The Comprehensive Program). The Fund supports an array of diverse projects each year. Grant projects, however, are local improvements which, if successful, usually continue beyond the period of fund support.

Each year administrators of the Fund identify a variety of priority areas where proposals are encouraged. One of the areas for the past several years has been the "Uses and Implications of the New Technologies," an area developed out of concern about the capacity of organizations to use technology appropriately and effectively. Many institutions seem to be treating these strictly as administrative questions without considering their educational implications. The Fund administrators envision the best proposals (in this area) to be those that create better visions about learning which reconceive the content and the students' mode of learning, and proposals about institutional arrangements that reflect understanding of how organizations can influence learning.

The FIPSE program has a two-stage submission and review process. The first stage consists of a 5- to 7-page preliminary proposal. This is reviewed by the Fund and about 10% of the applicants are requested to submit a final proposal. The final proposal should consist of 20–30 double-spaced pages and should address the following:
1. Problem identification;
2. Description of proposed project;
3. Statement of intended outcomes;
4. Discussion of the applicants capacity and commitment;
5. Discussion of plan for wider impact.

About 30–50% of the final applications are funded. Further information as well as guidelines and application forms can be obtained by writing: The Fund for the Improvement of Postsecondary Education, 7th D Street, SW, Room 3100, Washington, DC 20202.

National Science Foundation

The one program in the Foundation that might be applicable to the reader, depending on the nature of the institution or specialty of the individuals, is the Linguistics Program. The program supports studies of syntactic, semantic, phonological, and phonetic properties of individual languages and of language in general, psychological processes in the production and perception of speech, biological foundations of language, social influences on and effects of language and dialect variations, and formal and mathematical properties of language models.

The Linguistics Program of the Foundation is part of the Directorate for Biological, Behavioral, and Social Sciences, within the Division of Behavioral and Neural Sciences.

For further information contact Paul G. Chapin, Program Director, Linguistics, National Science Foundation, 1800 G St., NW, Washington, DC 20550.

State agencies

The possibility for obtaining funding from state and local agencies certainly exists. The number and types of programs are dependent on state and local governments and are too diverse and complex to specifically delineate in this chapter. The reader is urged to contact state and local educational and health agencies to determine the programs in their area (see Wilkins, chap. 4).

There is, however, one program that is common to all states. This program is a result of the 1981 Education Consolidation and Improvement Act (Chapter 2). The purpose of Chapter 2 is to consolidate a variety of previous federal programs, which include:
1. Titles II, III, IV, V, VI, VIII, and IX of the Elementary and Secondary Act of 1965;
2. the Alcohol and Drug Abuse Education Act;
3. part A and section 352 of Title V of the Higher Education Act of 1965;
4. the Follow Through Act;
5. section 3(a)1. of the National Science Foundation Act of 1950 relating to precollege science teacher training; and
6. the Career Education Incentive Act,

into a single authorization to states to be used in accordance with educational needs and priorities of state and local educational agencies as determined by these agencies. It is the goal of Chapter 2 that approximately 80% of these funds be distributed by the state to local educational agencies, while the remaining 20% may be used by the state to develop a competitive grants program. The reader is urged to contact the State Board of Education for the details.

CONCLUSION

The external funding process represents one means by which to obtain microcomputers. This mechanism is available to any nonprofit organization regardless of size, scope, purpose, or goals. The key ingredients are a worthwhile project, the right funding agency, writing and research skills, patience, and perhaps a little bit of luck. This mechanism will not meet the needs of all organizations.

This chapter addresses sources, procedures, and strategies to follow in obtaining funding for the purchase of microcomputer systems. The list that follows contains references which will be of help to the reader.

The reader is urged to use the information in the chapter as a guideline in determining the best combination of resources and skills necessary to be competitive in the "grants game." Exactly what these are will differ between individuals and institutions, and only the readers entrance into the "grants arena" will help in determining the successful combination.

REFERENCE NOTES

Corry, E. (1982). *Grants for libraries: A guide to public and private funding programs and proposal writing techniques.* Littleton, CO: Libraries Unlimited.

Duca, D. (1982, February). New strategy for writing proposals now necessary. *Fund Raising Management, 12:12,* 58.

Goldberg, L. M. (1982, November). Resources for successful grantseeking. *Perspective for Teachers of the Hearing Impaired, 1:2,* 22–23.

Heathington, B. S., Teague, G. V., & Heathington, K. W. (1982, Fall). Understanding the proposal review process. *Journal of the Society of Research Administrators, 13:2,* 41–47.

Lee, L. (1982). *The grants game.* San Francisco: Harbor Publishers; New York: distributed by Putnam.

Reif-Lehrer, L. (1982). *Writing a successful grant application.* Boston, MA: Science Books International.

Seldin, C. A., & Maloy, R. W. (1981). Public school grant writing: Educational innovation in times of retrenchment. *Clearing House, 54:7,* 330–333.

Sultz, H. A., & Sherwin, F. S. (1981). *Grant writing for health professionals* (1st ed.). Boston: Little, Brown.
Upshur, C. C. (1983, September). Life after a grant: Now the hard work begins for grantee. *Fund Raising Management, 14:*7, 26-30.
Urgo, L. A. (1978). *Models for money: Obtaining government and foundation grants and assistance* (2nd ed.). Boston: Suffolk University Management Education Center.
White, V. P. (1983). *Grant proposals that succeeded.* New York: Plenum.

Chapter 4

Informational Resources, Systems, and Services

Walter R. Wilkins

"Where do I find out about...?" is one of the most frequent questions asked by speech and language pathologists, or by audiologists trying to obtain information about microcomputer hardware, software, or applications. A variety of resources and services exist that can assist specialists in locating information needed for making decisions about microcomputers. Books, directories, journals, and other published material can be obtained from libraries. Information on microcomputers can in addition be obtained using online data bases, through dealers and users' groups, through professional associations, and from consultants.

Rarely will a single resource be fully adequate for every information need. Each of the different kinds of resources discussed here provides some types of information better than others. The purpose of this chapter is to explore the various kinds of resources and services available to specialists in communication disorders, so that those seeking information on microcomputer applications may become more fully aware of the information resources that are now available.

LIBRARIES

Accessibility of libraries

Libraries are convenient informational resources because they contain books, journals, other documentary material on a variety of subjects, and because they are *accessible*. Published information on microcomputers is becoming more and more plentiful in libraries. Libraries can be useful informational resources for speech-language pathologists and audiologists to locate information about microcomputers.

Almost every community of any size has a public library. Most community college, university, or college libraries are open to the public. Libraries of corporations, hospitals, schools, or government agencies are occasionally open to the public on a limited basis. In many cases these "special libraries" are also able to provide informational services *indirectly,* through public libraries, by means of cooperative arrangements between libraries within a municipality or region. Such cooperative arrangements make it possible to borrow material, or to obtain photocopies of pages from journals or reference books that are unavailable.

©College-Hill Press, Inc. All rights, including that of translation, reserved. No part of this publication may be reproduced without the written permission of the publisher.

Nearly every library is staffed to provide assistance to people. Reference librarians and paraprofessional staff assist people in locating publications, and can assist people in using bibliographies or indexes that identify useful microcomputer publications.

In each state capital there is a *state library,* the library of the state's government. Established to meet the informational needs of the state's legislature, and other governmental agencies, the state library contains books, journals, and other materials needed by officials.

State libraries are often a good source of *referral* information for those who need to know which state agency or agencies can best provide a specific service or answer a specific question. The libraries themselves often contain information on sources of state grants, or federal grants administered by the state. Where this is not available, the reference librarian can usually direct the query to the appropriate agency.

Using libraries

Libraries provide a number of different information sources and services. To use a library effectively, the specialist should try to use the library *systematically* when searching for information. Figure 4-1 illustrates how one might proceed in searching for information in a library.

First, the specialist should characterize the kind of information that is needed. This need not be complicated. The point is to match the library's resources to the type of information that is needed.

Second, relevant sources for locating publications should be selected and used. If the information needed is of a general, rather than a specific nature, then books are the most likely source of that kind of information, and the specialist can proceed to the *card catalog* to find appropriate books. If the information is specific, but brief in nature, an address, a definition, a price, then a *reference book* is probably appropriate. Again the card catalog should be consulted to find relevant reference books. Time need not be spent elsewhere if this approach answers the question.

More thorough queries usually mean that *indexes* may need to be consulted, perhaps in addition to the card catalog. *Data base search services* should be considered here, especially if the query is somewhat complicated, or if the indexes are not immediately productive.

The indexes and the card catalog should be used systematically as well. If appropriate subject headings cannot easily be found, the specialist should immediately begin looking through the index or card catalog to see if the index uses a synonym in the index for the term the specialist was looking for. If an appropriate subject heading cannot be found quickly, assistance should be sought from a librarian before abandoning the search.

Third, determine whether the library has material found in the card catalog or the indexes and decide whether to request an interlibrary loan or referral to another library, if the library does not have the particular publications needed.

Finally, if after consulting the publications more information is needed, repeat the search process. Assistance from the library staff should be sought whenever the search process does not proceed smoothly for any reason. The point is to proceed *deliberately* whenever searching, and to avoid wasting time in unproductive search procedures.

Types of informational services in libraries

Some commonly available library resources are particularly useful sources of information on microcomputers. Of particular value are:

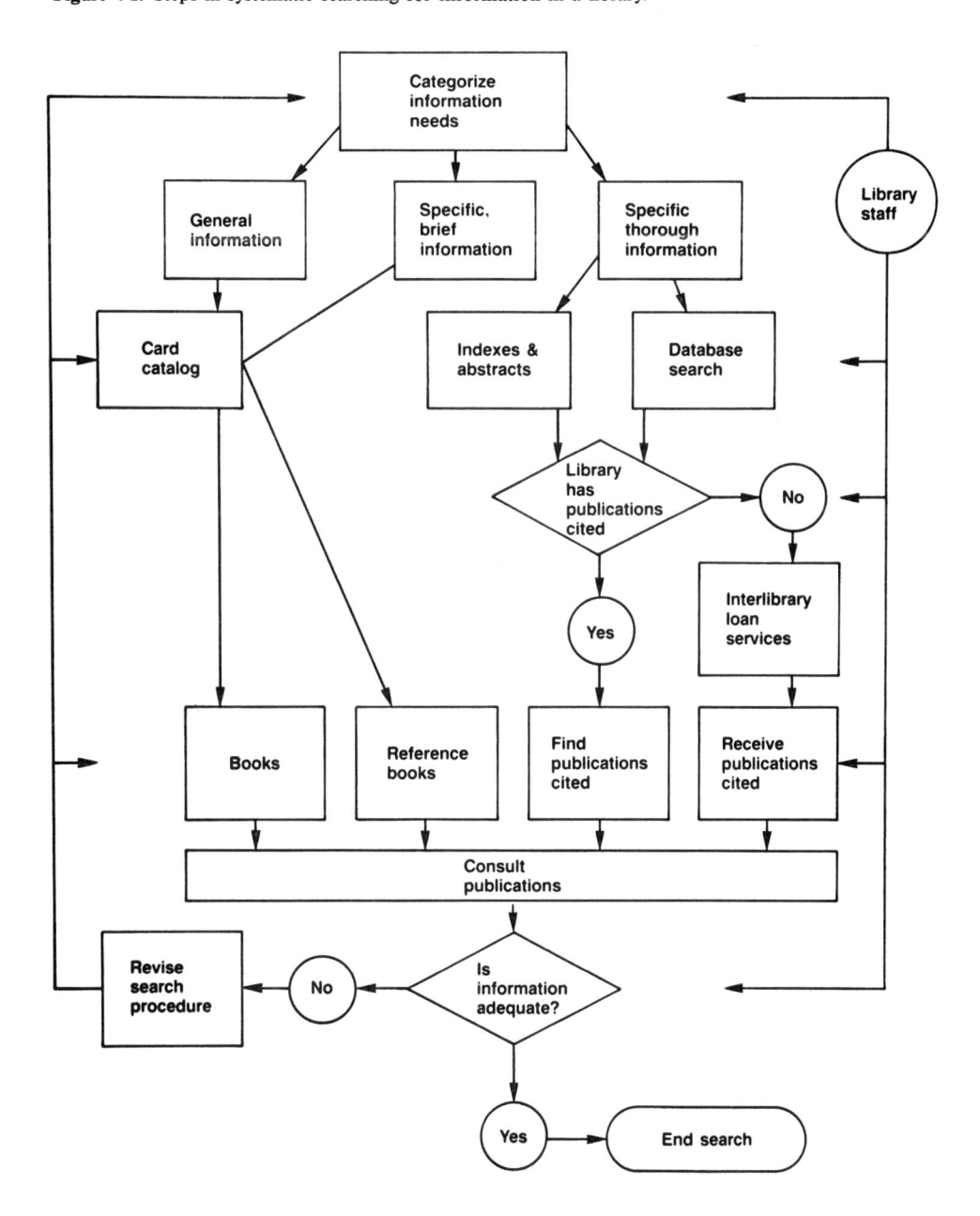

Figure 4-1: Steps in systematic searching for information in a library.

Reference Books and Directories Data Base Search Services
Books on Microcomputers Interlibrary Loan Services
Journals Microcomputers
Indexes and Abstracts

The procedures outlined in Figure 4-1 may help in choosing among the different types of materials and services available through a library.

Reference books and directories

References books and directories permit quick location of brief, basic, or detailed information. Some questions about microcomputers should not require a great deal of reading or perusal of books and magazines. Reference books are published with the idea of providing specific information, arranged in such a way that answers to a question can be found quickly, without reading through a great deal of text. Those needing brief, specific information may find their questions answered after consulting appropriate reference books. The library's card catalog (see Figure 4-1) can be used to locate reference books or directories by title, author, or subject.

Dictionaries and encyclopedias. Definitions of terms and concise explanations of specific facts, concepts, or ideas are given in dictionaries and encyclopedias. Galland's (1982) *Dictionary of Computing* is a good example of such a dictionary. Another is Sippl's (1980) *Computer Dictionary,* which contains over 12,000 definitions of terms. Where such dictionaries are not available, many introductory books, such as Hartnell's and Veit's (1983) *The Complete Buyer's Guide to Personal Computers,* and Blumenthal's (1983) *Everyone's Guide to Personal Computers,* include a glossary of over 100 definitions of commonly used microcomputer terms. Elsewhere in this book, Chial presents a glossary of over 500 common terms that are relevant to speech-language pathologists or audiologists using microcomputers.

Helm's (1983) *McGraw-Hill Computer Handbook* is a good example of the special encyclopedia devoted to computers. It presents, briefly, and in one volume, a wide variety of facts about computers.

Included in the encyclopedia category are *information services,* encyclopedias which provide highly detailed information, and which are regularly updated by monthly supplements. The *Datapro Management of Small Computer Systems* (Datapro Research Corporation, 1982) contains reports on microcomputer hardware, software packages, vendors, planning a microcomputer system, advice on using microcomputers, and a glossary. It is kept up to date with monthly supplements. Arrangements for *writing or telephoning* the Datapro staff for answers to specific questions are set forth in the introductory pages of this service.

Somewhat similar is the *Auerbach Data World* (Auerbach Publishers, 1978) which gives highly detailed reports on currently available hardware and software. Monthly supplements keep the information current. The *Auerbach Data World* also permits subscribers to telephone for answers to specific questions.

Directories. Specialty directories provide names, addresses, and brief descriptive information about people, organizations, or products. This may be helpful when trying to locate a source of microcomputer hardware or software. The cost of directories usually discourages purchase by individuals. But a good directory is often the best way to find out what sorts of equipment and software are available. The editors of *Personal Computing* (Answers, 1983b, p. 154) recommend consulting directories as one of the major ways to find appropriate hardware and software sources.

The *Online Terminal/Microcomputer Guide and Directory 1982-83* (1982) is one of several directories of equipment for microcomputers. Information is provided on manufacturers, sales outlets, brokers, service, and maintenance. A "guide" section includes specification of printers and terminals. The *Online Micro-Software Guide and Directory, 1983-84* (1982) is a microcomputer software directory. In addition to listing software packages and software producers, there is a section of the directory that lists software distributors, and the specifications of software packages.

Hardware and software are also listed in the *Microcomputer Buyer's Guide* (1983). *The Microcomputer Market Place* (1983) also lists both hardware and software sources, and it includes listings of computer associations and consultants. This may be helpful to individuals or organizations with unique questions or specific needs for microcomputers. Brubaker and Rolnick (1984) have developed a directory of clinical software which can be used for aphasia rehabilitation and cognitive retraining that includes a description of over 130 software programs in the public and proprietary domain that are indexed by areas of patient deficit.

Manufacturers and publishers usually offer their catalogs free of charge, and many dealers can supply an assortment of brochures. But directories display the offerings of several manufacturers or software publishers at once, simplifying comparisons and selection. Dewey's (1984) review of software directories may be useful in choosing an appropriate directory.

Books on microcomputers

Books on *microcomputers* provide a wide range of information, from general or introductory material to specialized or highly technical data. Some general books on microcomputers, however, do include information on specific microcomputers, peripheral equipment, or software relevant to those in the communications sciences. *Everyone's Guide to Personal Computers,* by Blumenthal (1983) and *The Complete Buyer's Guide to Personal Computers,* by Hartnell and Veit (1983) are examples of this sort of book. Many of these books also contain bibliographies, lists of other useful books or journals.

In addition to introductory or "survey" books on microcomputers, many libraries have more specific books that deal with programming languages, word processing, and other aspects of microcomputer applications. Some are user guides to specific equipment or software, such as *The Vic 20 User Guide* (Heilborn, 1983) and *The Apple User's Guide* (Poole, 1983). There are also "how-to-program" books, such as *Armchair BASIC* (Fox, 1983) which give step-by-step instructions in writing programs for a microcomputer in one of the available languages.

Some books focus on specific programs or specialized applications. *A User's Guide to the UNIX System* (Thomas, 1982) and *The Visicalc Home and Office Companion* (Castlewitz, 1982) are examples. Specific professions are the focus of some books, such as Taber's (1983) *Microcomputers in Special Education,* and Rienhoff's (1983) *The Computer in the Doctor's Office.*

There are so many books now available on microcomputers that, for those needed only occasionally or for a short time, borrowing them from a library may be the more feasible option. A library can also be of help in finding books that the library does not have, but which the specialist might want to purchase or borrow from another library. Book reviews that appear in many microcomputer magazines might be helpful.

Journals

Libraries provide a selection of current issues of magazines or journals. Older volumes, or backfiles, may be available. There are an increasingly large number of journals, magazines, newsletters, and so forth, becoming available, whose focus is on microcomputers.

These are some of the journals that are substantially or entirely devoted to information on microcomputers:

Byte (1975)
Compute! (1979)
Computers and Electronics (1982)
Creative Computing (1974)
Personal Computing (1977)
Popular Computing (1981)

The articles in these journals are general in scope, and usually do not require that the reader be expert with microcomputers. And frequently there are articles in such magazines that may be useful to those in the communications sciences.

There are also many journals that focus on a specific brand or model of microcomputer, such as *The Atari Connection* (1981) aimed at the Atari 400 or Atari 800 user, *80 Microcomputer* (1980) for the TRS-80 user, and also *Nibble* (1980) which is primarily for users of Apple computers. Nearly every microcomputer has its own journal or newsletter.

An increasing number of journals are being published that are devoted to the use of computers in specific disciplines. These are some of them:

AEDS Journal (1967)
AEDS Monitor (1962)
Computers in Biology and Medicine (1970)
Computers in Healthcare (1982)
Computers in Psychiatry/Psychology (1978)
The Computing Teacher (1979)
Educational Technology (1961)
T H E Journal (1973)

It is not uncommon for professional journals to publish occasional articles or devote whole issues to microcomputer applications in that particular discipline. Many highly specialized journals, such as *Behavior Research Methods and Instrumentation* (1968) include specific studies of computer applications in the clinical or educational professions.

Articles in many of these and other similar journals describe developments in microcomputer hardware, peripheral equipment, or newly released software. Some journals regularly publish *reviews* of microcomputer hardware and software, such as "Rating Micros for Word Processing," by Hannan (1983). Specialists considering purchasing new equipment or peripheral equipment may find the information in these articles useful, especially if the article is based on actual test use of the item.

Many of these magazines also have a regular column where the editorial staff attempts to answer readers' questions. Frequently these columns contain brief but valuable pieces of information, such as whether a surge protector really does any good, or what kinds of memory are useful for different graphics programs.

To get an idea of what microcomputer magazines are available, the specialist can consult an introductory book on microcomputers, such as Blumenthal (1983) or Hartnell and Veit (1983) which contain an annotated list of major microcomputer magazines. Some directories, such as the *Classroom Computer News Directory of Educational Computing Resources* (1982) provide a substantial listing of microcomputer journals. The *Ulrich's International Periodicals Directory* (1932) and *The IMS Ayer Directory of Publications* (1925) have for many years provided thorough listings of available magazines.

Current issues of journals are often available in stores and at computer dealers, of course, not only in libraries. But for older issues, the library may often be the only source.

Indexes and abstracts

Articles in magazines or journals may be located by subject in many of the indexes available in libraries. Those needing thorough and current information (see Figure 4-1) may need the sort of material published in journals. It is not difficult to find articles on microcomputers using indexes and abstract services such as these.

Almost all libraries have *The Reader's Guide to Periodical Literature* (1900) which covers articles on computers and microcomputers that appear in the weekly news magazines and in other popular magazines. Specialists may often find these articles useful, even though they are not highly technical.

A large number of journals on computers and data processing are indexed in the *Business Periodicals Index* (1958), making this index valuable even for those who do not consider themselves to be "in business." The *Education Index* (1929) indexes articles in professional education journals, as well as those in special education. Specialists working in an education setting, or who work with schoolage children would find the articles on microcomputers in this index relevant in many cases.

Some more specialized indexes, like *Index Medicus* (1879) cover a larger number of journals than those previously mentioned. Articles can be found here on new computer applications from a medical or health care perspective, in the professional journals. Indexes such as *Psychological Abstracts* (1927) provide summaries of the articles and documents indexed. It is not difficult to find material on microcomputers using professional-level sources. And the new index format in *DSH Abstracts* (1960) makes it easier to find articles in speech and hearing journals on microcomputers than it has been previously.

Data base search services

The indexes and abstracts held by a particular library can often be usefully supplemented by searching online data bases. Data base search services are provided by libraries to obtain references on a variety of topics. The data bases searched are simply computerized versions of printed indexes and directories. For instance, citations and abstracts in the ERIC indexes are available, as are the biographical entries in *American Men and Women of Science* (1982). With data base searching services, it is possible to search for references to journal articles simply on the basis of whether the word "microcomputer," or "Commodore" is present in the citation or abstract of the article.

Many libraries charge a fee for data base searching, to recover a portion or all of their costs. According to Roose (1983) many of the public libraries performing data base searches find that most searches done for their clients cost no more than $20.00. By using data base search services, indexes not available at a particular library can be searched via computer, eliminating the need to travel to another library just to use the more specialized indexes.

Interlibrary loan services

When, in following the procedure outlined in Figure 4-1, the indexes or data base search results cite a publication not available in the library, the next step is either to visit the library that has the publication, or to request an interlibrary loan.

Almost all libraries will borrow books or secure photocopies of journal articles for their own clientele. If, in searching an index or in going over the results of a data base search, an article of real interest is found, the library can probably send for a copy of the article, if it happens to be in a journal that the library does not own.

To facilitate interlibrary borrowing services, many libraries participate in state or regional cooperative organizations, whose purpose is to make interlibrary borrowing more reliable and effective among those libraries. In most states, public libraries are organized into regional cooperative organizations, often called "systems." Academic, school, and special libraries are often included in these systems. These organizations help set up detailed arrangements for interlibrary borrowing.

Many heath science libraries are organized into regional consortiums for similar purposes. Through the consortiums they, too, are able to arrange for regular interlibrary borrowing for their clients.

With effective interlibrary loan services, books and articles about microcomputers can usually be supplied without difficulty, even though the library does not actually own the publications.

Microcomputers

Although not directly related to the process of searching for information in a library, communication disorders specialists may be interested to know that some libraries are beginning to provide microcomputers for use, often charging a fee or, according to Kusak and Bowers (1982), providing coin-operated access. Such services, developed primarily to permit children and youth to become familiar with microcomputers, also provide a prospective buyer with a chance to try out a particular microcomputer or program.

Where public microcomputers are available in libraries, specialists may find them useful if there is a desire to try out the equipment or software without obligation.

There are, without doubt, a substantial number of published information sources on microcomputers and microcomputer applications. In many cases it will be useful to purchase some of the books and subscribe to some of the journals. But the specialist cannot possibly buy every publication that might be needed. Libraries provide an organized collection of many of these resources, along with the means to identify and procure publications not held by the library itself. Many libraries have *subject specialists* on their staff, familiar with the literature of data processing, or the health sciences, who can provide informed guidance to specialized resources. A library, properly used, can be quite helpful to the specialist seeking information on microcomputers.

AGENCIES AND ASSOCIATIONS

These are at present a large number of associations and agencies that have programs for providing information and assistance to microcomputer users.

National educational and professional associations

National organizations hold meetings and conventions, where new developments can be presented and discussed with colleagues. Some associations support publications on microcomputer applications; some sponsor workshop or seminars. Here are a few examples of these associations.

The *Association of Computer Users* (ACU) provides its members with newsletters, technical publications, and guides. It also offers a telephone reference service called SOFSEARCH whereby, according to Segal and Berst (1983, p. 100), members can request specific advice from Association staff on selecting software packages appropriate for their applications.

An example of an education association is the *International Council for Computers in Education* (ICCE) which publishes *Computing Teacher* (1979) as well as several booklets on instructional applications of computers. This association also encourages local and regional educational computing associations to affiliate. The *Association for Educational Data Systems* (AEDS) includes both educators and data processing professionals in its membership, and publishes articles of interest to administrators. This organization sponsors workshops and seminars and publishes two journals and a newsletter.

Consortiums

National and regional consortiums of organizations pool the resources of smaller organizations to provide evaluations of hardware and software, technical assistance, workshops, and other assistance to groups who are consortium members, and frequently to nonmembers as well.

The *Minnesota Educational Computer Consortium* (MECC) is a consortium of Minnesota educational agencies and institutions. It provides for group purchase of hardware for its members. This consortium also develops software, according to Marchionini (1981), and offers it for sale. Many consortiums in other states are affiliated with the MECC.

A number of teacher centers participate in *INTER—Informal Network for Technological and Educational Research* (Norwood, 1983), to keep up to date on research being done with educational software. The state of Illinois has at least three regional computer consortiums for school districts. Many other states have one or more such consortiums.

Clearinghouses

Clearinghouses facilitate the collection and distribution of information. Many organizations perform clearinghouse services for their members. There are also a few agencies which are clearinghouses specifically for computer information.

The *Microcomputer Software and Information for Teachers* (MICROSIFT) clearinghouse, begun in 1979, provides evaluations of instructional software for microcomputers (Williams, 1981). The *Microcomputer Education Applications Network* (MEAN) assists teachers in developing and selling software packages. It also provides information on microcomputer applications to school districts and state education agencies. The *National Association of State Directors of Special Education* (NASDSE) sponsors the SpEd Tech Center, which provides assistance on technology utilization to state education agencies, and which also conducts training programs for educators of the deaf on microcomputers and other applications of technology.

State education agencies

Most state departments of education have programs providing information and training on microcomputers for school district personnel. Here are some examples, taken from the *Classroom Computer News Directory of Educational Computing Resources* (1983).

Arizona's Department of Education sponsors a Resource Center, which has a library of software reviews and collection of software publisher's catalogs. The Center also provides referral services for teachers. A series of regional Teacher Education and Computer (TEC) centers has been established by the California agency to provide inservice training and to help answer individual requests for information from teachers. In Michigan, the State Library has set up a Microcomputer Resource Center to provide training for educators, librarians, and government employees.

Almost every state department of education designates a staff member to coordinate information on computer applications in education or related fields. Many of the states sponsor or co-sponsor an agency to serve as a clearinghouse or training resource within the state.

Finding agencies and associations

Most national associations may be found in the *Encyclopedia of Associations* (1984) which gives the address and phone number of each association listed, as well as a one-paragraph summary of the association's purpose and activities. Associations may be found by subject, using the encyclopedia's index. This encyclopedia is also accessible as an online data base.

The *Classroom Computer News Directory of Educational Computing Resources* (1983) has one of the better listings of state and regional agencies and associations in the area of applications for computers. Each listing includes a brief description of the organization's activities, as well as its address and telephone number.

Agencies and associations can be useful sources of current information on microcomputer applications and on microcomputer hardware and software. Both novices and experienced microcomputer users may find them helpful.

ONLINE DATA BASES

Commercially available online data bases include indexes, directories, and statistical data, all available in machine-readable form. The data base can be searched by computer; individual records or entries can be selected, displayed online, or printed offline. Data base *vendors* make the data base accessible to their customers by offering telephone access to the computers on which the data bases are loaded. Bibliographic Retrieval Service's *BRS,* Lockheed Corporation's *DIALOG,* and System Development Corporation's *ORBIT* are three of the major commercial data base services. Electronic mail services such as *EarNet* or *SpecialNet* facilitate the exchange of information particularly relevant to specialists in communications sciences.

Microcomputer information from data bases

A number of data bases are useful for providing references to information on microcomputers and data processing. *Microcomputer Index* (available through DIALOG) is an index to microcomputer journals. It is the machine-readable version of the printed index of the same title. Each citation in the data base includes a short abstract. This data base can provide citations to general information articles, hardware and software reviews, and other citations that could be retrieved by subject.

The *Computer Database* (DIALOG) is an index with abstracts to journals, newsletters, research reports, and books in the field of computers and telecommunications. This data base attempts to index publications "cover to cover," so that minor news notices are indexed and retrievable, as are major articles in the publications. This has no print counterpoint; it exists only as a data base.

DISC (available through BRS) is another index to microcomputer journals. The citations in this data base do not include abstracts. However, this data base has a feature that permits the entire table of contents of a magazine to be displayed. DISC is also available only as a data base.

The *International Software Database* (DIALOG) is a directory, rather than an index, of journal citations. It contains listings of commercially available software for microcomputers and minicomputers. The entries can be searched by subject and by the hardware with which the software happens to be compatible (Apple II, TRS-80, etc.). Entries for the software packages include a short description, as well as the price and the supplier's address. The *International Microcomputer Software Directory* (1982) and the *International Minicomputer Software Directory* (1982) are the print versions of this database.

The *Online Microcomputer Software Directory* (SOFT) (BRS) includes entries for commercially available microcomputer software, and the entries in the data base can be searched by subject and by hardware requirements. It is a data base version of a printed directory of the same title.

Speech and hearing information from data bases

A number of data bases may be useful information resources for searching professional literature relevant to speech and hearing. *Index Medicus (1879)* and *Psychological Abstracts*

(1927) are both searchable as online data bases. Articles in the field of education and special education are searchable in the *ERIC* and in the *Exceptional Child Education Resources* data bases.

In addition to online journal indexes, there are also a few online *directories* in the field of education. Some of these may be useful for specialists. *Resources in Computer Education (RICE)* (BRS) is a directory of educational software packages produced by the Northwest Regional Educational Laboratory. Directory entries may be searched by subject and by hardware requirements. The *School Practices Information File (SPIF)* (BRS) is a directory of educational programs and materials. Both curricular materials and instructional techniques, contributed by school districts from all over the country, can be found in SPIF. This data base is produced by the School Practices Information Network (SPIN). The citations include an ample descriptive abstract. Specialists interested in finding out about relevant materials or techniques developed at other schools may find this a useful data base.

Funding information from data bases

Some online data bases may be useful in seeking sources of grants or funding. The *Foundation Directory* (1983) and the *Foundation Grants Index* (1983) are available as data bases. In addition, there are *Grants Database* (DIALOG) and the *National Foundations* (DIALOG) data base, which provide similar information on funding sources. The *Commerce Business Daily* (1977) which includes announcements of federal grants available, contact persons, and deadlines for applications, is also a data base on DIALOG. Like the print version, it is updated daily.

Rockman (1983) gives some helpful suggestions for searching the grant directories as data bases. The chief advantage of having the directories available as data bases is that they can be searched by more than one subject (e.g., "stuttering" AND "computers"). Unfortunately, the subject indexing in these directories is often very broad, and the descriptive paragraphs in the directory entries are often very generalized. It may not be easy to retrieve many citations from a given term or subject heading. When searching these directories a wide variety of possible terms should be used, supplementing highly technical or specific terms with general, common language words. Rockman sees these data bases as a useful supplement to the grant literature, but really no substitute for checking the directories in print, by hand.

Relative merits of using data bases

One of the relative advantages of searching for information on a data base is *convenience*. Clinicians or researchers can access a data base at any microcomputer or terminal that has a MODEM. Few libraries have all the print indexes and directories available as data bases. If the specialist is searching directly, using a microcomputer, a trip to the library is not even necessary. Searching by data base takes less *time* than searching by hand. The search logic available with data base searching services makes it possible to search by *multiple categories*, such as two different subjects ("stuttering" AND "computers") or by subject and publication date, or by author and any term in the abstract. Searching using a data base can be done with much more flexibility.

On the other hand, data base searching costs money. Unless the specialist has regular access to a library that performs such searches at no charge, or for a minimal fee, the hourly rates charged by data base vendors for using the data bases can be formidable. The hourly rate for using *ERIC* is around $25.00; this is one of the less expensive data bases. The more common rate is around $65.00/hr, the rate for *PSYCHINFO*. Most searches can be done in 5 or 10 min. But frequent searching, or searches where many records are displayed online, can quickly run up quite a bill for those searching on their own equipment or obliged to pay the full charges.

Still, against these costs, according to Roberts (1981), must be laid the cost of the *time* it would take to make a search and take notes by hand.

Retrieving information from data bases

Searching

Data bases can be searched by entering a term, such as "Apraxia" into the computer, using a terminal or microcomputer. The data base then shows the number of records or entries retrieved by that term.

It is usually possible to *combine terms,* using Boolean logic, to retrieve only those citations that meet the specialist's specifications. For instance, the term "Apraxia" might retrieve over 400 citations. If the specialist is really interested only in articles about "Apraxia" that involve "Augmentative Communication," then the next step would be to enter that term. Suppose the data base retrieves around 80 citations on "Augmentative Communication." The next step is to find out if any of the 400 citations retrieved under "Apraxia" are also among the 80 citations retrieved under "Augmentative Communication." The data base searcher could then combine both "sets" of citations, to cause the data base to show what records were in BOTH the citations found under "Apraxia" and those found under "Augmentative Communication," which might come to approximately 13 citations.

In this way the specialist can retrieve a manageable number of records from a data base, and avoid looking through citations that were not on both "Apraxia" and "Augmentative Communication."

Displaying or printing

The data base user usually has the option of instructing the data base to display one or more records on the monitor, or to print the records through the printer of the terminal or microcomputer. There is also the option of displaying either full data base entry, or just those portions, such as the title and the abstract, that the specialist wishes to examine.

Offline printing

Most vendors also allow the searcher to instruct the data base service to print the records *offline,* that is, to be printed by the vendor's computer and mailed out to the searcher on the following day. This is much cheaper than displaying or printing the citations online, and is ideal when large numbers of records have been retrieved. On the other hand, the searcher must wait for the records to arrive in the mail.

Ordering documents

The entire text of a journal article or other document cited in a data base can be purchased through the services of some data base vendors. Lockheed's DIALOG includes a service called *DIALORDER,* whereby a data base user can place an order with any of the number of companies who supply copies of texts for a fee. Most of these companies supply documents from a specific group of data bases or just a single data base. It is also possible to order *software* from the *International Software Database* through DIALORDER. System Development Corporation's ORBIT also has arrangements for ordering documents online.

The cost of ordering documents online varies with the supplier, the type of document, and of course the length of the document. There may be many times when the specialist will be relieved to know that a particular reference displayed on the screen of the microcomputer can be purchased simply by hitting a few more keys on the keyboard.

Using data bases on a microcomputer

There may, then, be a real advantage for researchers in using a microcomputer for data base searching. Casbon (1983) believes that the main difficulty in getting started might be in selecting among the many hardware and software options that are available. A MODEM will certainly be needed, a printer, and possibly a disk drive and communications software. Later in this volume, Chial discusses in greater depth some of the peripherals needed to access data bases on a microcomputer.

Downloading

Disk storage capability is needed to "download" the data base search results and store them temporarily on a disk. Casbon (1983) considers this a real advantage, as downloading permits the transfer of records from the data base to a diskette at high speed. The records can then be printed later from the diskette, when no longer connected to the data base.

Data bases on disks

Downloading has become such a common practice that some data bases are beginning to sell portions of their records on diskettes. Microcomputer users can buy the disks and search them as long as they wish, without paying the hourly use rates. *ERIC* is already available this way, and recently it was announced that the National Library of Medicine is proposing to offer subsets of MEDLINE on disks (NLM to offer MEDLINE subsets, 1983). There are some other options that make data base searching on microcomputers very attractive.

Data base services designed for microcomputers

Some vendors are offering data base searching services specifically designed for use on microcomputers. Both BRS and DIALOG are offered in modified versions, which are cheaper and simpler to operate.

The service offered by BRS is called *BRS/After Dark*. According to Janke (1983), people who use it feel that it is not complicated. This service is available only on evenings through the early morning hours and on weekends, hence the name, "after dark." Only 23 of the BRS data bases are available on this service.

DIALOG's personal data base service is called *Knowledge Index*. It currently offers 16 of the data bases available on DIALOG, according to Ojala (1983). *Knowledge Index* includes the DIALORDER service, whereby full texts of documents can be ordered through the data base service. Neither service at present allows for offline printing of data base records. Search results must be displayed on the monitor, printed online, or downloaded onto disk.

The specialist who wants to use a microcomputer for data base searching may find these services both convenient and inexpensive. Using *Knowledge Index* or *BRS/After Dark* permits searching data bases such as ERIC, PSYCHINFO, OR MEDLINE at times when most libraries are closed.

There are a number of other sorts of personal data base services available. Rubin (1984) refers to them as "information utilities" and considers the ones most widely in use to include *CompuServe, Dow Jones News/Retrieval,* and *The Source*. All offer news reports online *CompuServe* and *The Source* also offer information on computer groups and clubs, information on computer programming, online shopping, and electronic mail. Microcomputer users have found them every useful. Of most interest to the speech and hearing specialist may be the electronic mail services, which permit exchange of messages and data files with colleagues, using microcomputers.

Electronic mail

Electronic mail services are available from many commercial sources. In her review of a number of these sources, Smith (1983) observes that what most services offer is the ability for a microcomputer user to transmit a message, via MODEM, to the electronic mail service's computer, where the message is placed in an online file created for the addressee. When the addressee logs on to the service, the system shows that a message is waiting. *MCI Mail,* one of the electronic mail services, permits users not only to transmit messages and documents to another microcomputer user; according to Smith, it also includes a feature whereby messages are *printed* and sent, via Purolator, Inc., to addressees who do not have computer addresses.

SpecialNet

For speech and hearing practitioners, SpecialNet may be a useful electronic mail service. SpecialNet is a communications network, developed by the National Association of State Directors of Special Education to provide for communication and information sharing among people involved with education of the handicapped. According to Gibbs and Nash (1983) SpecialNet includes a regular electronic mail service, enabling microcomputer users to send and receive messages from each other.

It also, however, provides a number of *electronic bulletin boards,* where people can place messages or announcements, and make them accessible to everyone in the network. Included are bulletin boards devoted to federal legislation, employment, consultants, conferences, and new products.

In addition to providing bulletin board information, microcomputer users may use SpecialNet to send messages by TWX, Mailgram, or Telex, much the same as with MCI Mail. There is also a feature providing for data transfer from computer to computer. Researchers who need to share information and data regularly may find that it can be done effectively on SpecialNet.

EarNet

Another similar network is called EarNet, an electronic mail service provided by And/Or Corporation, Golden, Colorado. This service offers an electronic bulletin board, where microcomputer users may leave messages or "post" announcements. A "calendar of events" bulletin board is planned for the near future. Specialists may also use this service to pose specific questions about microcomputers, to which other EarNet users may offer answers or suggestions.

EarNet is offered without charge by And/Or Corporation, as a means of promoting the use of microcomputers in the speech and hearing professions. The products catalog is also accessible through EarNet.

Microcomputer users whose information needs are often quite varied and unstructured may find these electronic mail services to be both less expensive and more directly useful than some of the other data base services.

Finding data base vendors, software, and equipment

Many of the hardware and software directories mentioned earlier list data base vendors, as well as hardware and software sources. *Communications Software for Microcomputers,* by Bruman (1983) is a concise, 25-page listing of such sources. Thé's (1983a) review of hardware and software in *Personal Computing* includes a similar listing.

The *Information Industry Market Place* (1980) is one of many good directories of data bases and data base vendors. Almost all data base vendors provide ample documentation and training. Grosswirth's (1983) article in *Personal Computing* includes a brief list of both data bases and vendors. Rubin (1984) supplies a brief list with his review, and also reviews *The Source, CompuServe,* and the *Dow Jones News/Retrieval.*

For the specialist who needs access to sophisticated information resources, the online data bases can prove to be both convenient and economical. Libraries can frequently provide data base searching services, but so can the specialist's microcomputer.

CONSULTANTS

Consultants can be valuable information resources for the microcomputer user, providing information, solving problems, and preparing evaluations. Most microcomputer hardware and software are designed for business or personal uses. Some are designed for educational applications. Very few are designed specifically for applications in the speech and hearing sciences. To adapt existing hardware and software for speech and hearing, or to organize the specialist's operations in order to take advantage of the features of microcomputer hardware or software, an outside expert, or consultant, is sometimes needed.

Services provided

The types of services that a consultant may be able to provide for microcomputer users include the following.

Needs assessment

A consultant can help determine with the client the various types of data processing or microcomputer applications that are needed for the client's particular situation. If the specialist does not know precisely how a microcomputer system might be used, a consultant can help (Birnbaum, 1983). The role of the consultant here would be to define needs in an operational fashion, and specify the kind of hardware and software needed.

Purchasing advice

A consultant can assist in evaluating and selecting hardware and software. Consultants may also assist in selecting vendors, or in evaluating lease versus purchase options. Where the proposed system is complex or requires special equipment, more than one dealer may be required to supply all the system's components. Or the system's specifications may be too technical to permit evaluation of specific hardware and software items without the benefit of the technical expertise of a consultant.

Operational training

A consultant can be retained to train staff in using microcomputer hardware and software. This is a rather expensive sort of training. But if the specialist has a complex microcomputer system, or if improper operation might damage or destroy valuable clinical data, customized training by a consultant might be the best option. If the consultant is already involved in designing the system, training at least assures the specialist that the consultant will not need to be called back simply because the specialist's staff was not familiar with some aspect of the system. Kafotou (1981) believes that training by the consultant is necessary in such cases, so that the client will not become dependent upon the consultant.

Design of applications

A consultant can assist in arranging ways of performing particular jobs or operations, unique to the client's situation, on existing hardware for the client's particular application, or even create customized software (Segal and Berst, 1983).

Program evaluation

A consultant can provide an analysis of the effectiveness of microcomputer utilization in a specialist's program and recommend modifications. Segal and Berst (1983, p. 64) suggest that if there is any substantial *data conversion,* it may be worthwhile to think about retaining a consultant to evaluate the conversion plan. It is also useful to ask the consultant to *test* the operation of the system.

These are the sorts of things that computer consultants frequently do. The specialist may need some or all of these services, depending largely on the complexity of the particular microcomputer system.

Is a consultant needed?

Consultants are usually retained because the client has a problem that cannot be easily solved. Sometimes the organization simply lacks information or knowledge, cannot readily acquire the information, or finds that hiring a consultant would be more effective than trying to acquire the information directly.

Specifically, according to Birnbaum (1983, p. 103), a consultant may be needed if:
1. No one on the staff has the time or skill to analyze the hardware/software needs and select appropriate material.
2. It is obvious that a great deal of special software must be selected.
3. The situation poses a problem that apparently cannot be dealt with by existing equipment or software.
4. There is need for independent evaluation of plans being made.

The key idea is that a consultant may be needed in cases where either the problem is too complicated to tackle or there is not enough time to solve the problem without assistance.

Although it is possible to retain a consultant to take care of the entire process of computerizing your operation, Segal and Berst (1983, p. 71) suggest that clients at least try to analyze their operation and do some planning first. Otherwise, the consultant may spend much expensive time trying to learning what is going on before making any recommendations.

Selecting a consultant

Once a particular need or problem is identified, and it is decided that a consultant is needed, the issue becomes one of selection. Technical qualifications may be difficult to evaluate, but there are some questions that an organization might ask a consultant, suggested by Birnbaum (1983, p. 105–106).

How long has the consultant been doing consulting?

A person who has been consulting only occasionally, or not for a long time, or who has begun only recently, may not be as qualified as one who has been consulting for a longer time. If the consultant is not directly familiar with speech and hearing sciences, a good bit of experience in consulting for different organizations may make it easier for the consultant to promptly grasp the situation.

How much does the person know about the client's line of work?

The more familiar the consultant is with the client's type of work, the less the client will have to explain, and the less the consultant will need to take time to learn about the client's situation. The consultant will have to be able to clearly see the problem, in order to solve it.

It may be that people with only moderate expertise in microcomputers, but with a good speech and hearing background, may be more helpful on some problems than an expert on computers with no prior knowledge of speech and hearing sciences.

What sorts of hardware and software is the person familiar with?

If the problem involves selecting or evaluating hardware or software, a consultant with wide experience is preferable. It may, on the other hand, be preferable for the consultant to have thorough knowledge of the hardware or software that the client already has, if that's the essence of the problem.

The main point that Birnbaum (1983) makes is that the client should be fully aware of the consultant's preferences and expertise.

What do previous clients think of the consultant?

Naturally it would seem preferable to find a consultant whose references include primarily satisfied customers; but it may be wise to look carefully. Each consulting problem is different. If deadlines are important, then a consultant who misses deadlines ought perhaps to be ruled out, even if past performance was rated high.

In summary, the more clearly the problem is specified, the easier it may be to select someone to help solve it. If there is uncertainty on this point, it may be wise to seek information through some of the other information resources first, before retaining a consultant.

How to find consultants

There are many ways of locating potential consultants. Some of the sources suggested below may be more appropriate than others, depending largely upon whether the client needs a fully professional consultant, or whether a knowledgeable amateur with specific experience in an aspect of speech and hearing might be preferable.

Directories and data bases

There are at least two directories that list consultants. Wasserman's (1982a) *Consultants and Consulting Organizations Directory* lists consultants in many fields. The directory is kept up to date with supplements. *Who's Who in Consulting* (Wasserman, 1982b) gives biographical and career information on consultants. This sort of information might be useful to the specialist who wants to make a preliminary selection, and wants to know a little about the consultants without engaging in a great number of telephone calls or interviews.

The *Computer Database* includes entries on consultants. Those with microcomputers and MODEMs could search this data base themselves. Many libraries will perform data base searches for their patrons. There is another data base, the *Electronic Yellow Pages—Services Directory*, with nearly two million entries on various sorts of services to business, including consultants. *SpecialNet* includes a "Consultant Resource Bank" as one of its electronic bulletin boards.

These sources may all be useful for identifying professional consultants, though it may not really be possible from these sources to learn how much they might be acquainted with the specialist's type of work.

Educational institutions

Higher education institutions, as well as elementary and secondary schools, may have qualified people on their staff who are able to serve as consultants part-time. This may be an especially good source if the institution employs speech or hearing clinicians, or in the case of higher education, communication sciences are taught there.

Dealers

Since computer dealers may have had occasion to deal with consultants as they work for their clients, they may know of consultants who regularly work in the area. Collopy (1983) recommends consulting dealers for this purpose.

Professional associations

Members of professional associations, engaged in similar work, may have had occasion to use consultants, and may be able to recommend a few. Some association members may be sufficiently experienced to serve as consultants themselves. They may be especially useful where it is important that the consultant be familiar with the type of work being done.

According to Malinconico (1983, p. 2032), there are a number of professional associations which will help identify consultants by specialty and location. These include the *Association of Consulting Management Engineers,* the *Data Processing Management Association,* which has many local chapters, the *Independent Computer Consultants Association,* and the *Institute of Management Consultants.*

Users' groups

At users' group meetings or in conversation with members, it may be possible to learn of people and firms who do microcomputer consulting. Some consultants may very likely be members of users' groups. As Collopy (1983) observes, since most consultants secure contracts through referrals, users' groups and special interest groups may be good sources of information on consultants.

Consultants can be a valuable source of information, especially when the solution to a problem is not readily apparent. Proper use of a consultant requires ample advance preparation and careful selection. A consultant may not be required in every case. The information that microcomputer users need can often be provided through more informal channels.

USERS' GROUPS AND COMPUTER CLUBS

Microcomputer users' groups and computer clubs can be a valuable information resource for both the novice and the experienced computer user. Most users' groups are organized around a specific brand of equipment, and many have the support and cooperation of the manufacturer, though as Metzger (1983) points out, users' groups are rarely affiliated directly with the manufacturer.

Benefits

Advice and troubleshooting

Club members are usually familiar with and concerned about solving minor difficulties that arise in using microcomputers. Sharing advice and experience is often a key purpose in the formation of users' groups. It is Hoffberg's (1980) view that users' groups can help the novice by giving advice on coping with minor defects in hardware or software which make the system difficult to operate. People who are using the same equipment can often help each other master minor but aggravating idiosyncrasies of a microcomputer system. Hoffberg believes that users' groups are an effective vehicle for registering complaints with the manufacturer or software producer when defects or poor designs are discovered.

New developments

Group meetings are often sources of evaluations of hardware, software, and peripheral equipment. For Metzger (1983) this is one of the main values of belonging to a users' group. In fact, Meilach (1983, p. 148) recommends very strongly that people attend some users' group meetings *before* buying a microcomputer. The advice available in such groups may save the prospective buyer time and money.

New equipment is often demonstrated at group meetings, as part of the meeting's program. Lieff (1980) observes that group members are unlikely to be acquainted with more than a few microcomputer models and does not recommend relying entirely upon such advice as a basis for purchase.

Discounts or group purchasing

Some clubs or users' groups are large enough to purchase equipment or supplies as a group, negotiating directly with manufacturers or wholesalers to obtain discounts. This, according to Meilach (1983, p. 149), can be an important reason for joining a users' group.

Swaps and dubs

Users' groups and clubs often arrange for members to swap equipment or trade software. Copies of software which is in the public domain, and not copyrighted, are sometimes available through users' groups, according to Lieff (1983, p. 80). Copies are usually available at the cost of a blank disk. Some users' groups maintain network or electronic mail arrangements that enable members to transfer software from one member's computer to another, using MODEMs.

Special interest groups

Many users' groups will form subsections or "special interest groups" (SIGs) which focus on specific applications, such as word processing, or a specific program, such as Visicalc. Swallow (1983) mentions that often separate users' groups will form around software, such as *CP/M*, or programming languages, such as *Pascal* or *LOGO*.

Such special interest groups provide the more experienced microcomputer user with colleagues using microcomputers for similar purposes. This makes the interchange of ideas and advice more germane.

How to find users' groups and clubs

Users' groups and computer clubs try not to be hard to find. There are usually a number of ways to locate these groups.

Dealers

Dealers are usually aware of the computer groups in their area. Though they may not know of all of them, dealers are generally considered to be a good local source. Professional acquaintances who have microcomputers may also be able to give information on some local groups.

Manufacturers

Manufacturers often sponsor users' groups, and usually try to keep aware of the groups that are focused on their equipment. Contacting the manufacturer is often a quick way to get a list of the groups in your area. Swallow (1983) and Metzger (1983) list addresses for use in contacting manufacturers about users' groups.

Journals

Microcomputer journals and magazines occasionally mention users' groups and clubs in their news pages. *Byte* and *Personal Computing* regularly feature notices regarding computer groups. Periodically, there are articles, such as those of Hoffberg (1980), Metzger (1983) and Swallow (1983), on users' groups.

Data bases

The electronic mail features of CompuServ and The Source make them useful for finding information about users' groups. Both data base services make electronic bulletin board services available, according to Rubin (1984) for notices about computer groups. Specialized electronic mail services, such as SpecialNet and EarNet, may also be worth consulting for information on users' groups in the communication sciences.

In summary, there is, of course, no way to tell whether the knowledge that can be gained from participation in a users' group will be worth the time spent there; however, it seems that the advantages of belonging to a users' group are too great for the specialist not to consider joining one, or perhaps starting one.

DEALERS

Since most microcomputer use revolves around hardware or software matters, the source of these items, the dealer, is perhaps the most frequently consulted source of information and assistance.

Services available from a dealer

In addition to selling equipment and software, dealers often offer information and other services. In selecting a dealer, the specialist may wish to consider the services that different dealers offer, in addition to considering which brands and what sort of prices are available. Here are some services frequently offered by dealers:

Maintenance and Repair
Training
Accessories
Information and Referral

Maintenance may be one of the most important services to consider in choosing a dealer. Lieff (1982, p. 89) recommends that a dealer's service agreement be given to the customer in writing. The prospective purchaser should also find out how long warranty service is available, who will provide it, and where it will be done. Looking for a dealer who makes repairs on site is what De Martino (1982) recommends, to avoid the delay in sending equipment away for repairs.

Training is often called "support" (Meilach, 1983, p. 146) when it refers to the initial instruction that dealers usually provide to purchasers of new hardware or software. Many dealers offer up to 2 hours of free support. Some also offer classes or training sessions for a fee. Meilach recommends thoroughly investigating the amount of free support that a dealer is willing to offer, and the availability of additional training.

Accessories should be available in adequate quantities from the dealer. There should be enough basic software, supplies, and peripheral equipment available promptly through the dealer. De Martino (1982) feels that the selection available from the dealer is one of the three most important factors to consider, along with maintenance service and price.

Information and referral to other sources of information are often available from good dealers. Meilach (1983, p. 151) considers dealers to be good sources of information on local users' groups and special interest groups. The editors of *Personal Computing* (Answers, 1984) point out that prospective buyers should find out if a dealer can recommend computer courses or workshops being offered in the area. The dealer's store ought to be used as a resource center, according to Blumenthal (1983, p. 86). Both before and after making a purchase, a good dealer ought to be a convenient first source for information.

The dealer with the best assortment of services may not always be the dealer with the lowest *prices*, but it may be wise to consider whether time and money might be saved by using dealer's services. Novices may need more assistance from a dealer than would more experienced users. The editors of *Personal Computing* (Answers, 1983a, p. 149) feel that a good dealer's services might make it worth paying higher prices. De Martino (1982) believes that it is important to pay a *little* more, but he suggests that customers shop around, become familiar with current prices before buying anything major, to avoid paying a *lot* more.

Retailer versus mail order dealer

The issue of price brings up the question of whether to buy from a retailer at all, or whether to buy a mail order dealer instead. Much equipment and software is sold through mail order outlets. Fuchs (1983) found in a survey of software distributors that 80% of those surveyed sell by mail. Buying by mail is obviously an option for the specialist.

Advantages of mail order

The chief advantage of the mail order option is a cheaper price than what would be available from a retailer. The *services* that a good retailer can provide are usually not available from a mail order dealer, but mail order dealers often offer other services.

Free trial or preview. Some mail order dealers may let customers try out equipment or software for several days, up to a month and a half according to Mason (1983), with full right of return for full refund. However, 20 to 25% of the companies surveyed by Fuchs (1983) do not permit returns of materials once purchased. This service does appear to be common enough, though, to be worth looking for.

Warranties and replacement. Some software products sold by mail are given extended warranties, in a few cases up to 2 years, according to Fuchs (1983). Some companies are experimenting with offering replacement diskettes at low prices, in cases where a diskette was purchased but now no longer works.

Online and telephone ordering. Several companies, according to Mason (1983), are experimenting with accepting orders by microcomputer, using an electronic mail arrangement. People with MODEMs can leave messages, request catalogs, or place orders using their microcomputers. Many dealers include in their advertisements a toll-free number for placing orders by telephone.

Risks of mail order

Delay. Even with online or phone ordering, customers may experience some delay in the actual receipt of the material ordered, according to Mason (1983). In cases where one is ordering frequently used supplies by mail, it is probably wise to keep an ample supply on hand, so as not to be shut down by a delayed shipment.

Lack of repair service. Not only do mail order dealers usually not offer repair service, retailers who do provide repair service may be reluctant or unwilling to repair items that they did not sell ("The Gray Market in Micros," 1983) or charge high fees for making such repairs.

When buying equipment by mail, the specialist might want to first determine the availability of repair service.

Damage. Ordering by mail always runs the risk that the item will be damaged in shipment, according to *Consumer Reports* ("Where and How to Buy a Computer," 1983). If the damage is not immediately obvious, it may be difficult to convince the mail order firm to make a replacement. Even with obvious damage, or a sympathetic mail order dealer, there is the delay and the nuisance of correcting the problem.

The advantage of buying from a retailer is generally the service and support that the dealer supplies. The advantage in buying from a mail order dealer is generally the lower prices. It is hard to say, in general terms, which is the better option. *Consumer Reports* ("Where and How to Buy a Computer," 1983) conducted a survey of buyers and found that those who bought by mail reported few if any difficulties. Nor were many complaints registered about computer retailers. It seems that the specialist should be encouraged to investigate and consider using both types of dealers, as long as they meet the specialist's requirements.

Locating dealers

Within a municipality, microcomputer dealers can easily be found in the telephone directory, but there are other sources as well.

Manufacturers
Manufacturers can frequently supply a list of dealers or provide referral to nearby dealers.

Directories and data bases
Microcomputer directories such as the *Classroom Computer News Directory of Educational Computing Resources* (1983) list some dealers. Since it is unlikely that many of the dealers listed in directories would be within normal shopping range, such directories and data bases would be used primarily to find mail order dealers. The *Datapro Management of Small Computer Systems* (Datapro Research Corporation, 1982) is another directory which includes a list of vendors, as well as *user evaluations* of some of them. The *Computer Database* and the *Electronic Yellow Pages—Retailers* provide access to listings of dealers. These data bases can be searched by those with microcomputers or terminals and MODEMs. For bargain hunters there is the *Directory of Discount Computer Suppliers* (1983).

Journals
Microcomputer journals and magazines are probably the best source of information on mail order dealers. Local newspapers, of course, frequently carry advertisements for local retailers. Professional journals also often carry dealer's advertisements.

Users' groups
Members of users' groups are a source of information on dealers in the local area, since many of them are likely to be regular customers. Informal conversations among group members, or among friends or colleagues, are a convenient source of information on local dealers.

Dealers may be the one type of resource most frequently consulted by the microcomputer user. If chosen carefully, the dealer may also be one of the most useful information resources available to the microcomputer user.

TRAINING SOURCES

Some sources of training have been mentioned in various sections of this chapter. Here are some of the major sources of training.

Dealers

Most dealers are willing, at the very least, to explain how a piece of merchandise works, but many also sponsor training sessions and classes on a regular basis. Adequate training is one of the services that should be considered when selecting a dealer (Segal & Berst, 1983, p. 140). Dealers vary in their ability to provide training and instruction, although 1-hr training sessions on specific topics, such as word processing or spreadsheets, are not uncommon (Rothfeder, 1983). Taber (1983, p. 41) found that manufacturers and software publishers occasionally sponsor classes held at retail stores. Dealers may also be able to refer the specialist to local courses or workshops.

Self-instructional resources

Manufacturer's manuals are often quite elaborate. A great deal can be learned by patiently following these manuals. However, Fawcette (1983) observes that the manuals and instruction booklets that are supplied with new hardware and software are generally not adequate for novices.

Several companies sell software specifically designed for self-instruction in aspects of microcomputers. Thé (1983b) reports that CDEX Corporation has designed a manual and disk package that provides introductory training for the Apple IIe, another for the IBM Personal Computer. Bonner (1983) mentions over 16 sources of self-instructional tutorial packages that teach programming languages. Self-instructional resources may be preferred by the experienced user. However, Rothfeder (1983) points out that lack of human feedback or interaction with an expert may make this sort of material less useful for novices.

Workshops and courses

Educational institutions and professional associations frequently sponsor workshops or institutes on microcomputers. The *Classroom Computer News Directory of Educational Computing Resources* (1983) lists over eight such conferences in the month of October alone. Many of these conferences offer "hands-on" workshops in microcomputer applications. Where there are microcomputer *consortiums* active, they frequently sponsor workshops and training (Norwood, 1983).

Colleges and universities frequently offer both formal courses and extension or adult education courses on microcomputers. For elementary orientation to microcomputers, such courses may be quite useful.

Consultants

When specialized training is needed and a consultant has already been retained, it may be worthwhile to include training as part of the consulting service. Kafotou (1981) believes that the client should, in fact, insist on thorough training whenever a consultant has been retained, to make sure that the client can fully understand and operate any system developed by the consultant.

Arranging for customized training can be costly. Dight (1983) points out that, however, when the alternative to customized training involves travel to attend a workshop or institute, the cost of customized training on the premises may not seem overly expensive. Dight lists 99 organizations that conduct on-site training. Such training may be costly, but apparently is not scarce.

Users' groups

Users' group members may not only mutually educate each other at their meetings, but may also sponsor workshops or demonstrations. Some group members may have already participated in various training programs, or taken courses. They may be able to give a personal evaluation of some of the available training programs.

The specialist may discover that finding appropriate and affordable training sources may not always be easy. Training needs will vary depending upon the complexity of the microcomputer system and the prior experience of the specialist. A number of different training resources are available, however, to meet various needs.

SUMMARY

There are many potentially useful sources of information and assistance available to microcomputer users. Proper use of these resources requires first that the user *select* those resources likely to provide relevant information, and second that the particular resources chosen be used *deliberately*, taking into consideration both the assets and the limitations of a particular resource.

Many of the information resources mentioned provide *referral* to other sources of information, facilitating the process of selecting appropriate resources. The microcomputer user with direct access to *data base* searching and to electronic mail services can easily consult any of several different sources, facilitating the use of information resources.

Finding useful information on microcomputers may be at times expensive, and not infrequently tedious, but rarely nonfeasible.

REFERENCES

AEDS Journal (1967). Washington: Association for Educational Data Systems.
AEDS Monitor (1962). Washington: Association for Educational Data Systems.
American men and women of science (1982). New York: Bowker.
Answers (1983a, December). *Personal Computing,* 7(12), 149.
Answers (1983b, December). *Personal Computing,* 7(12), 154.
Answers (1984, January). *Personal Computing,* 8(1), 174.
The Atari Connection (1981). San Jose, CA: Atari Home Computer Division.
Auerbach Publishers (1978). *Auerbach data world.* Pennsauken, NJ: Author.
Behavior Research Methods and Instrumentation (1968). Austin, TX: The Psychonomic Society.
Birnbaum, M. (1983). *How to choose your small business computer.* New York: Addison-Wesley.
Blumenthal, H. J. (1983). *Everyone's guide to personal computers.* New York: Ballantine.

Bonner, P. (1983, August). Computer programming: What's in it for you. *Personal Computing, 7*(8), 128-137.
Brubaker, S., & Rolniek, M. (1984). *Compilation of clinical software for aphasia rehabilitation and cognitive retraining.* Birmingham, MI: Clinical Software Resources.
Bruman, J. L. (1983). *Communications software for microcomputers.* San Jose, CA: CLASS.
Business Periodicals Index (1958). New York: H.W. Wilson Co.
Byte (1975). Peterborough, NH: Green Publishers.
Casbon, S. (1983). Online searching with a microcomputer—getting started. *Online, (*7(6), 42-46.
Castlewitz, D. M. (1982). *Visicalc home and office companion.* Berkeley, CA: Osborne/McGraw-Hill.
Classroom computer news directory of educational computing resources. (1983). Watertown, MA: International Education, Inc.
Collopy, D. (1983, April). Made to measure software. *Personal Computing, 7*(4), 80-86.
Commerce Business Daily (1977). Washington: US Govt. Printing Office.
Compute! (1979). Greensboro, NC: Compute Publications, Inc.
Computers and Electronics (1982). New York.
Computers in Biology and Medicine (1970). New York: Pergamon.
Computers in Healthcare (1982). Englewood, CO: Cardiff.
Computers in Psychiatry/Psychology (1979). New Haven, CT: CP/P.
Computing Teacher (1979). Eugene, OR: International Council for Computers in Education, University of Oregon.
Creative Computing (1974). Morris Plains, NJ.
DSH Abstracts (1960). Washington: Deafness, Speech and Hearing Publications.
Datapro Research Corp (1982). *Datapro management of small computer systems.* Delran, NJ.
De Martino, M. (1982, January). Selecting your computer and your computer dealer. *Personal Computing, 6*(1), 109-110.
Dewey, P. R. (1984). Searching for software: A checklist of microcomputer software directions. *Library Journal, 109,* 544-547.
Dight, J. (1983, November). A guide to DP training. *Datamation, 29*(11), 202-216.
Directory of discount computer suppliers (1983). New York: Discount America Publications.
Education Index (1929). New York: Wilson.
Educational Technology (1961). Englewood Cliffs, NJ: Prentice-Hall.
80 Microcomputer (1980). Peterborough, NH: Wayne Green.
Encyclopedia of associations (1983). Detroit: Gale.
Fawcette, J. (1983, December). Finally, some help for documentation. *Personal Computing* 7(12), 141-145.
Foundation directory (1983). New York: The Foundation Center.
Foundation grants index (1983). New York: The Foundation Center.
Fox, A. (1983). *Armchair BASIC.* Berkeley, CA: Osborne/McGraw-Hill.
Fuchs, V. E. (1983). Software publication considerations and the hearing impaired. *American Annals of the Deaf, 128,* 600-604.
Galland, F. J. (1982). *Dictionary of computing.* New York: Wiley.
Gibbs, L. K., & Nash, K. (1983). SpecialNet: Instant information/communication. *American Annals of the Deaf, 128,* 631-635.
The gray market in micros. (1983). *Computing Teacher, 10*(9), 33-35.
Grosswirth, M. (1983, May). Getting the best from databanks. *Personal Computing, 7*(5), 111-117.
Hannan, J. (1983, December). Rating micros for word processing. *Infosystems, 30*(12), 30-34.
Hartnell, T., & Veit, S. (1983). *The complete buyer's guide to personal computers.* New York: Bantam.
Heilborn, J. (1983). *The Vic 20 user's guide.* Berkeley, CA: Osborne/McGraw-Hill.
Helms, H. (Ed.) (1983). *McGraw-Hill computer handbook.* New York: McGraw-Hill.
Hoffberg, A. (1980). ED perspective: User groups play vital role in realizing full benefits of microcomputer systems. *Administrative Management, 41*(7), 74.
The IMS Ayer directory of publications, (1925). Philadelphia, PA: Ayer Press.
Index Medicus (1879). Bethesda, MD: US Dept. of Health and Human Services.
Information industry market place (1980). New York: Bowker.
International microcomputer software directory (1982). Fort Collins, CO: Imprint Editions.
International minicomputer software directory (1982). Fort Collins, CO: Imprint Editions.
Janke, R. V. (1983). BRS/After Dark: The birth of online self service. *Online, 7*(5), 12-29.

Kafotou, T. (1981). Controlling consultants the professional way. *Data Management, 19*(4), 18-19, 37.
Kusak, J. M., & Bowers, J.S. (1982). Public microcomputers in public libraries. *Library Journal, 107,* 2137-2141.
Lieff, J. D. (1982). *How to buy a personal computer without anxiety.* Cambridge, MA: Ballinger.
Malinconico, S. M. (1983). Managing consultants. *Library Journal, 108,* 2032-2033.
Marchionini, G. (1981). Educational computing resources. In B. R. Sadowski (Ed.), *Using computers to enhance teaching and improve teacher centers* (pp. 85-89). Houston, TX: Houston University (ERIC Document Reproduction Service, No. ED 205 478).
Mason, M. (1983). More bargains and Osborne's executive. *Library Journal, 108,* 981-982.
Meilach, D. Z. (1983). *A practical guide to computer shopping; Before you buy a computer.* New York: Crown.
Metzger, E. (1983, March). The helping hands of computer clubs. *Personal Computing, 7*(3), 142-147.
Microcomputer buyer's guide (1983). New York: McGraw-Hill.
Microcomputer market place (1982). New York: Dekotek.
NLM to offer MEDLINE subsets. (1983, November). *National Library of Medicine News, 38*(11), 1-2.
Nibble (1980). Lincoln, MA: Micro-Sparc.
Norwood, D. C. (1983). Hold the hardware: Here's a logical way to plan for microcomputers. *Illinois School Board Journal, 51*(2), 22-24.
Ojala, M. (1983). Knowledge Index: A review. *Online, 7*(5), 31-34.
Online micro-software guide & directory 1983-84. (1982). Weston, CT: Online, Inc.
Online terminal/microcomputer guide & directory 1982-83 (1982). Weston, CT: Online, Inc.
Personal Computing (1977). Rochele Park, NJ: Heyden Publishing Co.
Poole, L. (1983). *Apple II user's guide.* Berkeley, CA: Osborne/McGraw-Hill.
Popular Computing (1981). Peterborough, NH.
Psychological Abstracts (1927). Washington: American Psychological Association.
The Reader's Guide to Periodical Literature (1900). New York: Wilson.
Rienhoff, O. (1980). *The computer in the doctor's office.* New York: Elsevier.
Roberts, S. K. (1981, December). Online information retrieval: Promise and problems. *Byte, 6*(12), 452-461.
Rockman, I. F. (1983). Money online: How to search the grant literature. *Online, 6*(2), 26-33.
Roose, T. (1983). Online database searching in smaller public libraries. *Library Journal, 108,* 1769-1770.
Rothfeder, J. (1983, February). Striking back at technological terror. *Personal Computing, 7*(2), 62-66.
Rubin, C. (1984, January). Touring the on-line databases. *Personal Computing, 9*(1), 82-85.
Segal, H., & Berst, J. (1983). *How to select your small computer...without frustration.* Englewood Cliffs, NJ: Prentice-Hall.
Sippl, C. J. (Ed.) (1980). *Computer dictionary.* Indianapolis: Sams.
Smith, A. E. (1983, December). Electronic mail goes first class. *Business Computer Systems, 2*(12), 84-91.
Swallow, L. (1983, Fall). Users groups, a valuable resource. *Buyer's Guide to Small Computers, 1*(3), 19-22.
T H E Journal (1973). Acton, MA: Information Synergy, Inc.
Taber, F. M. (1983). *Microcomputers in special education.* Reston, VA: Council for Exceptional Children.
Thé, L. (1983a, March). Data communications: A buyer's guide to modems and software. *Personal Computing, 7*(3), 96-175.
Thé, L. (1983b, June). Comprehensive disk-based training courses for Apple IIe and IBM Personal Computer. *Personal Computing, 7*(6), 202-205.
Thomas, R. N. (1982). *A user guide to the UNIX system.* Berkeley, CA: Osborne/McGraw-Hill.
Ulrich's international periodicals directory (1932). New York: Bowker.
Wasserman, P. (Ed.) (1982a). *Consultants and consulting organizations directory.* Detroit: Gale.
Wasserman, P. (Ed.) (1982b). *Who's who in consulting.* Detroit: Gale.
Where and how to buy a computer (1983, September). *Consumer Reports, 48*(9), 485.
Williams, A. (1981). Instruction and microcomputers. In B. R. Sadowski (Ed.), *Using computers to enhance teaching and improve teacher centers* (pp. 49-53). Houston, TX: Houston University. (ERIC Document Reproduction Service No. ED 205 478).

Chapter 5

Evaluating Microcomputer Hardware

Michael R. Chial

COMPUTERS AND OTHER INFORMATION PROCESSORS

Computers are representational engines: they manipulate symbols representing events, quantities, or ideas. Because events and ideas are represented symbolically, computers can be considered symbol processors; to the extent that those symbols convey information, computers are *information processors*. Other machines and systems serve similar functions.

A "machine" example: the vending machine problem

A machine that dispenses candy bars can be viewed as an information processor that replaces and (in a limited way) simulates the behavior of a human clerk. To operate the machine, coins are inserted and a choice is made. The machine must determine whether the coins are valid, whether enough money has been inserted, whether the choice selected is available, whether change is required, and whether change can be provided. It "behaves" differently depending upon available information and a simple set of rules leading to a limited number of alternatives. Such machines can dispense almost any kind of candy bar, but they cannot (without intervention) change the rules they use to select behaviors. Although candy machines have physical existence, they have also a functional existence independent of any particular machine.

A "human" example: detection of middle-ear infection

A more complex task faces the audiologist who tests a child with the goal of diagnosing hearing loss. Otoscopic, audiometric, historical, and other data are gathered, the validity of those data is assessed, decisions are made about the need for additional information, and test results are evaluated with a set of rules about relations between test outcomes and physiological state. Some rules are highly formalized (e.g., determining whether a loss exists); others are "fuzzy" in the sense that unambiguous rules have not been stated or do not exist (e.g., predicting the effect of a given loss upon subsequent language acquisiton). A small set of alternative etiologies are available, each with an associated a priori and a posteriori probability; the diagnostician

©College-Hill Press, Inc. All rights, including that of translation, reserved. No part of this publication may be reproduced without the written permission of the publisher.

entertains alternative options, including the option to "keep looking." The diagnostic process is essentially a system for gathering, interpreting, and acting upon information. Unlike the candy machine, the "diagnosis machine" can recruit additional information, reacquire information, resolve paradoxical data, and revise rules for processing information. Like the candy machine, diagnostic systems have a functional existence that transcends any particular case history form, audiometer, or diagnostician.

Characteristics of information processing systems

The examples just noted differ in complexity, but are similar in that both (1) require external information, (2) contain rules for manipulating information, and (3) exhibit definable classes of "behavior" determined by the results of applying rules to information. Together, information (data) and rules (operations) make up the events of information processing systems.

Data

Generally, *data* are reports of observations of things that happen in the world—of phenomena apprehended by the senses or by instrumentation. Data may be cast in the form of virtually any symbol system—numbers, spoken reports, or written descriptions. Both the observations and the symbols have existence distinct from the phenomena they describe. When data are organized and reorganized, they can reveal relations that otherwise would be obscure: the informational value of data derives from the structure or pattern of symbols used to represent phenomena.

Two worlds: Analog and digital

Most of the physical phenomena relevant to human communication vary in amount from small to large in a continuous manner. The level of a speaker's voice, the mechanical force exerted by an articulator, the magnitude and spectrum of a masking signal, the duration of a stutterer's hesitation—all of these can assume values that differ by infinitely small amounts. Such phenomena are called *analog*. Others are essentially quantal in nature, varying in amount in a steplike manner. Examples include binary (two-state) events such as single-nerve action potentials and the presence or absence of voicing, as well as other phenomena that assume discrete numerical values. These are called *digital* events. Just as there are analog and digital phenomena, there are machines that accept or produce such phenomena. An example of an analog machine capable of storing and producing sound is the audio tape recorder; a digital machine with similar functions is a music box. Contemporary microcomputers employ digital signals and circuitry; if analog signals are to be acted upon or produced by a microcomputer, some form of conversion is necessary.

Operations

The symbols representing phenomena (be they analog or digital) can be manipulated in mathematical, logical, or procedural ways to produce new data. These manipulations are events in the same sense that real-world occurrences are events: the operations themselves can exist independent of any particular data; a set of operations can be represented symbolically. Some operations may involve transduction or conversion of data; others may involve description, classification, summarization, decision making, and control or physical manipulation of symbols or actual events. The recipes by which operations are performed are called *algorithms*. Algorithms can be expressed as verbal instructions, as equations, as sequences of written or graphical rules, or as computer programs.

Computers as information processors

The data and operations of an information processing system act together to accomplish functions that can be viewed as distinct from any particular implementation of function. In the most general terms, these functions entail acquisition (*input*), manipulation (*processing*), and production (*output*) of data. Many systems (people, calculators, vending machines, computers) can perform such functions. What makes computers special as information processors is their ability to store, recall, and modify *both* data and operations. Like vending machines and some people, computers can perform only the operations they have been "told" to perform (someone must do the telling). Those operations can be performed only on the data specifically made available for processing (someone must provide data). Consequently, computers are extremely sensitive "error amplifiers." If data are biased, contaminated, or insufficient, or if operations are logically flawed, poorly structured, or incomplete, mistakes will occur.

In the context of computers, operations are referred to as *software*. *Application software* is designed to service the needs of particular end-users (the people who buy computers); *system software* serves the needs of the computer itself; *utility software* occupies a middle position, helping users manage the computer system in tasks that transcend particular applications (see chap. 6 for a detailed discussion of software). The physical devices which input, process, and output information are *hardware*. For microcomputers especially, the distinction between hardware and software becomes obscure because (inevitably) some software is permanently stored in hardware (*firmware*). Assemblages of hardware and software are called *systems*. Subsystems which specialize in data input, output, or mass storage of information are peripheral to other subsystems which effect basic operations on data (the central processor unit or CPU). The variety of hardware, software, and systems (and of peripheral and central processing subsystems) makes it necessary to systematically assess alternatives.

EVALUATING HARDWARE SYSTEMS

Buying a computer is easy: find a store, write a check, and walk out with a box. Acquiring a computer that solves more problems than it creates is quite another matter. The difference is that of making a choice versus making a decision. A useful decision strategy is to (1) *identify* particular needs, (2) *determine* system requirements (both hardware and software) arising from those needs, (3) *investigate* available alternatives, and (4) *select* the alternative that best meets requirements and needs. Effective statements of needs and requirements necessitate an understanding of what is feasible. Therefore, it is appropriate to begin by noting some general ways in which microcomputers and microcomputer systems differ.

General evaluation parameters

Function
Microcomputers are a class of computers based upon large scale integration (LSI) manufacturing techniques capable of placing the equivalent of thousands of transistors on a single integrated circuit. Microcomputers can be classified as *general purpose* or *special purpose* systems (more a continuum than a bipolar distinction). Specialization of function involves trade-offs between speed and flexibility: general purpose systems tend to be slower, but more flexible; special purpose systems tend to be faster, but less flexible.

A major distinction in function relates to the type, form, and quantity of data that can be acquired, processed, and produced by a computer. Some microcomputers (or subsystems) optimize data input (e.g., grocery store cash registers that read standard product bar-code marks on packages, graphic tablet systems for quantifying images captured by video cameras in oral pendoscopy and speech-recognition systems). Others optimize simple processing of large bodies of data (e.g., high-speed form-letter generators and computerized systems for auditory brainstem response audiometry) or complex processing of smaller amounts of data (e.g., language analysis systems, text-to-synthetic speech translators, digital signal analyzers). Still others optimize output functions (e.g., computerized audiometers that generate and control test tones and masking noise, laboratory process control computers, "game" computers that generate sounds and animated images).

"Minimum" function general purpose microcomputers require a way to enter commands, data, and programs (e.g., a keyboard), a way to store data and programs (e.g., memory), a way to process data (the computer itself), and a way to display results (e.g., a video monitor and/or a printer). In some cases, general purpose systems can be optimized for particular tasks through addition of hardware (see expandability).

Capacity

Capacity refers to the amount of information (both data and programs) that can be stored and accessed by a system, usually expressed in *bytes*. One byte (eight binary digits treated as a unit) is equivalent to one typed character (e.g., a letter or space). One index of capacity relates to the *primary memory* of a computer: capacities between 16,000 and 256,000 bytes are common. Primary memory capacity is limited by the design of the central processing unit. Another index of capacity relates to the *secondary memory* or bulk storage of a system: capacities range from 0 to about 30,000,000 bytes. Secondary memory is limited by recording technology and other factors. Large programs and/or large bodies of data require large memory capacity.

Speed

For the majority of end-users, the most useful index of computer speed is *throughput:* the time required to complete a task, beginning with the first input and ending with the last output. Obviously, throughput will vary with the task. Tasks standardized for purposes of comparing computer systems are called *benchmarks*. Throughput rates for nominally similar systems may vary by ratios of 10 to 1, depending upon the performance of components (hardware and software, central and peripheral subsystems). For most tasks appropriate to microcomputers, throughput is determined largely by input and output operations. In cases requiring complex computations or logical operations, throughput is determined largely by the central processing unit itself.

Flexibility

Flexibility (the ability to do different tasks to an acceptable—and similar—level of quality) is largely related to system software, but has implications for hardware because system software is hardware dependent. Flexibility is also a function of expandability and compatability.

Expandability

Relative to hardware, expandability is the capacity to add memory or other hardware devices (e.g., printers, plotters, manipulanda, color video displays). Expandability implies an increase in functions that are available simultaneously, rather than sequentially. Some microcomputers allow no expansion; others permit modest additions (four to eight hardware subsystems) in the form of plug-in circuit boards; still others accommodate hundreds of additional hardware devices through special communication devices called *interfaces*. When microcomputer systems are acquired piecemeal, or when users "grow" into new applications, expandability becomes a crucial factor. Ideally, this should be taken into account before a basic system is acquired.

Portability

Some microcomputers are designed to be moved from place to place; others contain mechanical components (e.g., "hard disk" subsystems—see below) whose designs are generally incompatible with frequent movement. Portable systems tend to be smaller (in capacity and physical size) than nonportable systems.

Portability has another meaning relative to software; the ability to operate a program on different hardware configurations. Software portability depends significantly upon issues of hardware–software compatability.

Reliability and service

Microcomputers differ in quality of design and construction, and in "robustness," the ability to survive unintentional abuse. These differences are reflected by the performance index mean time between failures (MTBF—a statistical estimate of minimum use-life), by the durations of warranties offered by vendors, and by the service histories of systems. Subsystems with few or no moving parts (e.g., video monitors) are generally more reliable than mechanical systems (e.g., disk drives). Most early hardware failures are related to poor manufacturing quality control. Later difficulties are usually related to misuse, heat build-up, static or electromagnetic shielding problems, improper cleaning, or poorly conditioned electrical power sources (Mau, 1983).

Servicing microcomputers requires special equipment and skills, both of which are expensive, and neither of which is standardized or regulated. Intelligent use and maintenance by the end-user can minimize service costs (maintenance planning is an important part of acquisition—see Schneider, 1981; Perera, 1982; Whitaker, 1982; Margolis, 1983; Stephenson and Cahill, 1983). Some systems and subsystems are inherently easier to service than others. The most expensive aspect of service is usually problem diagnosis; repairs are effected by replacement of parts or entire subsystems because hardware is less expensive than labor. The availability of local service should be a significant factor in purchasing decisions. The vast variety of hardware designs (and of expendable supplies such as printer ribbons and disks) can create problems of supply that also should be considered prior to acquisition.

Cost

Microcomputer system costs range from about $100 to more than $10,000. These are "entry" costs for minimum integrations of hardware and software. The total cost of implementing an application can be many times greater, depending upon the need for additional hardware, software, personnel training, maintenance of both hardware and software, expendable supplies, and losses of productivity ("down time") due to system failures. Site preparation, an additional expense associated with large computers, is seldom an issue with microcomputers. Where computer systems are used by single individuals to accomplish only one or two applications, hardware tends to be the major cost factor. Where systems are used by several people for several kinds of tasks, application software and personnel training become the principal costs. In either case, when custom software must be devised to solve problems, programming costs predominate.

Compatibility

This issue eclipses all of the above, simply because incompatibility results in a loss of function. Compatibility involves both hardware and software; it is especially important in the expansion of computer systems.

Hardware compatibility.
The microcomputer industry is intensely competitive. Some hardware manufacturers seek to control competition by designing proprietary physical interconnection schemes which force buyers to purchase subsystems and hardware additions from a single source. Very popular computers quickly produce "second sources" of hardware. These manufacturers claim (with differing validity) that their products are compatible with some or all microcomputers built by other firms (Montague et al, 1983; Welch, 1983). Although

some technical standards exist, claims of compatibility are often more a matter of marketing than engineering design. Physical compatibility (e.g., among connectors and cables) does not guarantee functional compatibility, nor does software compatibility guarantee hardware compatibility (e.g., inconsistencies between the physical configurations of secondary memory storage media and the hardware devices which read such media). The only sensible test of hardware compatibility is observation.

Software compatibility. Hardware and software do not always work together. Some word processing programs will not work with some printers, even when both are designed for the same microcomputer; some application software cannot be copied to large-capacity disk systems, even when both work independently; some system software is incapable of supporting special control devices (e.g., a "joystick," a touch-sensor, or a "mouse"), despite compatibility with other hardware. Again, the best test of hardware–software compatibility is empirical.

Operator compatibility. Some hardware is friendlier than other hardware, depending upon who uses it and how they use it. This is especially the case with hardware subsystems designed to let people tell computers what to do. Keyboards and other input devices differ in efficiency, speed, accuracy, and ease of use. Users (including clients with neuromotor disorders, children, and the elderly) differ in their ability to manipulate control devices. Output devices such as speech synthesizers and video monitors differ in capacity, flexibility, accuracy, intelligibility, resolution, and overall quality. Beyond simple preference, user compatibility can be assessed through *ergonomic* studies of systems and subsystems, which focus on the use of human energy (see Dillon, 1983).

A crucial aspect of operator compatibility is documentation (see chap. 6). Although casual users may be satisfied with cute, glossy instructions about unpacking, plugging in, and playing games, persons who use systems for professional purposes require sufficient technical information to be able to accomplish first-echelon maintenance and (as their backgrounds allow) understand how the system works. Professionals should understand the technical limitations of the tools they use to benefit their clients; a microcomputer is simply another tool.

Information sources

A vexing feature of the current technological revolution is the explosive speed with which both the technology and the marketplace are changing. This is reflected not only in a burgeoning number of periodicals devoted to specialized aspects of the technology (even *Playboy* magazine features articles about computers—see McWilliams, 1983a,b,c), but also in the increasing rate at which new products (hard and soft) are being promoted to professional and lay audiences. Effective use of available information is complicated by the fact that much of it is simply "sales talk."

Popular periodicals respond quickly to technological innovation and occasionally contain competent comparative reviews of hardware. Stilwell (1983) offers a reasonably current annotated list of periodicals dealing with microcomputers and microcomputer applications. Professional journals respond less rapidly, but are credible sources of information and experience. Unfortunately, journals in communication disorders offer slight information pertinent to microcomputer hardware. Four exceptionally good sources from related disciplines are *Behavior Research Methods and Instrumentation, IEEE Computer, The Computing Teacher,* and *Speech Technology.* All offer articles directly pertinent to instructional, clinical, and research applications in communication disorders.

Some specific resources are especially noteworthy in the context of hardware (see chap. 4 for additional suggestions). Raskin and Whitney (1981) review the development, problems, and probable future of microcomputers. Toong and Gupta (1982) and Blodgett (1983), writing in *Scientific American,* introduce technical issues related to microcomputers and microelectronics, respectively. Bailey (1980) overviews computers and their application in psychology; Durrett and Zweiner (1981), Kolotkin, Billingam, and Feldman (1981), Flowers and Leger (1982), Reed (1982), Poltrock and Foltz (1982), Gordon, Foree, and Eckerman (1983), and Lowe (1983) note experiences in using small computers in divergent areas of behavioral research; Thomas (1981) and Vanderheiden (1981) discuss microcomputers as augmentative communication devices; Schwejda and Vanderheiden (1982) give a design for an adaptive interface for handicapped computer users; Popelka and Engebretson (1983) describe computer-augmented hearing-aid assessment; Bull (1983) discusses application of microcomputers to a university curriculum in speech–language pathology; and Kamm, Carterette, Morgan, and Dirks (1980) describe applications of computers to audiological research involving speech stimuli. Kieras (1981) and Mayer (1981) give detailed and humorous accounts of their efforts to apply microcomputers to problems in behavioral research. Reed (1980) offers more positive (but dated) suggestions for selecting a microcomputer for experimental research. Willis and Miller (1984) give competent, nontechnical introductions to microcomputer hardware and systems. *Data Sources* (Ziff–Davis Publishing Company, New York), a quarterly publication directed at computer consultants and retailers, gives brief company profiles and product data (features and prices) on computer systems, subsystems, peripherals, and software for the entire computer industry.

The role of hardware in selecting microcomputer systems

Chapter 2 discusses procedures for identifying appropriate and feasible applications of microcomputers. Once the details, priorities, and phasing of application needs are identified, they must be translated into hardware and software (i.e., system) specifications. This is a highly formal activity for large computers because the financial risks of error are significant. Financial hazards are less with microcomputers, but (at the level of the end-user) operational risks associated with bad decisions are just as significant. The hardware component of system analysis can be very straightforward if applications are simple and limited to "garden variety" problems such as word processing, modest data base management, statistical analysis, routine telecommunications, or financial management. In such cases, the result of system analysis is a set of functionally similar alternative systems, each of which meets minimum specifications for the tasks to be "computerized."

Most serious acquisitions involve some effort to trade benefits and costs in order to arrive at an optimal choice. Where applications are simple, decisions can and should be made primarily in terms of commercially available software and the general hardware parameters of function, compatibility, capacity, speed, expandability, reliability, and cost. When applications are uncommon, however, hardware issues may assume a more important role. This is most often the case where user or data characteristics dictate special requirements for input and output operations, or where the requirements for processing speed and complexity predominate. Professional advice and technical assistance from unbiased sources are crucial in these situations.

End-users are often more comfortable dealing with a single vendor and a single manufacturer, even if less expensive options exist through "distributed" purchasing. This trade-off of dollar costs for the benefits of proven compatibility is often preferred by users with little previous experience.

Some "trap avoidance" advice for the would-be buyer: Allow adequate time to learn about hardware and about computers in general. Deal with established vendors selling established products. If a particular system satisfies needs without modification (of either the system or the intended application), state-of-the-art and obsolescence issues should not be taken too seriously. Be wary of claims about compatibility, especially relative to "work-alike" computers.

Don't expect hardware to perform faster, quieter, or better than advertised: it won't. Current users of candidate systems can be valuable sources of information, but "missionaries" for particular systems may not be objective. Verify claims of hardware performance through observation. Attend to details such as connecting cables, hardware and software reference manuals, and the availability of expendable supplies (disks, printer ribbons, paper). Finally, recognize that microcomputers are like cars, audiometers, and other utility devices; if there is a good reason to purchase one now, there will almost certainly be a better reason to buy another in the future.

A GENERAL ARCHITECTURE FOR MICROCOMPUTERS

Computer "architecture" refers to the physical and functional design of hardware. Although computers differ in size, speed, complexity, and other characteristics, most share a functional structure similar to that shown in Figure 5-1. A central processing unit (CPU) accomplishes logical and mathematical operations and communicates with memory devices and peripheral devices by means of a set of electrical connections called a communication bus. There are two categories of memory devices: *primary memory*, which provides fast, short-term storage of programs and data, and *secondary memory*, which offers slower, but larger capacity storage. The communication bus is an "information channel" that allows a CPU to communicate with other subsystems housed within the computer (internal bus), and with devices physically separated from the computer (external bus). Peripheral devices permit entry and display of information (programs, data, and results of processing), as well as control of the computer and its attendant devices.

CENTRAL PROCESSING UNITS (CPUs)

The old days

The earliest electronic computers were monsters of size, power consumption, and complexity of use. They were designed, built, and programmed by engineers for purposes largely related to military applications. The earliest of these was ENIAC (Electronic Numerical Integrator and Calculator), completed at the University of Pennsylvania in 1946. ENIAC required 800 ft^2 of floor space, contained 18,000 vacuum tubes, weighed 30 tons, and cost half a million dollars (Borko, 1962). It was less powerful, much slower, and vastly more difficult to use than the Timex–Sinclair 1000 microcomputer, released in 1982 at a list price just under $100.

Since the mid-1940s, computer technology has gone through several "generations." First-generation systems used vacuum tubes for storing and processing information. Second-generation systems (introduced in 1958) were based upon individually packaged transistors. In 1966 integrated circuits (ICs) gave rise to third-generation systems. Fourth-generation computers emerged in 1971 with the development of large-scale integration (LSI) manufacturing methods. ("Fifth-generation" computers are in planning stages, but will require an order of magnitude's improvement in IC technology—see Lemmons, 1983).

Modern CPUs

Contemporary microcomputers are based upon *microprocessors* contained in a single IC, the physical area of which is usually less than 2 cm^2 (most microprocessors require several

Figure 5-1. Generic architecture of a computer.

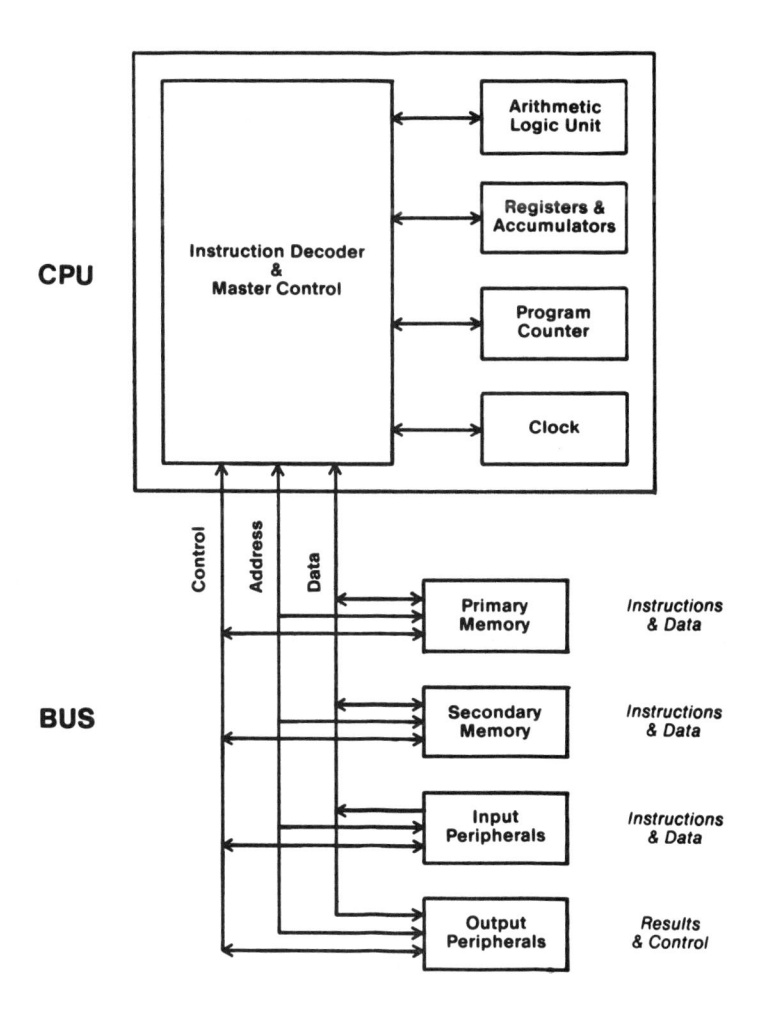

The central processing unit (CPU) steps through program instructions, including mathematical and logical operations on data. The bus allows communication between the CPU and memory devices. Primary memory provides fast access to programs (both system software and application software) and to data. Secondary memory is slower, but accommodates larger bodies of information. Most primary memory is volatile (information is lost when electrical power is removed); secondary memory is not. The bus also lets the CPU communicate with input devices (e.g., a keyboard) for entry of programs, data, and commands to the system, and with output devices (e.g., a printer, display screen, or mechanical manipulator) to display results and/or control the external environment. See text for further explanation.

additional "support" ICs). Microcomputers continue a general trend in size reduction that saw its first major jump with the introduction (in about 1965) of the *minicomputer*, a late second-generation development of Digital Equipment Corporation. The principal advantages of microminiaturization are conservation of space, electrical power, and "waste" heat, increased operating speed (because shorter distances separate components), simplified design of support circuits, improved isolation from electrical noise, and reduced cost (due to mass production).

CPUs are *hardwired* with limited repertoires of fairly primitive operations called "instruction sets." Particular operations or instructions (e.g., "fetch the number stored in memory location X") are coded as numbers; a sequence of instructions constitutes a program. Programs written directly in the number codes of the CPU instruction set are in the "machine language" of the CPU. Although the CPU requires that these numbers (called "operation codes") be expressed in binary notation, machine language programs are usually written in *assembly language*, a class of fast, low-level, computer language that allows the use of mnemonic abbreviations to designate operation codes.

Microprocessors typically contain control subsystems to carry out operations and manage communication with other devices in the system, accumulators and registers to temporarily store information, a device that sequences operations, and a timekeeper to ensure that operations proceed in proper "rhythm."

The *master control unit* (MCU) of the CPU translates operation code numbers into actions affecting the rest of the system. The MCU also controls the flow of information to and from the CPU via the communication bus. The *arithmetic logic unit* (ALU) effects instructions involving mathematical or logical operations. A set of *registers* and *accumulators* store addresses of memory locations and the rsults of ALU operations. Some registers are organized as *stacks* that accept and release information on a last-in, first-out (LIFO) basis; others serve as *buffers* that temporarily hold incoming or outgoing information on a first-in, first-out (FIFO) basis. The *program counter* (PC) is a stack register that keeps track of current "position" in a sequence of operations by remembering the memory addresses of the last, current, and next instructions. The *system clock* acts as a pacemaker for the CPU, ensuring that data, operations, and memory locations (and the functions affecting them) interact smoothly.

Variations in central processor designs

Microprocessor designs differ in several ways that influence total computer system performance. Major differences include the number of bits used in storing information (the memory bit width), the number of bits used in data manipulations (the data bus bit width), and the number of bits used in memory addressing (the address bus bit width). Other important differences include processing speed (determined by clock speed and size of instruction set), the precision and modes of computation, the number of internal registers, the ability to handle "interrupt" signals from other hardware, and cost (Artwick, 1980). Of these, cost is probably the least significant: most microprocessor chips themselves cost less than $25 and account for less than 10% of the cost of an integrated microcomputer system. Table 5-1 summarizes features of several common microprocessors.

Bit width

A *bit* is a single "chunk" of binary information, the value of which may be 1 ("on") or 0 ("off"). Bit width (also called "bit length") refers to the number of parallel binary information channels the processor can manage for computations, storage, and addressing memory. Bit width limits the magnitude of the largest and smallest numbers a computer can accommodate, overall computational accuracy, the number of bits in each uniquely addressable "chunk" (*word*) of memory, and the capacity of a computer's primary memory. Contemporary microprocessors have nominal bit widths of 8, 16, or 32 bits. Single-number designation of bit width can be misleading, however, because virtually all CPUs employ different bit widths for computations, memory addressing, and memory cell size. For example, most "8-bit" CPUs use 16 bits for memory addressing, 8 bits for computations, and 8 bits for each chunk of memory (e.g., the

Table 5-1. Comparison of selected features of five common central processing units (CPUs)

CPU	Manufacturer	Bit width Mem/Addr/Comp	General registers	Memory capacity (bytes)	Clock speed (MHz)	Used in
6502	MOS Technology	8/16/8	1 (8 bit)	64K	1-2	a
Z80	Zilog	8/16/8	7 (8 bit)	64K	2-6	b
8086	Intel	16/20/16	4 (16 bit)	1M	5-10	c
8088	Intel	8/20/16	14 (16 bit)	1M	5-8	d
68000	Motorola	8/24/32	17 (32 bit)	16M	8	e

Notes. The majority of microcomputers sold in the United States use one or more of these five common CPUs, but not all integrated systems utilize their respective CPUs fully, or even to the same degree. Clock speeds shown apply to entire families of CPUs (e.g., Z80, Z80A, Z80B), not just to a single version.

[a] Apple II, II+, IIe; Commodore VIC 20, CBM-8032, Pet, SuperPet; Franklin 1000; Olympia Portable Computer; Panasonic Link.

[b] Radio Shack Model II, Model III, Model 16; Franklin 1200 (also 6502); Acorn (BBC) computer (also 6502); North Star Advantage, Horizon; Hewlett-Packard 100; Sony SMC-70; Sanyo MBC-1000, -1200; Eagle II, III, IV; Televideo Systems 802, 803, 806, 816; Kaypro II, 10; Timex 1000, 2000; Telcon Zorba; Epson QX-10.

[c] Eagle 1600; Zenith Z-100 (also 8085); Wang Personal Computer.

[d] International Business Machines (IBM) Personal Computer, XT, Peanut; Eagle Personal Computer: Columbia MPC; Compaq Portable Computer; Corona Personal Computer; Digital Equipment Corporation (DEC) Rainbow 100 (also Z80); Compupro 816 (also 8085); Hewlett-Packard 150; NCR Decision Mate V (also Z80); Victor 9000; Vector Graphic 4 (also Z80); Texas Instruments (TI) Pegasus; Televideo Systems 1602, 1603; Seequa Chameleon (also Z80).

[e] Apple Lisa, Macintosh; Radio Shack Model 16; Cromemco Systems One-D (also Z80); Hewlett-Packard 200-16.

8-bit MOS Technology 6502 CPU found in the Apple II computer); others use different bit widths for these functions (e.g., the Intel 8088 employed in the IBM Personal Computer which uses 20 bits for addressing, 16 bits for computations, and 8 bits for memory).

Recall that a *byte* is 8 bits treated as a unit. Memory capacity is expressed in *kilobytes* (2 to the 10th power or 1,024 bytes, usually expressed as 1K) and *Megabytes* (2 to the 20th power, 1,048,576 bytes, or 1,024 Kbytes). (By way of illustration, a typed character requires 1 byte of memory; assuming five letters per word, one typed page of 300 words—and spaces—requires about 2 Kbytes.) Processors with 8-bit widths can directly address only 256 words of memory, but sequential addressing schemes (e.g., using two 8-bit bytes for addressing) push this number up to 64 Kbytes (65,536 bytes). Those with 16-bit widths (and the equivalent 2.5-byte addressing schemes) typically address 0.5 Mbyte (512 Kbytes or 524,288 bytes); some can address up to 1 Mbyte of memory. One 16-bit CPU (the Zilog Z8000) can directly address 8 Mbytes and a common 16/32-bit processor (the Motorola 68000) uses a 24-bit address bus to access up to 16 Mbytes (2 to the 24th power). CPUs with larger bit widths also have potential for greater numerical precision and range (these factors are also influenced by other details of architecture and by instruction sets.)

Processing speed

One factor influencing microcomputer speed is the system clock. These operate at speeds ranging from 1 to 10 MHz, limited largely by the ability of IC packages to dissipate heat (faster operating speeds generate more "waste" thermal energy). The same or very similar microprocessors may be assigned different clock speeds. Faster speeds reflect improvements in packaging and competition in the marketplace: speed is more a matter of how long a particular processor has been available than of inherent potentials of design (King & Knight, 1983).

Native instruction sets for microprocessors differ widely in the number of instructions in the set, in details related to the number and modes of addressing options, in the types of variables directly supported by the set, and in the complexity and power (capacity for work) of individual instructions (Artwick, 1980). Instruction sets are incompatible across CPUs with different bit widths (e.g., 8-bit vs. 16-bit). CPUs which share a common architecture constitute a "family," within which instruction sets tend to be "upward compatible," that is, the sets of less advanced CPUs are included within those of more advanced CPUs (e.g., the Intel 8085 uses an instruction set that is a superset of that used by the Intel 8080).

Processing speed (the rate at which a CPU executes a program) is directly related to clock speed, but different operations (e.g., loading the contents of a memory address or adding the contents of registers A and B) require different numbers of clock cycles. Depending upon the particular CPU, processing speed may be directly or inversely related to the size of the machine language instructions set (30–200 discrete operations are common). Although larger instruction sets usually mean greater efficiency, some high-speed, large repertoire CPUs actually take longer to complete a task than slower CPUs with fewer, more powerful instruction sets (Artwick, 1980). Thus, clock speed or the size of an instruction set alone is not a good index of CPU quality.

Precision and modes of computation

At bottom, all CPUs perform mathematical operations in the "ones" and "zeros" of *binary* (base-2) arithmetic. Other number bases are used for intermediate coding of data, instructions, and addresses, the most common being the hexadecimal (base-16) number system in which the digits 0–9 and the letters A–F represent the base-10 values 0–15. Although these alternative systems of numeration are not particularly difficult to understand (see Ashley, 1980), most users are more comfortable with the *decimal* (base-10) system. Fortunately, CPU software (or firmware) translates base-2 and base-16 values into more familiar form. This is accomplished by coding systems for numbers, letters, and other characters which usually employ successive segments of 4 bits each. Each 4-bit segment can accommodate numbers ranging from 0000 (decimal 0; hexadecimal 0) to 1111 (decimal 15; hexadecimal F). Thus, the byte 0001 1110 is equivalent to decimal 114 or hexadecimal 1E.

Precision of computation is typically limited by errors (of rounding or truncation) that may occur in the least significant digit of a coded number (the right-most digit in the examples above). CPUs that use 2-byte (16-bit) systems for computation offer accuracy of 1 part in 65,536; those using 4-byte (32-bit) systems are accurate to 1 part in 4,294,967,300. These numbers may seem impressive at first, but are less so in the context of common physical constants and the very large (or small) values that can occur in statistical analyses.

Most CPUs enhance their inherent potential for accuracy by offering optional "double-precision" modes that double the number of bytes normally used for computation (trading precision for speed and capacity); other CPUs employ special internal coding schemes (e.g., exponential notation) to more efficiently manage very large or very small values, as well as real numbers, that is, those with both integer and fractional parts.

Registers

Registers are specialized memory cells located within a CPU that provide rapid access and temporary storage for computations, for addressing, for indexing operations, and for stacks which keep track of where the CPU "is" in programs containing routines nested within other routines. A practical processor must have at least three registers, one for the current operation code, one for the memory address of that code (i.e., the program counter), and one general register for the datum (operand) currently being acted upon. Beyond these, CPUs differ in the number, type, and bit width of registers. Processors such as the MOS Technology 6502 reserve only one 8-bit register for computations, while the Motorola 68000 has sixteen 32-bit registers (King & Knight, 1983; Starnes, 1983). CPUs with fewer registers can accomplish essentially the same operations as CPUs with more registers (the use of registers instead of primary memory is a philosophical issue), but with less speed and precision. Processors with more registers also tend to feature more powerful computation modes.

Interrupts

Once a CPU begins a set of instructions, it continues until it is finished, or until it encounters a message to stop while some other event is completed. Such messages (called "hardware interrupts") might signal that an input peripheral has data to send to the CPU, or that an output peripheral is momentarily occupied and cannot accept additional information. When an interrupt occurs, the CPU jumps to a specified memory address to initiate an "interrupt-handling" subprogram (see Leibson, 1982b, 1982c, and Artwick, 1980, for more detail). Some CPUs have priority interrupt systems that allow several devices to stop processing, and then "service" those devices in an order determined by importance of the interruption. Levels of priority vary from 2 (e.g., the MOS Technology 6502 CPU) to 16 (e.g., Texas Instruments 99000 CPU). The larger the number of priorities, the more flexible the CPU (see King & Knight, 1983).

Other features

Some microprocessors have the ability to control the flow of information from one location to another without passing that information through the registers of the CPU. This feature is called "direct memory access" (DMA) and makes possible extremely high-speed transmission of data. DMA subsystems are common in the acquisition and processing of external signals that vary in real time, that is, at rates independent of the CPU system clock (see Leibson, 1982b).

CPU selection

Most end-users buy integrated computer systems, not central processing units. For these users, variations in CPU design are relevant only to the extent that they influence memory capacity and processing speed. Even these differences may be minimized by other hardware factors that degrade the performance of more advanced microprocessors. Furthermore, software designers often modify their products for newer CPUs in order to retain customers, rather than to take advantage of improved CPU performance. Sadly, many of the glowing reports of features of newer CPUs (Heywood, 1983a,b,c; Zinagle, 1983) do not materialize in ways that benefit users directly.

CPU variations can become quite critical in specialized applications, however. This is especially true where the bulk or complexity of mathematical operations predominate, where an application requires very rapid processing of information, where a very large amount of data must be directly available to a processor, or where an especially efficient operating system, computer language, or dialect of a language is required. For example, applications involving analysis of speech signals, rapid physiological events (e.g., electromyological or electroneurological signals) or fast laboratory animals (e.g., rats and chinchillas) may require faster processing and greater memory capacity than would be necessary in behavioral studies of people or in routine word processing applications. Similarly, a task requiring manipulation of large data matrices (i.e., 250 columns by 1000 rows) via *spread sheet* or *data base* programs will require a CPU capable of addressing more memory than the 64 Kbytes common to 8-bit machines.

Benchmark comparisons of CPUs can help resolve issues related to processor speed, precision, and efficiency. An example of a benchmark comparison is given by Monahan (1983) for several computers nominally running the same BASIC program to generate prime numbers. Four systems performed as follows: Apple II+ (CPU: MOS Technology 6502), 241 sec.; IBM personal computer (CPU: Intel 8088), 190 sec.; Radio Shack TRS-80, Model II (CPU: Zilog Z80), 189 sec.; and Hewlett-Packard Model 200-16 (CPU: Motorola 68000), 19 sec. Differences in processing speed of this magnitude (10 to 1) are not uncommon.

It must be remembered, however, that such tests are influenced by factors in addition to the CPU itself, such as the language used for the benchmark and the implementation of that language for a particular CPU. Further, the problem addressed by a given benchmark test may not exercise features of a CPU relevant to a particular class of applications. Critical comparisons of CPU (and total system) performance are probably best approached with benchmark programs designed or selected by the prospective buyer (Houston, 1984).

CPUs: One or many?

Computers need not be limited to a single microprocessor. In fact, most contain second or third processors which service specialized functions such as decoding keyboard signals. A few others (e.g., the IBM personal computer and the Apple Macintosh computer) are capable of accepting specialized "coprocessors" to speed up mathematical operations. These are not really "multiple CPU" systems because a single CPU controls the entire system. Other microcomputers are designed with two or more CPUs to allow user access to more than one library of processor-dependent software (e.g., the Zenith 100, Digital Equipment Corporation Rainbow 100, British Broadcasting Corporation, and Franklin 1200 computers). Still others with "open bus" designs (e.g., the Apple II and the IBM personal computer) can accept separate components that contain their own CPUs and (thus) simulate entirely different computer systems. These are also not "multiple CPU" systems because only one CPU is active at one time.

Some computers *are* multiple CPU systems because they contain from 2 to 16 separate and independent combinations of CPUs and primary memory. These multi-user systems usually let several users share secondary memory; they also use a single communication bus and power supply. Cromemco, Altos, and several other firms offer systems of this type.

COMMUNICATION BUSES

The internal communication bus of a microcomputer consists of three functionally separate channels: an *address bus*, a *control bus*, and a *data bus*. Although Figure 5-1 represents each of these channels with a single line, an actual system would reserve several wires for each channel.

The communication bus can be thought of as a system of city streets. In this analogy, data and operations are represented by people. The address bus is akin to a city directory that designates street addresses, the names of residents at each address and (by implication), routes between locations. The control bus is similar to the stop lights and flagmen that control the direction of traffic flow. The data bus is represented by the streets that carry traffic to and from the center of the city. In most microcomputers, the "streets" are eight or 16 "lanes" (bits) wide. "Street signals" or "flags" on the control bus allow data to flow in only one direction at a time. The control bus also manages the speed of information flow. "Service lanes" are included for electrical power and ground signals.

In actual microcomputers, internal communication buses are implemented via conductive traces of metal placed on the main circuit board or "motherboard" of the computer, or by electrical connectors soldered to the motherboard and designed to accept "daughter boards" (peripherals). Bus systems differ between microcomputers as a function of the requirements of particular microprocessors and as a function of the philosophies of manufacturers about proprietary hardware design (see Artwick, 1980; Leibson, 1982a,b). An exception is the *S-100* bus (so-named because 100 electrical connections are used), now standardized as *IEEE-696* (Garetz, 1983). This bus evolved during the late 1970s for use with the Intel 8080 and Zilog

Z80 families of microprocessors and enjoys wide use in business and scientific microcomputers. Other exceptions include the internal bus designs of the Apple II computer (Titus, Larsen, & Titus, 1981) and the IBM personal computer (Eggebrecht, 1983). The manufacturers of these machines intentionally disseminated details of bus schemes to stimulate development of peripheral products by other firms, thus enhancing the viability of their products in a mass market.

An entirely different class of communication bus exists to allow microcomputers to communicate with peripherals physically separated from the computer system (see the section on interfaces to follow).

MEMORY SYSTEMS

Figure 5-1 indicates two classes of memory: primary and secondary. Primary memory is housed within the computer itself and is used to store currently active data and programs that must be directly available to the CPU. Secondary memory systems are often housed separately from the computer and are used to store larger bodies of information. These systems are *online* with the CPU, in other words, data and programs can be stored and recalled under CPU control. Secondary memory is also used to store information after the computer is turned off, and to physically transport information from one computer to another.

The old days

The first commercial electronic computers produced in the 1950s used cathode-ray vacuum tubes as primary memory devices. Tubes approximately 3 inches in diameter "remembered" information by placing electrostatic charges on grids containing 256 points (bits). At about the same time, vacuum tubes filled with mercury vapor and fitted with crystal transducers at either end were used to store information by means of ultrasonic propagation delays. A delay line 2.5 ft long could store several thousand bits (Borko, 1962). Both systems were cumbersome, slow, fragile, and extremely limited in capacity. During the 1960s, magnetic core memory came into use. This technology employed tiny rings of ferromagnetic material woven into matrices with several sets of wires that coursed through the holes of the rings. "Write" wires stored information by changing the polarity of the magnetic charge of individual rings. Charges could be "read" by another set of wires. Early core memory frames stored about 4,000 bits in an area approximately 1 ft^2 (Borko, 1962). Magnetic core memory was cheaper, faster, more compact, more robust, and required less electrical power than tubes; increasingly compact core memory was used in large and small computers through the early 1970s. It became so common in mainframe computers and minicomputers that "core memory" is still used as a synonym for primary computer memory of any technology.

Secondary storage methods can be traced back to the US census of 1890 and the development of the punched card by Herman Hollerith. Hollerith cards (also called "IBM cards"), based on a still-earlier technique used to program weaving machines, store information in the form of holes placed in a matrix of 80 columns and 12 rows. This represents a "raw" capacity of 960 bits on an area slightly larger than a modern dollar bill. Punched-paper tape, used for many years with teletype (TTY) machines, uses 5 rows and an indefinite number of columns to store information. Manual and computer-driven punching, listing, and reading machines are used to generate, print, and retrieve data stored on these media. Magnetic tape, magnetic drum, and magnetic disk memory systems emerged during the 1960s as faster, larger capacity alternatives to cards and paper tape. These devices (and their attendant technologies) offered peak memory capacities between 0.25 and 30 Mbytes.

Primary memory

Modern primary memory employs integration techniques that improve on earlier storage systems by several orders of magnitude in speed, density, and cost. In 1970, core memory cost about a dollar per byte; in 1983, a less-valuable dollar could buy a kilobyte of memory. Primary memory is used for two different purposes: (1) to retain systems software that must be available to the CPU every time the computer is used, and (2) to store programs and data required by a user for a particular task. It is available in three forms: as part of an integrated computer system, as part of a subsystem added to a computer after purchase ("add-in" memory), and as individual ICs ("add-on" memory).

Characteristics of primary memory

Volatility. Nonvolatile primary memory retains information permanently (even when the computer is turned off). It is typically used for low-level programs that service the needs of the computer itself. Volatile primary memory holds information until a user (or program) modifies it, or until the computer is turned off.

Access speed. The time required to "put" or "take" information from memory is called access speed or cycle time, typically measured in nanoseconds (ns—there are a billion ns in 1 s). Access speed varies with memory circuit design and device technology. Microcomputer primary memory speeds range from 200 to 500 ns.

Density. This refers to the amount of memory in a single IC package, expressed in Kbytes. Some primary memory "chips" have bit widths of 4 or 8 bits; most are 1 bit wide. Greater density translates into faster, smaller, cooler, more efficient (in power consumption) and ultimately less costly computer systems. Early primary memory for microcomputers used ICs containing 1 Kbyte (by 1 bit); 4-, 16-, and 64-Kbyte/IC densities are now common. In 1983, Bell Laboratories announced an IC with 256 Kbytes (by 1 bit). Most contemporary microcomputers employ chips with 16 or 64 Kbytes per IC. An 8-bit computer capable of addressing 64K of memory would be "fully populated" by eight, 64-Kbyte ICs.

Cost. In chip form, primary memory is relatively inexpensive, usually less than $100 for 64 Kbytes of 8-bit memory. Subsystem (e.g., daughter board) memory is more expensive because communication bus circuits and mechanical support are necessary. Prices vary widely: 8-bit add-in memory ranges between $5 and $10 per Kbyte.

Types of primary memory

Random-access memory (RAM). RAM is volatile, high-speed, high-density, low-cost memory used for working programs. New information is placed in RAM simply by writing over old information (RAM is similar to audio tape). RAM is "random" because a given cell of memory can be identified directly by what amounts to a coordinate address, rather than by sifting through a sequence of other cells. Thus the same time is required to access any cell in an array of RAM. Most RAM is based upon *MOS* (metal oxide semiconductor) technology capable of holding information for only a few microseconds. "Refreshing" schemes are used to retain data for as long as necessary. This type of memory is called *dynamic.* Less common (also faster and more expensive) is *static* RAM which requires no periodic refreshing. Static and dynamic RAM cannot be interchanged.

Read-only memory (ROM). ROM is nonvolatile, high-speed, lower density memory used for system programs. Permanent information is placed in ROM during manufacture (much like a phonograph record). Like RAM, ROM is accessed randomly by coordinate address.

Virtually all microcomputers contain ROM. ROM is cheap for manufacturers (who buy it in vast quantities), but excessively expensive for end-users.

Programmable ROM (PROM). PROM is a kind of ROM that can be written to after it is manufactured (i.e., in the field). This is done by passing relatively high voltages to the device, burning away portions of circuits. Once encoded, PROM cannot be reprogrammed.

Erasable PROM (EPROM). EPROM is PROM that can be erased in the field by exposure to ultraviolet light. Thus, it can be encoded and reencoded as often as necessary. EPROM is used in professional products (e.g., computerized audiometers) to reduce the cost of "updating" system software.

Electronic EPROM (EEPROM). Yes, EEPROM is a kind of EPROM that can be erased electronically, rather than optically. Otherwise, it is the same as EPROM.

Magnetic bubble memory. This is a relatively new technology offering the advantages of EEPROM (nonvolatile, reprogrammable), and is very high density. The major disadvantages are cost and access speed. Magnetic bubble memory is also used as secondary memory.

System implications

Microcomputers usually contain a "mix" of RAM and one or more of the varieties of ROM. Regardless of the proportions of each, total primary memory normally cannot exceed the addressing capacity of the CPU. If a large proportion of ROM is present, less capacity is available for user programs (in a sense, the memory space occupied by such software represents an "overhead expense"). Some systems use very little ROM for system software. Instead, these programs are stored in secondary memory and automatically loaded into RAM (by means of a short "bootstrap" program held in ROM) whenever the system is turned on. This also reduces the amount of RAM available to the user for application programs, but is somewhat more flexible because it is usually not necessary to load all system software for all application programs.

As RAM has become less expensive, software developers have worried less about the memory efficiency of programs. This has produced some exceptionally powerful software, most of which requires more than the minimum memory provided with a computer when it is purchased. Adding memory to accommodate such programs is not particularly difficult, but it should be done by someone experienced in the handling of ICs and printed circuit boards. Not all computers permit addition of primary memory; of those which do, added memory may not be accessible to all application programs otherwise compatible with the computer system.

Serious users are advised to purchase a microcomputer with at least 64 Kbytes (for 8-bit systems) or 128 Kbytes (for 16-bit systems) of primary memory (Wolf, 1983).

Secondary memory

Secondary memory serves two major functions: (1) it provides for mass storage of data and programs that are only occasionally required by the CPU, and (2) it makes possible the transportation of programs and data between computers. Relative to primary memory, this type of storage trades speed, cost, and density for bulk and portability.

All systems for secondary memory (except magnetic bubble memory) include a communication bus interface, some medium to store information, and a mechanism that physically manipulates the storage media.

Characteristics of secondary memory

Organization and access speed. Functionally and physically, secondary memory subsystems may be classified as either *sequential access* or *random access*. To reach a particular datum stored in sequential access memory, all of the data prior to the focal datum first must be processed. In this sense, sequential access memory is similar to an audio cassette tape: to replay the fifth song on a tape, songs one through four must pass the reproduce head. Random access (strictly speaking, pseudo-random access) secondary memory can be thought of as a rectangular or polar matrix. Any cell of the matrix can be located (addressed or accessed) by a system of coordinates. Random access memory is faster and more expensive than sequential access memory.

Recording technology. Most secondary memory systems store and recall digital information using analog magnetic techniques similar to those used in audio tape recording. A few employ digital magnetic (see bubble memory) or digital optical (see video disks) methods to store digital or analog data.

Capacity and density. Depending upon recording technology, data organization, and the physical size of storage media, the capacities of secondary memory vary from a few thousand Kbytes to several Gigabytes (1 Gbyte = 1024 Mbytes).

Other features. Most secondary memory systems employ removable media capable of erasure and reuse, but some media are inherently nonerasable, nonremovable, and nonportable. Most (but not all) secondary memory hardware is light weight and robust enough to permit some regular movement from place to place. The coding schemes used to record and recall information (which, of course, involve software as well as hardware) are generally incompatible across the various secondary memory technologies and across brands of computers.

Cost. The cost of secondary memory varies in direct proportion to capacity, density, and speed of access. Subsystem costs range from about $50 for cassette tape systems to more than $10,000 for high-density hard disk systems.

Types of secondary memory

Magnetic tape. Early microcomputers used audio cassette recorders as storage devices. Information was coded in the form of audio tones of different frequencies for the binary states 1 and 0. Advantages included low cost and ready availability of recording media. Major disadvantages were limited capacity and extremely slow access speed. Audio cassettes have been replaced by floppy disks in virtually all serious applications. Specialized, high-capacity tape systems are now used to "back up" hard disk systems, that is, to protect investments of money, time, and effort associated with stored programs and data.

Floppy disks. This is the most common form of secondary memory for microcomputers. Floppy disks (so called because they use thin, pliable platters of Mylar or similar recording media) are essentially audio tape in circular form. The Mylar disk is permanently sealed inside a protective plastic envelope. A drive mechanism activated by the CPU (via an interface called a "controller") causes the disk to rotate at a moderate speed (e.g., 360 rpm) whenever necessary. Information is magnetically placed on (written) and recalled from the disk (read) by means of a tiny record-playback head mounted on a movable arm. The head rides on the surface of the disk and is positioned along a radius of the disk by a small stepper motor. Disks are logically (i.e., with software) organized into concentric tracks and radial sectors: thus, they are psuedo-random access devices.

Floppy disks are similar to audio tape in that old information is erased whenever new information is recorded; reading information from a disk leaves that information unchanged. In other words, all writing is destructive and all reading is nondestructive. Accidental erasure can be costly. For this reason, disks are equipped with a notch at the right front of their protective envelopes. Disk drives contain a microswitch that senses whether the notch is covered (e.g., by a piece of tape) or uncovered. If the notch on a 5.25-thick disk is covered, the disk is *write-protected*, in other words, new information cannot be recorded. If the notch is uncovered, the disk is *write-enabled,* that is, new data can be recorded (exactly the opposite logic is used on standard audio cassette tapes and 8-inch disks). The status of the notch has no effect on reading information from the disk. As with any magnetic medium, accidental erasures can occur through exposure to motors, earphones, power cords, or other devices that generate magnetic fields. Therefore, backup procedures (making copies of disks) are necessary.

Floppy disks (and disk drives) are available in two incompatible dimensions (8-inch diameter floppy disks and 5.25-inch diameter) in three "upward compatible" densities (single, double, and quad), in two "side" configurations (single or double), and in several sectoring formats. Single-sided, single-density disks can store about 180 Kbytes, equivalent to about 90 pages of text; double-sided quad-density disks can store up to about 720 Kbytes. Because disks must be formatted with "housekeeping" information (analogous to a table of contents) before use, the actual memory space available to the user is somewhat less. "Soft" sectored disks use magnetically recorded information to designate sector boundaries; "hard" sectored disks indicate sector boundaries with holes punched in the Mylar medium. The different sectoring schemes are not compatible.

Although disk manufacturers certify the performance of their products, disks do wear out (good quality disks should last a year); poor handling and storage practices can cause early failure. Similarly, the heads of disk drives accumulate magnetic particles and require periodic cleaning.

Floppy disks, disk drives, and disk controllers are available from many sources for many microcomputers. Systems currently range in price from a few hundred dollars to over a thousand dollars, depending upon number of recording sides and recording densities.

"Firm" or microfloppy disks. This memory system uses recording and playback techniques similar to floppy disks, but with a 3.5-inch diameter "shirt pocket" medium contained in a rigid plastic case. Microfloppy drive systems are smaller, lighter in weight, and less expensive to manufacture than those used with floppy disks. Some rotate at speeds twice that of standard floppy or 5.25-inch floppy disks (Moran, 1983). The disks themselves are more robust and have greater capacity than single- or double-density floppy disks: 500 Kbytes is typical (Jarrett, 1983). Originally developed by Sony for that company's microcomputers, microfloppy disks and drives are also used in newer Hewlett–Packard and Apple computers. They are rapidly becoming available as add-on or replacement systems for other machines. Several other diameter systems have been developed or proposed, usually as proprietary subsystems (e.g., 3-, 3.25-, or 4-inch), but these are unlikely to become common (Jarrett, 1983).

Hard disks. Like floppy and microfloppy disk systems, hard disks employ analog magnetic recording techniques. Unlike floppies, hard disks use a rigid medium and a record-play head that floats a microscopic distance above the media (to limit head wear). The disks themselves are mounted on precision bearings and packaged in a sealed cartridge which protects the disk from dust. The most common size is 5.25 inches. Hard disks have much faster access speeds and storage capacities than other magnetic disks: they rotate at speeds up to 3600 rpm and can store from 2 to 40 Mbytes, depending upon diameter and other features. These advantages are the result of very strict tolerances in design and manufacture, factors which also significantly increase cost: hard disk systems range in price between one and several thousand dollars. The precision that makes possible such dramatic increases in capacity is also the reason why most hard disk systems employ nonremovable media and why most are nonportable (Moore, 1981; Sarisky, 1983; Thé, 1983).

Microcomputer hard disks were originally designed as part of a system containing 30 Mbytes of removable storage and 30 Mbytes of nonremovable storage. Hence, they were dubbed "Winchester" drives after the 30-30 rifle made by Winchester Arms (Sutton, 1983).

Hard disk systems are appropriate to applications where very large bodies of data are required. Because most of these systems use nonremovable media, additional devices (magnetic tape, floppy disks) are required to produce backup records of data. Because they store much more information than floppy disks, they require special controller interfaces and system software not compatible with floppy disks. Hard disk systems also can be effectively used as a shared resource, in which case several users have access to large-capacity secondary memory via a *network* of some sort.

Video disks. This type of secondary memory differs from other disk technologies. Although video disks (more precisely, optical reflective video disks, as opposed to the capacitive video disks offered as alternatives to video tape) are not in wide use, they are included here because they have already found application in education and the entertainment industry (Bejar, 1982; Hon, 1982). Video disks record information in digital form by means of a high-intensity laser that burns microscopic pits in the surface of a rigid, metal platter. The recording process permanently changes the surface of the disk: thus, reflective video disks are "read-only" devices. Information is retrieved with a low-intensity laser whose reflected image (or unreflected image in the case of a pit) is sensed by a photodetector.

Because lasers can be aimed very precisely, because the disk surface area is very large relative to the space required by a single datum, and because the disk is rigid enough to rotate at high speed, video disks are capable of storing thousands of Mbytes (i.e., Gigabytes). Further, they can store color video images and extremely high-fidelity audio signals, as well as text and more conventional data (Moberg & Laefsky, 1982). Disadvantages of this technology include high cost of recording (Daynes, 1982; Wicat Systems, 1982), nonerasibility, slow access times, and a lack of standards for encoding–decoding, recording, medium size and material, and rotation speed (Rothchild, 1983). Read-only drive systems are slightly more expensive than floppy disk drives, but less costly than similar capacity hard disk drives. Optical reflective video disks already have been used in communication disorders and will undoubtedly see greater use as repositories for standardized tests and test stimuli (both visual and auditory).

System Implications

Hardware compatibility. Secondary memory systems are controlled by central processing units via interfaces called "controllers." These hardware–software subsubsystems are specialized for particular technologies and for particular versions of a given technology. They also are designed for particular internal communication buses, particular CPUs, and particular system software. Thus, the disk, disk drives, and disk controllers suitable for, say, an IBM personal computer will not work with an Apple IIe computer, a Radio Shack TRS-80 computer, or a Kaypro computer.

Software compatibility. Sizes and some other features of secondary storage media are relatively well standardized. There are no recognized standards for support hardware (i.e., drives) or for encoding–decoding schemes. Indeed, the lack of standardization is often a hardware marketing tactic designed to take advantage of very popular software distributed in disk form. Thus, programs on disks configured for use with one brand of computer are almost always incompatible with other brands, even though the disks and disk drives share common dimensions and designs.

Protection and security. In a sense this is more an operational issue than a hardware issue, but it should be noted nonetheless. As a practical matter, secondary storage media are less valuable than the information they hold. Increasingly, commercial software distributors seek to protect their investments in development by "copy-proofing" their products. This practice has no effect on the needs of users to backup their own data and programs. Smaller capacity systems (e.g., floppy disk or "firm" disk systems) usually allow this, but it is feasible only if the system includes two identical drives. Very large capacity hard disks represent a different level of risk if, for example, they are used to retain clinical records on a large number of clients. If there is no backup procedure (including personnel time and necessary additional hardware), a "head crash" could have disastrous consequences. Similarly, if several users share secondary memory resources, "privileged" information may be compromised.

Serious buyers are advised to look very carefully at immediate and future needs for mass storage. A minimum configuration consistent with the goals of portability and protection would include two secondary memory devices, at least one of which employs removable media (e.g., two floppy disk drives sharing one controller or one hard disk and one floppy disk, each with its own controller).

GENERAL PURPOSE PERIPHERALS

Input devices

General purpose peripherals are those developed for routine use in routine applications. General purpose input devices serve two functions: (1) they allow the user to enter data (text, numbers, other information) for processing by the computer, and (2) they let the user send "metaprocess" information to the system to control the execution of programs and the behavior of the computer itself.

Keyboards and keypads

The most common input devices for microcomputers are keyboards. Although most computer keyboards resemble those of typewriters, they inevitably contain specialized keys not found on conventional typing machines. The functions of special keys are straightforward and fairly standard. Many of these harken to the operational terminology of teletypewriters (TTYs), used in telecommunications for over 40 years and in computer applications for at least 30 years.

Some special keys are used to control the computer or the devices attached to it. Several of these are described in the glossary (e.g., see control key, escape key, repeat key, return key, cursor control keys, and function keys). The remaining keys are similar in purpose to the number, letter, shift, and symbol keys of a typewriter: they allow entry of alphanumeric data (text and numbers).

QWERTY keyboards. Typewriter keyboards place letters, numbers, and the space bar in standardized locations. Punctuation marks, special symbols, (e.g., @, &, %) and control keys are far less standard. So it is with microcomputer keyboards. These keyboards also differ in the size, shape, and feel of keys, the switch technology and use-life of keyboard mechanisms, and whether they can be detached from the rest of the system. Inspection of even two or three keyboards reveals very obvious differences in the way keys are grouped (separate number pads, function keys, cursor position keys, etc.). Some keyboards let a single key serve three or more functions, depending upon the use of shift, control, and "supershift" (alternate) keys. A few microcomputers feature proprietary, dedicated-function keys to clear the display screen, to print entire pages of information, to allow editing, to invoke different application programs, or to produce reminders of keyboard or program functions (i.e., "help" keys). More subtle differences include the angle of successive banks of keys, the presence of audible "keyclicks" (for feedback to the typist) and something called "rollover" —the number of key strokes the keyboard subsystem can "remember" prior to display. Rollover memory varies from one keystroke to many and is particularly important to fast typists who can outrun many microcomputer keyboards.

Most of these variations are intended to help people use a particular computer as efficiently as possible. This is often the case, but skilled touch typists are just as often frustrated by the differences between computer and typewriter keyboards, as well as differences among keyboards of different computers. Because keyboards are so important, many criticisms of specific microcomputers have focused on peculiarities of key size, placement, and comfort.

Specialized keyboards. Several firms offer add-on keyboards for specific microcomputers. Some of these are simply remote numeric keypads or "improvements" of the units originally supplied by the computer manufacturer. Others are "smart" systems with their own ROMs or EEPROMS capable of being "taught" character sequences frequently employed by the user.

Keyboards are normally supplied as an integral part of a computer system and interfaced to the CPU via the internal (parallel) communication bus (Leibson, 1983c). Replacement or add-on keyboards usually cost less than $300.

Other control devices

Keyboards are not the only way (nor necessarily the best way) to tell a computer to do something. One alternative is the *light pen*, a device used in conjunction with a video screen. Light pens contain circuits that sense the scanning electron beam of the display screen and convert that information into *X-Y* coordinate data. Another is the *touch sensor*. One type of touch sensor—the touch screen—uses a system of light-emitting and light-sensing diodes positioned around the periphery of a video screen. When a stylus or finger interrupts (invisible) light beams, positional information is sent to the computer. A similar touch sensor is the touch pad—a small tablet separate from the display screen which senses finger or stylus position on a flat, electronically sensitive surface. A fourth control device is the *mouse*, a small box about the size of a deck of playing cards that can be moved across a flat surface, thus "pointing" a display screen *cursor* at locations on the screen. Assuming appropriate software, positional information from light pens, touch sensors or a mouse can be translated into actions. Because they require special interfaces and integration with software, such control devices are normally sold as part of a complete computer system. They are available as add-on subsystems for a small number of computers at prices ranging from less than $25 to more than $500.

System implications

Hardware compatibility. Because microcomputers are (almost) always sold with keyboards, there are seldom problems of compatibility with the CPU or the memory systems of the computer. Similarly, add-on keyboards (QWERTY or specialized) are designed for particular computers. Incompatibility can arise, however, between *other* add-on devices and existing keyboard systems. For example, some supplemental video display systems (see below) that add the ability to display lower-case letters will function only after hardware modification of the keyboard. Add-on special control devices (touch sensors, light pens, etc.) may present compatibility problems if they produce interrupt signals not "recognized" by other hardware or by system software.

Software compatibility. Just because a keyboard contains a useful special key (e.g., "help") is no guarantee that all programs written for that computer will use that function, nor that programs will use that function in the same way. Special problems may arise with systems whose keyboards have undergone revisions (e.g., the Apple II+ and IIe). Programs written for an older system could not anticipate a newer system: modification of the program (or of the way the program is used) may be necessary. Likewise, the benefits of special control devices may be unavailable to particular software, even though both the device and the program are designed for the same microcomputer. Integrating the features of these special devices into existing software is always difficult and sometimes impossible.

Where microcomputers are used primarily for word processing or numerical data processing, the feel of a keyboard and the presence and layout of a numeric keypad assume obvious importance. As a general rule, more keys mean greater flexibility—thus, more is better, at least for those who use the system often enough to remember the meanings of special keys. Exceptions to this generalization are computers equipped with a mouse. These systems typically have very sparse keyboards because the mouse (and its associated software) replaces most of the functions of special keys.

Output devices

General purpose output devices serve to (1) present results of processing operations, and (2) display status and feedback information about the computer system. These outputs may be in the form of "softcopy" (i.e., relatively transient, electronic signals or displays) or in the form of "hardcopy" (i.e., on paper).

Video terminals

Video terminals (more generically, "computer terminals" or simply "terminals") are stand-alone, general purpose devices designed for use with micro-, mini-, or mainframe computers. They are integrated systems consisting of a keyboard, a video display screen, and memory circuits that remember some number of characters (typically, 25 lines of 80 characters each). Video terminals may or may not be physically packaged as one unit, but they function separately from any computer they may be connected to (usually with help from one or more local microprocessors, communication interface hardware, a modest amount of dedicated primary memory, and a self-contained power supply). Some are *smart terminals* in the same sense as some specialized keyboards. Veit (1981) reviews these and similar units. Stand-alone terminals range in price from a few hundred dollars for very simple, general-purpose devices to several thousand dollars for high-resolution, color graphics display devices. Video terminals are generally more expensive than video display controllers and their associated video monitors or receivers.

Video display controllers

Most microcomputers include circuit boards that generate and store characters and other images to be displayed on a video monitor or video receiver. Visual information of this type consists of matrices of dots, each of which can be turned on or off. Dots are grouped in discrete patterns (called *pixels* or picture elements) to represent alphanumeric characters. Similar methods are used to display graphical images (i.e., any noncharacter visual information).

Characteristics. Display controllers differ in the number of dots used to form the pixel matrix and in the number of pixels remembered by the local memory of the controller. The number of dots per pixel (typically from 5-by-7 to 9-by-14) partially determines the legibility of the display, and the number of pixels per screen image determines the character density of the display (typically between 640 and 1920). Video display controllers also differ in their ability to display lower-case letters, specialized symbols, alternative character fonts, multiple pages (screen images) of characters, and multiple colors for alphanumeric symbols. The typical display mode is light letters on a dark field; many systems permit the reverse, plus flashing or blinking characters. Most display controllers are designed so that as new lines of characters are added, the oldest lines scroll off the top (or bottom) of the display.

Virtually all microcomputers can display some form of graphics in addition to alphanumerics. Video display controllers or separate video graphics controllers implement this through the use of *character graphics, raster graphics,* or *vector graphics.* The former reserves groups of dots in pixels to represent building blocks of larger images (e.g., an upper left-hand corner or a thick horizontal bar). Character graphics can be placed anywhere in the matrix of cells reserved for alphanumeric characters. Raster graphics build original images from individual dots. These can be placed at will on the screen by means of coordinates. The resolution of raster graphics (also called "bit-mapped graphics") varies widely across computers. Some high-resolution raster graphics systems use *sprites,* discrete images that can be defined and moved about independently of each other and of the background image. Vector graphics, a more sophisticated form of bit-mapped graphics, permits placement of lines and arcs through specification of starting and stopping coordinates.

Graphics display capabilities differ widely in terms of resolution and the number of different colors that can be shown. Although alphanumeric and graphic displays are found on virtually all microcomputers, not all systems allow simultaneous display of both kinds of information.

Display controllers are designed to work with particular classes of video monitors and receivers. Early microcomputer designs featured limited character display densities and limited resolution graphics; more modern designs (and second source add-on subsystems) have established the 80-character, 24-line display as a minimum for serious work with textural information. Compatibility problems among add-on display controllers and commercial software are fairly common.

Video monitors and receivers

The most common display devices used with microcomputers are video monitors and video receivers. Both are analog devices containing cathode-ray tubes (CRTs) and both are physically separated from the computer and the keyboard. Both resemble television sets, but only video receivers include the tuner sections required to sense radio frequency broadcasts. (When receivers—TV sets—are used as computer displays, the electrical video signal from the computer must be converted to radio frequency with an *RF modulator.*) Unlike video terminals, monitors and receivers are designed to accept (not store) video information generated elsewhere (i.e., by a TV camera, a video tape recorder, or a video display controller). Storage of characters or graphic images is managed by a video display controller of the microcomputer itself. Monitors generally produce better quality images and generally cost more than receivers of similar size and function. Most portable computers and some desktop computers contain integrated video monitors (or liquid crystal displays—see below); other microcomputers accept external video displays. Receivers and monitors are available from a host of sources.

Characteristics. Some obvious differences distinguish video display devices (both monitors and receivers): screen size (9 to 25 inches), chromicity (color vs. monochrome), and cost (typically between $150 and $3,000). Monochrome systems have CRTs with a single gun (electron source); color CRTs have separate guns for red, blue, and green signals. Some color monitors (RGB monitors) accept separate signals for each gun; all color receivers, as well as all monochrome monitors and receivers, are designed for standardized composite video signals that combine RGB information. Many color monitors are designed to accept both RGB and composite signals. RGB monitors produce better images (for both characters and graphics), but may cost several times more than monochrome devices or composite color systems.

The most important factor associated with video displays is image quality (Powell, 1984), determined largely by bandwidth, resolution, and registration. Bandwidth refers to the rate at which a display can accept video signals from a computer or display controller. The greater the bandwidth, the better (5 MHz may be sufficient for low character-density display, 15 MHz is a minimum for 24-line, 80-character displays, and color graphics may require bandwidths of 30 MHz or more). Resolution (the pixel density of the tube) is influenced by bandwidth and by details of CRT design. Registration (in a color system, convergence) refers to the accuracy with which the CRT electron beam is aimed—in how "true" vertical and horizontal lines appear.

Early monochrome displays used white letters on a black field; current monochrome units more often use green or amber to reduce glare and visual fatigue. Transparent cloth screens and tube shades also are used for these purposes.

Liquid crystal displays (LCDs)

Used for years in calculators and watches, LCD technology also has found application with microcomputers. LCD systems have advantages of low cost and robust, solid state design. They are limited in image resolution, legibility, resistance to ambient light, speed, and display capacity. LCDs are used in several portable microcomputers because they require little current and are compatible with battery operation.

Printers

Printers are used to generate hardcopy results for processing, to document programs during and after development, and to generate correspondence in word processing applications. Printers are also used to produce hardcopy graphics (i.e., charts, graphs, drawings, and figures). These uses suggest different (often incompatible) priorities for speed, image quality, and other parameters. Because these and other characteristics are determined by printer technology, it is desirable to summarize the various ways printers place images on paper.

Printer technologies. Alphanumeric shapes are formed for printing in one of two ways: as discrete, fully formed characters (similar to a typewriter), or as matrices of dots (similar to video display controllers—see above). The most common character printers use interchangeable type elements called *daisy wheels* because characters are placed on petal-like projections deployed radially about a hub. *Character printers* place images on paper by causing a particular symbol to strike an inked ribbon, which in turn leaves an inked impresson on paper. Thus, character printers are also *impact printers*. Character printers offer good print quality, but sacrifice speed (10 to 60 characters per second) and the ability to produce graphics.

Dot-matrix printers employ matrices of 5-by-7 to 13-by-18 dots to form characters. Dot patterns for individual characters are remembered in ROM and recalled as needed. Images are placed on paper by one of three major methods. One of these uses inked-ribbon and impact methods similar to character printers. In this case, the dots are actually tiny wires, each activated by a microsolenoid. The wires and solenoids form a "print head" which is moved back and forth across a page. Some dot-matrix impact printers have multiple print heads (matrices) and/or special ribbons to allow color printing. Two other dot-matrix printing methods are nonimpactive in nature. *Thermal printers* use temperature-sensitive paper and dots formed by print head of electric wires. When a current is passed through a given wire, heat is generated and a dark image is left on the paper. A variation of thermal printers uses paper coated with aluminum or other metallic substance, which is oxidized by current passing through the wire elements of the print head. Thus, ink and ribbons are not used for thermal or electrographic printing. A third printing method uses dots that are actually tiny pens, each fed by a separate ink supply. These *ink-jet printers* use special solutions and control systems to activate ink flow from individual dots or pens. A variation of this method uses a single pen and directs ink flow aerodynamically. Some ink-jet systems can produce multicolor output. The major advantages of dot-matrix printers are speed (50 to 600 characters per second) and flexibility.

Paper is moved through a printer by means of a tractor-feed mechanism or a sheet-feed mechanism. *Tractor-feed* systems require paper with perforated edges to accept alignment pins. After printing, the edges are removed by tearing along a finer perforation. Such paper is available in various weights and qualities and is in the form of a long series of single pages, joined by perforations (continuous, Z-fold paper). *Sheet-feed* mechanisms use a friction system like that of a typewriter and are suitable for single sheets of paper (called "cut-sheets"). Printers offer one or both of these feeding systems. Some printers designed mostly for cut-sheet work can accept accessories that automatically insert single sheets of paper, but they are significantly less reliable than tractor-feed systems.

Other printer technologies employ laser techniques to directly or indirectly burn images on paper, electrostatic transfer techniques (such as those used in office copy machines) or line printing (as opposed to character printing) methods to achieve very high quality at very high speeds. Because these printers are quite expensive, they are found only in large computer installations. A final printer type is the teletype (TTY), a slow, noisy character printer equipped with a keyboard and used as a general purpose input–output device. Readers old enough to remember TTYs will understand why they are ignored here. Younger readers can classify them with wood stoves, washboards, and other tools they would just as soon not know too intimately.

Regardless of technology, virtually all printers designed for use with microcomputers contain their own microprocessors and ROM to manage decoding of incoming signals as well as placement and (for dot-matrix printers) formation of characters. Except for a few very inexpensive dot-matrix units, most printers can provide at least 80 columns of characters (across a page). Because printers are mechanical devices with greater inertia than the electronic devices that drive them, most also have RAM buffers to temporarily store incoming information until it can be printed. Among other things, buffers allow printers to output information as the print mechanism moves from right to left, as well as from left to right (i.e., bidirectional printing). Printers contain either parallel or serial interfaces (or both) and require a cable and a compatible interface in the computer that drives them.

Characteristics. Print quality is influenced by the kind of ink used for ribbons (for impact printers), the density of dots (for dot-matrix printers), and the texture and weight of paper used for printing. Except for the least expensive models, character printers (sometimes called *letter-quality* printers) generally produce copy indistinguishable from that produced by a typewriter. Dot-matrix printers exhibit great differences in quality, largely as a function of the number of dots used to form the matrix. A touchstone of quality in dot-matrix printers is the presence of "true descenders" on letters with segments that drop below the line of type when produced by a typewriter (e.g., "p," "q," "g"). Several of the better dot-matrix printers produce typewriter-quality images; some allow selection of printing resolutions—coarse matrix for fast, draft copies and fine matrix for slower, final copies. Ink-jet printers produce excellent quality characters, but cost more than comparable character printers and dot-matrix printers employing other technologies.

Printing speeds range from about 10 characters per second (cps) for the slowest character printers to about 600 cps for the fastest dot-matrix printers. (By comparison, a good typist—90 words per minute, error-free—produces about 7.5 cps.) Generally, as speed increases, quality decreases, even within printing technologies, but the trade-off is far from linear.

Printers also differ in the number of characters that can be stored in the local buffer memory. Because most microcomputers can do only one thing at a time, and because printers are slower than computers, printing operations tend to be inefficient in terms of overall computer use. Large RAM buffers in printers (or in accessory devices installed between the computer and a printer) let the computer finish its output before the printer does, thus freeing the computer for other uses. Most printers contain buffers big enough to hold one line of type; some can hold a full page (about 2 Kbytes). Several companies offer accessory print buffers with up to 0.5 Mbytes of storage and a variety of special features.

Printers differ greatly in flexibility, that is, the ability to print different sizes of type, different character spacing, different type fonts (character sets), and graphics. The quality of graphic images depends upon the density of the printer's dot-matrix system and (in the case of direct "screen-dump" graphics) the resolution of the video display controller. Some dot-matrix printers are able to produce different styles of type. This can be accomplished with alternate character sets stored in printer ROM, or by *downloading* dot-matrix patterns for special fonts from the computer to a special RAM in the printer. Although the type elements of character printers can be changed to provide different fonts, this can become cumbersome if different character sets are required on a single page. With even medium-cost dot-matrix printers, it is possible to invoke several type styles or sizes on a single page by sending control sequences from the computer to the printer (i.e., under program control). Most character printers and dot-matrix printers allow simple selection of character spacing with options including 10 characters per inch (10 pitch or pica) and 12 characters per inch (12 pitch or elite). Most also allow proportional printing in which spacing is controlled by the different widths of individual characters.

A final major technical characteristic of printers is interfacing. The most common (and cheapest) interface is an 8-bit parallel system originally designed by the Centronic Corporation for that firm's printers. This has become a de facto standard in the industry. Another common type of interface is the RS-232C serial asynchronous interface (see below). Printers typically are designed for one or both of these protocols. Some computers are sold with compatible parallel or serial interfaces built into the computer system. Most are not: these require an additional interface (for the computer, not the printer) at additional cost. Most interfaces are "dumb" and relatively transparent to the user; others are designed for particular combinations of computers and printers and contain their own low-level software to optimize special features of the printer.

Printers differ in reliability, size, noise, and the availability of supplies (ribbons and type elements) and replacement parts. Impact printers are noisier than nonimpact printers; character printers tend to be larger than dot-matrix printers. Systematic redesign favoring electronic components has increased the reliability of printers: a moderately priced unit should function trouble free for at least 3 or 4 years. Although printers are not rated as "light duty" or "heavy duty," they differ in life expectancy and heavy use may cause early failure. Local repair services are less common for printers than for typewriters because of the large number of firms that manufacture printers and because designs change frequently. Printer ribbons are not standardized and local availability of the proper ribbon for a particular printer may be problematic if the printer is an uncommon one.

Other characteristics that distinguish printers include the ability to produce different colors (usually at reduced speed and increased cost), the ability to accept wider than normal paper (at increased cost), the ability to produce subscripts and suprascripts (possible with some character printers and some impact dot-matrix printers), the ability to print duplicates of display screen graphics (possible only with properly interfaced dot-matrix units), and the ability to print ditto masters and multiple forms (impact printers only).

Printers range in price from less than $150 for a 40-column, low-resolution, nonimpact printer to more than $4000 for a high-speed, ink-jet printer. Cost is directly related to print quality, speed, and the availability of special features. Interfaces for printers cost as little as $50 and as much as $300.

System Implications

Compatibility. Monochrome receivers, color receivers, and some RGB monitors normally cannot be used with "full" displays of 1920 characters; displays with even fewer characters may be illegible on color receivers because of color fringes on letters and numbers. Most monochrome monitors and the better RGB color monitors provide sufficient resolution for graphics and full text displays. Video displays and display controllers must be compatible in terms of bandwidth, resolution, and the number of electrical signals needed to drive the display.

Printer compatibility is more an issue of software than hardware, assuming reasonable care in matching computer interface, cable, and printer. Software compatibility problems occur because different printers require different special-character command sequences to activate features such as underlining, subscripts, type size, and font changes. Application software designed with printing in mind (e.g., word processing and presentation graphics programs) may or may not take account of variations among printers. Better programs have configuration routines (run once when the software is installed) capable of recognizing specific printers.

Applications limited to text processing and simple graphics are probably best served by nonglare, amber or green monochrome monitors, 12 or 15 inches in size (Wolf, 1983). In these cases, the choice of a printer is largely a function of who will get hardcopy and for what purpose. If low-volume, formal communications with external agents are required, and if no graphics are necessary, a character printer may be best. On the other hand, if large volumes of printed material are needed, and if graphics and special type styles are necessary, a moderate-cost ($500–$2,000) impact dot-matrix printer may be best. If hardcopy is required only for internal use, a low-cost ($200–$600) dot-matrix unit may be sufficient.

Communication devices

Communication devices allow computers and computer terminals to exchange data and other information over small and great distances. The most common communication device is the *MODEM* (MODulator–DEModulator), a system that converts digital information into analog form for transmission along dedicated lines or common carriers such as telephone lines. MODEMs allow individuals to communicate with each other via point-to-point linkages, with mainframe computers in a timesharing mode, with commercial data base services, and with groups of individuals via dial-access "electronic bulletin boards."

MODEM technology

MODEMs accept digitally coded information from a computer (via an asynchronous serial interface—see below) or a computer terminal and convert that information into tone pulses. For a MODEM that originates communication, the binary value 0 (called a "space") is equated to a tone of 1070 Hz and the binary value 1 (called a "mark") becomes 1270 Hz. Thus, the MODEM encodes information by frequency modulation (the space tone serves as a carrier signal). These coded tone pulses are then set over a communication channel to another MODEM. The receiving MODEM decodes (demodulates) the tones, converting them back into binary values. These are sent through another serial interface to the receiving computer. The answering MODEM also can send coded information to the originating MODEM, using 2025 Hz for binary 0 (space) and 2225 Hz for binary 1 (mark). In a system consisting of two MODEMs, four frequencies, and one channel, three communication modes are possible: *simplex*, in which one MODEM does all the "talking" and the other only "listens," half-duplex, in which two MODEMs take turns talking and listening, and *full-duplex*, in which two MODEMs talk and listen simultaneously. Most MODEMs are designed to let the user select either half- or full-duplex modes.

Mark and space frequencies, other technical issues, and most of the terminology of MODEMs were standardized by the Bell Telephone System at a time when only Bell equipment could be connected to telephone lines. Although this policy has changed, MODEMs using telephone lines as communication channels still conform to one of the Bell standards (103, 203, 212).

MODEMs can be connected to telephone systems acoustically (in which case an acoustic coupler is required for the telephone handset) or electronically (in which case the MODEM is plugged into a telephone base unit with a four-conductor modular plug). They are available as stand-alone units, or as separate circuit boards designed for specific computers.

An entirely different category of MODEMs exists to provide access to communication lines independent of voice-grade telephone systems. These communication systems include *baseband* and *broadband* networks organized for private use as "local area networks" (LANs). They are capable of extremely high-speed data transmission (millions of bits per second) and require MODEMs very different from those described here.

Characteristics

Speed. MODEMs send and receive information as a series of bits. A letter, for example, might be represented as a start bit, followed by eight data bits, followed by a stop bit (additional bits, called "parity" bits, may or may not be used to check the integrity of signals sent from one place to another). Thus, about 10 bits are required for a single character. Transmission speeds are expressed in bits per second, colloquially referred to as "baud" rate. The most common baud rates are 110, 300, 1200, and 2400 bits per second, or 11, 30, 120, and 240 characters per second, respectively. Acoustically coupled systems usually do not operate reliably at rates above 300 baud. Specially conditioned telephone lines or dedicated lines are required for transmission rates above 1200 baud.

Compatibility. The ideal MODEM is totally transparent to the user; it also does not exist. Originate or "calling" MODEMs must have the same baud rate as the answer MODEM they communicate with. Some (not all) MODEMs capable of acting as answer units can automatically sense the baud rate of calling MODEMs and adjust themselves accordingly (as long as the baud rate of the originating unit does not exceed their own). Daughter board MODEMs designed to be plugged into computers usually contain their own interfaces. Stand-alone units normally do not. For these, signal and connector compatibility with interfaces become important and (because technical standards are unclear—see Witten, 1983) occasionally problematic. Finally, MODEMs require specialized software programs called "communication packages." Some MODEMs and some communication packages are incompatible.

Other features. Some directly coupled MODEMs are capable of automatically dialing telephone numbers entered at a computer keyboard. Most of these accommodate both touch-tone and pulse-code dialing protocols. All MODEMs act as originate devices; a few also act as answer units, automatically responding to incoming calls. Some "smart" MODEMs contain (or can be interfaced with) real-time clocks to automatically dial a number, exchange logging information with another computer, transmit and/or receive information, and disconnect (Durham, 1983).

Cost. Some integrated microcomputer systems contain MODEMs and associated communication firmware (software in ROM). Simple acoustically coupled MODEMs without serial interfaces or software are available for less than $200. Stand-alone, direct-connect units range from $250 to $400. Add-in MODEMs with their own serial interfaces are somewhat more expensive.

System implications

Successful use of a MODEM depends in large part upon the quality of the telephone line it is used with. Noise (acoustical or electrical) can interfere with communication. Therefore, the telephone lines used with MODEMs should be single-phone types without extension sets or local intercoms. Long distance communication is not difficult if a moderate transmission speed is used.

Inter-MODEM compatibility and efficiency in communication suggest that a 300-baud MODEM will be suitable in most cases. It is recommended that communication software and any necessary cables or interfaces be acquired at the same time (and from the same source) as a MODEM in order to avoid problems of hardware and software incompatibility.

Real-time clocks

Although CPUs contain a system clock to synchronize computer operations, that clock cannot easily be used to monitor, oversee, or manage events that occur at real-world rates. *Real-time clocks* (RTCs) are peripherals that can make human calendar and time-of-day information available to computer programs. In addition, they can be used to "time stamp" program and data files stored in secondary memory, measure the durations of external events, and cause programmed actions at predetermined times.

RTCs can be part of an integrated computer system, a plug-in peripheral, a single-function external peripheral, or part of some other peripheral (e.g., a MODEM or speech synthesizer). Most contain batteries (recharged when the parent system is turned on) that keep the clock "ticking" and ROMs which manage the vagaries of months with different numbers of days, leap years, and military time (2400 hours per day).

Characteristics

Resolution. RTCs are based upon high-speed timing crystals and are very accurate (e.g., within 1 minute per month as long as power is available). Most display time in units as small as 1 second, some in milliseconds. Single-second resolution is sufficient for many applications, but not for measuring reaction time or controlling peripheral laboratory equipment (Goldband, 1979).

Compatibility. "Bundled" RTCs (those designed as part of a computer system) seldom present problems for other hardware or for system software. Add-in units sometimes employ interrupt signals that may create problems for some application programs. Add-on RTCs are usually supplied with sample programs that demonstrate their use in common applications and suggest ways users can incorporate RTC functions into their own programs. Obviously, this requires some programming skill.

Cost. Separate add-on RCTs are available for most open-bus computers for less than $200.

INTERFACES

As mentioned previously, interfaces are devices through which computers communicate with other machines. They differ from internal communication buses in that interfaces "talk to" devices located apart from the computer itself. Such devices include printers, computer terminals, MODEMs, and a host of specialized machines.

Classes of Interfaces

Parallel

Interfaces can be classified in terms of how many channels carry information from one point to another and how information is deployed across those channels. Internal communication buses use parallel communication in which 8 wires (usually) are reserved for data, rather like a one-way highway, 8 lanes wide. The digital pattern for a letter or number can be transmitted by sending a byte down the highway, such that one lane is reserved for each bit. The bits start their journeys the same time and successive bytes are "launched" at predetermined intervals (i.e., they are synchronized). A few additional wires are used for timing and control purposes. Parallel interfaces are organized in exactly this manner, but they differ from internal communication buses in the voltages used to represent binary zeros and ones and in speed of data transmission. Parallel interfaces can be made to operate at very high speeds (a major advantage), but they require several channels or wires (a major disadvantage). Because they are susceptible to electrical noise, they work well only over a few meters. Normally, parallel interfaces are simplex systems, supporting one-way communication, to a computer from a peripheral, or vice versa.

Serial

Serial interfaces are generally slower than parallel interfaces, but are more immune to noise and work well over longer distances (many meters). Instead of a one-way, 8-lane highway, serial interfaces are somewhat like a two-way, 2-lane street. Data are sent in packets of pulses, one pulse after another, down one lane of the "street." Each packet consists of a "start" bit, 7 or 8 data bits, and none, 1, or 2 "stop" bits. The start and stop bits bracket the data bits; as long as the intervals between these bits and the data bits are consistent, successive packets can be sent at random (asynchronous) intervals. Synchronous serial communication is also possible, but is limited to circumstances that exclude people as direct information sources. With a "2-lane street," data can be sent in both directions simultaneously. As noted in the discussion of MODEMs, the lanes might actually be different pairs of tones for sender and receiver, rather than different wires. Thus, serial interfaces offer the advantage of requiring only a single channel (one wire for signal, one for ground).

But if internal communication buses (where all of this must converge) are inherently parallel in structure, how can a serial signal ever get started? Parallel-to-serial and serial-to-parallel conversions are accomplished with specialized ICs called "universal asynchronous receiver-transmitters" (UARTs). During transmission, the sole task of this circuit is to capture and store a parallel byte of data, then dump that byte, one bit at a time, starting with the most significant bit (the one with the largest number value) and ending with the least significant bit. The reverse happens during reception (see Artwick, 1980).

Standards For Interfaces

The RS-232C interface

Serial transmission protocols (both synchronous and asynchronous) are standardized by RS-232C, a standard originally issued by the Electronics Industry Association (EIA) several decades ago. It is now the most commonly used scheme for connecting computers to other devices. The RS-232C standard specifies electrical signal characteristics, plug and socket dimensions, signal functions, and subsets of signals for particular types of serial interfaces (Witten, 1983). Signal functions are assigned to specific connector pins and include data lines (transmit and receive), grounds, and "handshaking" signals such as "request-to-send," "clear-to-send," and others.

This standard supports several discrete transmission speeds between 50 and 19,200 bits per second, including those of 110, 300, 1200, and 2400 baud common to MODEMs. A format for data is defined (start bit, data bits, stop bits) and the durations of bits and spaces between bits are specified.

RS-232C also defines two types of devices supported by the standard: *data terminal equipment* (DTE) and *data communication equipment* (DCE). The former is represented by computer terminals, the latter by MODEMs. The standard assumes the following communication system: a computer terminal (DTE) gets information from a person or a computer and sends it to a MODEM or other DCE. (The MODEM then sends the information to another MODEM via a single-channel network, but RS-232C is not particularly concerned with details of MODEM–MODEM communication.) Information received by a DCE over a single-channel line is then sent to another terminal (DTE). Thus, the standard focuses on how to pass information back and forth between terminals and communication equipment.

Signal functions assigned to individual pins of connectors are different for DTEs and DCEs. Therein lies a serious source of confusion and incompatibility among modern microcomputers and supporting devices that use serial protocols nominally compatible with the EIA standard. The problem has several aspects. First, RS-232C was designed assuming communication between DTEs and DCEs, not between two DTEs or between two DCEs. Second, the standard was intended to support point-to-point communication of digital signals over single-channel analog lines such as telephone lines, not quite the same as (for example) a microcomputer sending information to a printer, a speech synthesizer, or both at the same time. Third, although the standard specifies 25 pins (electrical connections) and signal functions for DTE–DCE and DCE–DTE communication, most signals are not mandatory. Some are downright obscure. Finally, the flexibility of contemporary hardware sometimes blurs the distinction between DTEs and DCEs in ways that could not have been anticipated when RS-232C was drafted. As a result, it may be difficult to determine whether an interface or other device is configured as a DTE or a DCE (the choice is arbitrary) and what should be done with data and control wires (one machine's transmit line is another's receive line). Leibson (1982d), Ciarcia (1983), and Witten (1983) provide cogent explanations of the RS-232C dilemma and solutions to the problems attendant upon this standard.

The IEEE-488 (HPIB) interface

As the technology of integrated circuits made digital processing easier, communication capabilities were added to electronic devices unknown at the time RS-232C was conceived. Many of these were signal generating, measurement, and analysis instruments used in laboratories or factories, environments that often require interconnection of several instruments to accomplish control or measurement. It became obvious that serial interface methods were ill-suited to such tasks. Hewlett–Packard Corporation developed a parallel interfacing scheme in 1972 that permitted data and control signal communication between a computer and as many as 16 peripheral devices, all on a single bus. This interface not only allowed instruments to talk to computers (and vice-versa), but it also let the instruments on the bus talk to each other. This scheme became known as the *HPIB* (Hewlett–Packard interface bus) or the GPIB (general purpose interface bus) and was formally standardized by the IEEE in 1978 as *IEEE-488*. Several other firms have adopted this interface scheme, and although it is not as widely used as RS-232C, it is far superior to the serial interface in applications limited to local communication. It is used with common peripherals (e.g., printers, plotters, graphic tablets) and laboratory equipment, and is standard or available as an add-in circuit board for many microcomputers.

This standard specifies a 16-conductor cable and assigns signal names and functions to connector pins. Several instruments can be connected to each other in a daisy-chain manner (i.e., in parallel). Each instrument on the bus can be assigned the role of "talker," "listener," or "controller." A given device can be both a "talker" and a "listener," but only one can serve as a "controller" at one time. Because an instrument may begin "talking" at any time, IEEE-488 is an asynchronous system. Each device on the bus is assigned an address, and data can be passed from one to another as directed by the controlling device. The controller is usually a microcomputer running an application program written to supervise movement of information from one instrument or peripheral to another.

The IEEE-488 standard reserves 8 lines for data, 3 for data control, and 5 for general management of the bus. It has the advantages of high speed, excellent noise immunity, and operational simplicity approaching transparency (Leibson, 1982c).

Parallel interfaces

Aside from IEEE-488, no formal standards exist for general purpose parallel interfaces (Artwick, 1980). A de facto standard, based upon the Centronic Corporation printer interface, has emerged for connecting computers to output devices. This scheme uses a 36-pin connector, 8 lines for data, and several lines for handshaking signals, grounds, and power. It is used primarily with general and special purpose output devices.

Other proprietary parallel interfaces exist to convert internal communication bus signals for use by output or input devices "outboard" from the computer. Most of these are of no real significance because they are dedicated to specific peripherals and, hence, transparent to both the host computer and the user.

System implications

If a computer system is limited to a small number of general purpose peripherals, the whole issue of interfaces and interfacing may become moot.

Selecting an interface system can be important, however, if different peripheral devices are to be used with a computer on a "part-time" or "shared-resource" basis, and if there are reasons to minimize unnecessary interface boards (e.g., to limit costs, reduce heat inside the computer, keep space free for other subsystems, or simplify programming).

Interface compatibility problems are exceedingly common, at least with respect to serial interfaces. Solutions to these problems are not difficult (they often involve reversing wires in cables), but they can be time consuming and frustrating. One way to avoid interface difficulties is to buy bundled systems in which everything is supplied by one manufacturer. This works, but may be expensive and may unnecessarily limit the functions of a computer system. A more reasonable approach is to insist that vendors who supply and configure add-on cables and devices meet a performance criterion before they are paid for their services. A third approach is to "cut and try," preferably with help from a "breakout box" such as that described by Ciarcia (1983).

SPECIAL PURPOSE DEVICES

Special tasks, special data, and special users

Keyboards, video monitors, printers, and general communication devices are sufficient for most computer applications involving entry and display of alphanumeric characters. Not all tasks or data are compatible with this relatively simple form of information, however. Many of the data to be manipulated by computer are inherently graphical (e.g., audiograms, tympanograms), or are tied to real-world analog events (e.g., acoustic, aerodynamic, electromyographic, or movement signals associated with speech production), or occur at times and rates determined by factors independent of any computer. Some forms of "presenting" information are far simpler—whether a listener did or did not hear a signal, which of four alternatives a child selected in a picture vocabulary test, whether a vocal response occurred within a particular time interval, and so forth. Similarly, the results of some computations are graphical, while others are in the form of control signals which operate reinforcement devices, electronic switches, signal attenuators, tape recorders, or other peripheral devices. Still other special purpose output signals include tones, tonal patterns, speech signals, and other auditory stimuli.

Some users are special, too. Most obvious among these are motorically impaired, nonvocal persons for whom computers (and related gear) may augment communication. Perhaps less obvious are those with grossly normal neuromotor function, but with temporary or chronic dysfunction of laryngeal or articulatory systems, or with language problems related to head trauma or stroke. Even less obvious as special users are young language-delayed or language-distorted children who are physically and mentally intact, but who cannot easily operate keyboards and other devices designed for trained typists and persons with mature perceptual-motor skills. Finally, developmental research with highly specialized sensory aids (e.g., cochlear implants, tactual stimulation systems) which require extensive machine processing of signals to supplement deficient decoding capacities (organic and otherwise) suggest entirely new subsystems of computer output devices.

A few specialized control (input) devices have been noted above. Although it is not possible to discuss all current or potential specialized input and output devices, it will be useful to note the major categories of each. Chapter 8 discusses several of these in the context of research applications.

Input devices

Switch closures

A switch is an extremely simple (but powerful) way to send binary information to a computer. Switches vary in configuration (numbers of contacts and positions) and in mechanism (direct vs. indirect activation; momentary vs. nonmomentary operation; mechanical vs. electronic; solid contact vs. liquid- -mercury- -contact), but usually involve physical movement of an electrical contact called a *rotor* relative to a fixed-position contact called a *stator*. When contact occurs, a signal is present. Switches can be arranged in arrays of one, two, or more dimensions. Information capacity is limited only by the imagination of the user and the number of switch channels available to the user.

Switch inputs can be interfaced to open-bus computers with little effort and often are provided as part of general purpose "game" manipulanda. They should be electrically isolated from computer circuitry to prevent damage to computer components. Gordon, Foree, and Eckerman (1983) and Poltrock and Foltz (1983) describe simple switch inputs as part of more extensive interface systems; Schwejda and Vanderheiden (1982) present a design for a "smart" input switch system for use by persons with limited motor skills.

Game paddles, joysticks, and trackballs

Intended primarily for gaming applications, these devices are essentially low-resolution position sensors. Game paddles (so called because they were first used with a video game that simulated table tennis) are simply potentiometers wired as voltage dividers: as the position of a rotor is varied, the voltage drop between the rotor and a stator varies. This voltage is digitized and periodically updated as required by an associated program. Joysticks and trackballs use similar methods, but with two channels of information (i.e., two independent potentiometers) instead of only one. Commercial devices of this type are usually combined with two or more switch inputs.

Joysticks and related controls differ in resolution, linearity, reliability, and (of course) cost. Many microcomputers are designed to accept game paddles and joysticks, but because digitizing circuits and connectors differ, most are not interchangeable. Although game controls are easy to incorporate into programs, they are typically nonlinear (equal intervals of displacement do not produce equal intervals of digitized output) and of limited resolution (e.g., one part in 256). Joysticks, game paddles, and trackballs for microcomputers are available at prices ranging from about $35 to $150. Higher precision systems designed for military, industrial, and scientific applications typically cost 10 times as much. These employ encoding techniques (often optical) offering greater resolution and mechanical components selected for use in adverse environments.

Graphic tablets

Graphic tablets are two-dimensional position sensors designed to allow entry of free-hand drawings or traced images. Although a variety of resistive, capacitive, and sonic sensing methods are used with different brands of tablets, most employ a nondrawing stylus which is moved across a flat surface. The surface is calibrated in units of length, and the position of the stylus is digitized as isolated pairs of X-Y coordinates, or as a continuous "stream" of points. Coordinate data can be stored and processed as numerical arrays, or stored and displayed as video images. More sophisticated graphic tablets are supported by software routines which facilitate construction of simple geometric shapes (rectangles, circles, squares) and compute distances between points, lengths of irregular curves, and areas of regular and irregular shapes. At least one graphic "tablet" is capable of digitizing positional information in three dimensions.

These features make possible a variety of applications involving printed, plotted, or projected images generated by any of dozens of analog methods. Examples include quantification of speech spectrographs, oscillographic records of waveforms, results of Bekesy-type audiometry, and measurement of articulatory dynamics as captured in fiberoptic or cinefluorographic studies.

Graphic tablets designed for small computers vary in resolution, surface area, and the sophistication of support software. Costs range between $500 and $2500.

Speech recognition systems

Speech recognition has the ultimate goal of machine understanding of the oral discourse of people (see Levinson & Liberman, 1981; Flanagan, 1981b). That goal is years away because of problems associated with the variabilities among speakers and the complexities of language, but limited-capability systems are available that offer interesting possibilities.

Characteristics. Microcomputer-based speech recognition (more precisely, word identification) systems are based on the idea of template matching. An individual talker first "trains" a system by repeating a particular utterance several times. Each utterance is analyzed by some relatively simple procedure (e.g., filtering the signal into high and low frequency components, then counting the zero amplitude crossings in each component as a function of time). The resulting data are combined to produce a single target template for that utterance. The template conveys information about variability as well as central tendency across training utterances. Target templates are generated for some number of words. Subsequently, when a talker utters a sample word to be recognized, the pattern of that word is compared to each of the target templates available to the system. A measure of distance is computed for each comparison. Assuming that at least one distance measure is small enough to satisfy "minimum match" rules, the system identifies ("recognizes") the new word as being "the same" as that associated with the target template yielding the smallest distance measure.

The comparison just described is a *direct* comparison between target and sample patterns. A *dynamic* comparison approach employs time warping of the target template to accommodate differences in speaking rate between target and sample utterances (Levinson & Liberman, 1981).

These approaches are fairly successful in identifying moderate numbers of words produced by a single talker. If several talkers contribute to target templates, performance deteriorates rapidly because of increased template variance associated with vocal tract differences. Depending upon analysis and comparison strategies, performance also decreases as the number of targets increases. Large computers can manage these problems because they are relatively fast and because large blocks of memory can be made available for target templates. Multiple talkers can be accommodated by using talker-identification procedures that do not involve speech.

Word identification systems for microcomputers are limited to relatively small recognition vocabularies (32-128 words) and performance on the order of 90% correct. Improvements in signal analysis algorithms (target "construction") and sample-target comparison methods may make it possible to use these devices in articulation and voice therapy, and in "measuring" the oral responses of subjects tested by speech audiometry.

Costs. Prices for microcomputer speech recognition subsystems begin at about $300.

Analog-to-digital converters

Position sensors, graphic tablets, speech recognizers, and some touch sensors are all examples of systems which convert analog (continuously variable) signals into digital (discretely variable) signals. More generally, analog-to-digital converters (ADCs) can be used to translate signals or events originally expressed as graded voltages or currents into digital signals.

Characteristics. ADCs are available as separate modular devices, as components of integrated data acquisition systems, and (in very limited versions) as game manipulanda. They can be used with virtually any signal that can be represented with a voltage (e.g., intraoral air pressure, nasal air flow, jaw position, heart rate, blood pressure, body temperature, galvanic skin response, electromyologic signals, or acoustical events). Application of ADC methods in any given situation depends largely upon characteristics of the signal to be converted (amplitude, dynamic range, temporal characteristics, and spectrum) and the processing to be done on the digital version of the signal. An analog voltage produced by some physical event is preamplified (to isolate the signal from its source), low-pass filtered (to eliminate high-frequency noise), amplitude weighted (to minimize conversion errors), and then sampled at some speed or rate. The sampled voltage is momentarily held, then converted to a binary-coded number (see Kamm, Carterette, Morgan, & Dirks, 1980). All of these operations are performed by the ADC under control of a computer. ADCs "built into" microcomputers are usually managed by the central processing unit of the computer; separate, modular ADCs are often controlled by dedicated, high-speed central processors. In either case, the quantized version of the signal is placed in a buffer memory, from which it can be sent (via an interface) to the primary memory of a computer for processing.

Several different methods are used to accomplish the actual conversion from analog signal to numeric representation (counting, integration, successive approximation, parallel comparators). The benefits and limitations of these are discussed by Artwick (1980), Goldsbrough, Lund, and Rayner (1983), and others. Regardless of conversion technology, the factors of sampling speed, dynamic range, signal-to-noise ratio, resolution, linearity, and accuracy determine the quality and utility of ADCs.

Sampling rate is determined by the signal to be converted and by the performance of the ADC itself. Sampling theory suggests that in order to maintain accuracy in the frequency domain, a signal must be sampled at a rate at least two times the highest frequency component of interest in the signal (assuming components above this frequency have been eliminated via filtering). Thus, to retain information up to 5 kHz in a speech signal, we must low-pass filter the signal at 5 kHz, then sample the filtered signal at a rate of 10 kHz or more. ADC systems currently available for use with microcomputers operate at sampling speeds ranging from 100 to 200,000

Hz (slower systems are more common); most allow sampling of 2, 4, or 16 channels of analog data. When several channels are used simultaneously, reduction in sampling speed (per channel) is necessary.

The dynamic range, resolution, and signal-to-noise ratio of an ADC system vary as a function of the number bits in the digital output of the converter. An 8-bit system has an inherent resolution of 1 part in 256 (0.39%) and a dynamic range of about 48 dB; a 10-bit system has a best-case resolution of 1 part in 1024 (0.1%) and a dynamic range of about 60 dB; a 16-bit system has a resolution of 1 part in 65,536 (0.002%) and a dynamic range of about 96 dB. Commercially available ADCs are commonly designed as 8-, 10-, or 12-bit systems.

ADC systems offer several advantages not possible with analog equipment, especially in applications involving acoustical or physiological signals. First, systems with 10-bit (or more) resolution are capable of better signal-to-noise ratios than even the best audio and instrumentation recorders. Second, because the output of ADCs is in numerical form, the quantitative description and manipulation of data is facilitated. Third, because ADC systems can be operated under computer control, acquisition, processing, and display of data can be managed conditionally, that is, in ways that vary as a function of the state of a process or the values of the converted data. This disadvantages of ADCs and ADC systems are related largely to the need for software support and issues of compatibility.

Compatibility. Successful use of ADCs depends very much upon compatibility with hardware, software, and the signals to be converted. A major hardware compatibility issue relates to the primary memory capacity of the host computer. Sampling rates greater than 5000 Hz and observation intervals greater than a few seconds can easily outstrip the capacity of 8-bit and 16-bit microcomputers with minimum memory, even with single-channel data. Higher resolution ADCs (12- and 16-bits) fill memory twice as fast as 8-bit converters. Chapter 8 discusses alternatives for dealing with the problems peculiar to the use of ADCs with microcomputers.

Some add-on ADC systems are provided with extensive utility software, but most require significant programming to manage the data acquisition and processing needs of particular applications. High-speed ADC data acquisition may not be compatible with relatively slow, interpreter-oriented computer languages such as BASIC. In such cases, it may be necessary to write specialized "driver" programs in low-level assembly language and/or resort to more complex compiler-oriented languages such as FORTH and FORTRAN.

Costs. Costs of ADC systems range from a few hundred dollars for slow, low-resolution "board-level" devices to over $10,000 for fast, high-resolution peripheral systems.

Output devices

Lamps and relays

Lamps, relays, and kindred devices are essentially reciprocals of input switches. Instead of sending single-bit information to a microcomputer, they output such information. They are most often used to signal discrete events, to convey limited information through patterns of discrete events, or to control external devices such as modular stimulus programming gear (e.g., attenuators, electronic switches, audio mixers, token reinforcement dispensers) and tape recorders capable of electronic (rather than mechanical) function selection.

Characteristics. Most microcomputers contain (or can support) at least a few channels of single-bit outputs accessible to the user under programmed control. These are often called "annunciator" outputs. Optional peripheral systems are available which allow more channels of discrete (single-bit) digital output, from 8 to 16, 32, or 64 bits. These are often combined with analog-to-digital and digital-to-analog subsystems to form integrated sensing and control systems for industrial and laboratory applications. In most cases, binary outputs are designed for low-current, low-voltage operation and must be electronically buffered (isolated) from external devices. This can be accomplished with solid state or low-power electromechanical relays, or with optical isolation systems (sealed pairs of light-emitting and light-sensing diodes which send information by light transmission rather than electron flow). Some systems designed to support microcomputer control of home appliances (including on–off operation of machines powered by house current) use ultrasonic isolation and relays to switch electrical power, or place control signals on the wires which carry electricity to fixtures and wall sockets. A special receiver (decoder) is necessary for each device to be controlled.

Compatibility. Complex control or signal operations based upon discrete digital outputs may present problems of speed, programming complexity, and compatibility. Simple operations involving eight or less channels of binary output are far more tractable, in terms of both hardware and software.

Costs. Add-on (or add-in) systems of this sort range in price from less than $50 to several thousand dollars. More expensive systems vary in cost as a function of isolation methods, number of discrete channels, and compatibility with other sensing and output options.

Print spoolers and buffers
   Microcomputers can output data much faster than mechanical peripherals such as printers and plotters can accept them. Interfaces gate the flow of data to peripherals, but essentially force the entire system to operate at the speed of the slowest single component device. Print buffers (or spoolers) are supplemental memory systems interposed between a microcomputer and an output peripheral to solve this problem. Because they are RAM-based FIFO devices, they can absorb data at microcomputer speeds (fast), then output the data at peripheral speeds (slow). In this manner, print buffers can free single-task computers for other work while the buffer drives the printer.
   Most print spoolers are stand-alone systems with their own internal power supplies. They vary in capacity from 8 Kbytes to 128 Kbytes or more. Some offer several combinations of input and output interfaces, but most employ simple parallel disciplines. Certain "smart" buffers accept data in marked segments which may be reordered via control commands from the microcomputer. Most buffers allow the user to load the buffer once, then output the contents of memory as many times as desired. Prices begin at about $200 and increase by about $100 for each 64 Kbyte increment in memory.

Speech synthesis systems
   Speech synthesizers are of special interest to specialists in communication disorders because they represent engineering implementations of the accumulated knowledge base in acoustical and physiological phonetics, because they provide practical tests of the linguistic rules thought to link written language to spoken discourse, and because they can be used therapeutically with individuals who would otherwise remain nonvocal. The reader may wish to consult Flanagan (1981a), Hansen (1982), Milich (1982), and Munro (1982) for nontechnical summaries of speech synthesis technologies and specific products. Carter (1983) and Sclater (1983) offer "pop-tech" treatments of the subject. Flanagan (1972), Rabiner and Schafer (1978), and Witten (1982) give comprehensive scientific and engineering reviews.

Characteristics. Contemporary synthesis systems compatible with microcomputers vary in synthesis technology, size and flexibility of vocabulary, ease of use, intelligibility, quality, and other respects. Some are available as integral subsystems of microcomputers (e.g., the Acorn computer); others are optional plug-in boards for particular computers. Several are configured for interconnection with virtually any computer via parallel or serial interfaces. Still others are designed as stand-alone devices for clinical applications. Synthesizers intended strictly for use as voice-output communication aids (VOCAs) employ the same technologies and often the same integrated circuits as more generic units. For this reason, and because dedicated devices do not illustrate the variety of the engineering arts, what follows will be limited to synthesizers as peripherals of microcomputers.

Speech synthesizers allow control at the level of phrases, words, or individual speech sounds. Many employ "firmware" programs to translate textual material into speech. Some also employ programs which add prosody (primarily pitch changes) based upon the punctuation normally found in written language. Elovitz, Johnson, McHugh, and Shore (1976) report a text-to-speech algorithm upon which most subsequent work is based. Allen (1981) discusses the problems and potentials of such routines. McHugh (1976), Nakatani and Schaffer (1978), Pierrehumbert (1981), and Hertz (1982) report attempts to develop and evaluate prosody (intonation and stress) algorithms.

Speech synthesis technology. Three technologies (with variations) are in common use: pulse code modulation (PCM), linear predictive coding (LPC), and formant coding (FC). Developments in speech synthesis have been guided by the design goals of high intelligibility and quality (including distinguishing one "talker" from others) and low data transmission rates and data storage requirements.

PCM synthesis is essentially digital recording and reproduction of the speech wave with little effort to optimize transmission rates or storage. Recording is accomplished via analog-to-digital conversion (see above) and reproduction is effected by digital-to-analog conversion (see below). The unit of synthesis is the arbitrary duration required for any particular utterance. Subject to memory limitations, any desired phrases or words can be recorded, but only a very limited number of utterances can be available for reproduction at any one time. To obtain intelligibility comparable to analog recording methods (i.e., a bandwidth of 6 kHz and dynamic range of at least 45 dB) it is necessary to digitize the signal at 12 kHz with an 8-bit ADC. This gives a data transmission rate of 96,000 bits per second (bps). Assuming an 8-bit (memory width) computer with 64 Kbytes of memory available for speech data, no more than about 5 seconds of speech can be retained at one time. Thus, PCM places stringent demands on transmission rates and storage. Although PCM can provide excellent fidelity, it ignores redundancies in the speech wave that could increase efficiency. (Adaptive differential pulse code modulation offers significant improvements in transmission speed and memory use. See Carter (1983).

LPC synthesis (Atal & Hanauer, 1971; Rabiner & Schafer, 1978) increases efficiency by abstracting parameters of vocal tract physiology such as sound source (e.g., laryngeal source vs. frication source), amplitude, and filter properties of the tract. Parameters are derived from analysis of speech produced by a particular talker, or from analysis of the utterances of many talkers. Vocal tract parameters are modeled mathematically as a function of time. Thus, LPC synthesis is actually synthesis by analysis.

The unit of analysis (and subsequently of storage and retrieval) may be the word, the phoneme, or the frame. *Frames* are ordered sequences of LPC parameters similar to the individual images of a moving picture. Frame data can be stored in ROM, RAM, or secondary memory for later synthesis. From a few dozen to several thousand words may be accommodated, depending upon available memory. One widely used synthesis circuit, the Texas Instruments 5220, controls a total of 13 parameters with about 50 bits. Ten parameters refer to filters analogous to the vocal tract; the rest deal with amplitude change and sound sources. Frames are updated 40 times a second. For 50 bits of data (nearly seven 8-bit bytes or 56 bits) and a frame rate of 40 Hz, this LPC system yields a data transmission rate of 2240 bps. For an 8-bit computer, each second of speech requires 280 bytes. With 64 Kbytes of available memory, synthesizers of this type can store about 225 seconds of speech. LPC systems offer fair to excellent fidelity, as well as transmission rates and data storage requirements much better (less) than PCM.

Still further economies are possible with formant coding (FC) techniques. Here, synthesis involves idealized mathematical analogs of individual phonemes and allophones. Unlike LPC synthesis, the FC approach does not simulate any particular talker. The unit of synthesis is the phoneme, rather than an arbitrary chunk of time or a frame of parameter values. Thus FC synthesis can support unlimited vocabularies. The most common FC synthesizer is the Votrax SC01 integrated circuit (see Fons & Gargagliano, 1981). This chip can produce 64 phones and allophones and requires 8–12 bits (i.e., between one and two 8-bit bytes) of control information: 6 bits select a speech sound, 3 select pitch, 1 controls amplitude, and 2 control rate. Assuming a phoneme rate of 5 per second and 2 bytes of control data per phoneme, FC synthesis requires 80 bps (ten 8-bit bytes per second of speech). A microcomputer with 64 Kbytes of "speech" memory could accommodate up to 6400 seconds of speech. In terms of transmission rates and memory efficiency, FC systems are an order of magnitude better than LPC systems and two orders of magnitude better than PCM systems. Formant coding is the most flexible speech synthesis method now available for microcomputers, but it offers poorer intelligibility than moderate-speed PCM or talker-specific LPC methods.

In summary, current speech synthesis technologies trade fidelity for capacity and data transmission speed. Systems featuring unlimited vocabularies typically offer less intelligibility than those with finite vocabularies.

Compatibility. The major compatibility issues of speech synthesizers relate to speech quality and intelligibility, in other words, compatibility with people, rather than with hardware or software. Much of the motivation for speech synthesis derives from military and industrial applications in which the problem of limited intelligibility can be compensated by listener training, constrained vocabularies, signal repetition, or the use of linguistic redundancy in message design. These constraints are acceptable in some circumstances, but where there is interest in supporting less structured communication, such accommodations are impractical and actually may be undesirable. The problem is complicated by the effects of variations in acoustical environments, the auditory abilities of users and listeners, the emerging language skills of users, and probable interactions between signal factors and message factors.

Formal evaluations of synthesized speech intelligibility often use assessment models, materials, and listeners more appropriate to the measurement of transmission lines (see Voiers, 1983), than to gauging the amounts, rates, or types of language interaction, or the efficiency of communication. These and other issues should be addressed relative to the use of speech synthesizers as VOCAs.

Costs. Assembled speech synthesizers for small computers range in price from one hundred to several thousand dollars, depending upon technology and performance factors. More expensive units offer more flexibility or better intelligibility, but not necessarily both.

Sound effects and music

Most microcomputers contain at least minimal sound generation capability, usually for gaming or musical applications. These vary in frequency range, amplitude range, the ability to control amplitude dynamics (attack, sustain, decay envelopes), numbers of channels (voices), and the ability to control the spectrum of individual channels. Most such systems cannot produce sinusoidal signals and offer very limited dynamic ranges. Therefore, they are ill-suited to routine audiometric applications. They may, however, prove useful in generating tonal patterns for studies of auditory perception and in producing audible reinforcers for therapy drillwork.

Optional sound effect and music subsystems range from simple pulse generators ($25 or less) to highly sophisticated musical instruments equipped with full piano keyboards and foot controls ($1500 and up). More expensive systems are accompanied by software capable of performing music from scores and generating printed musical scores from real-time performances (keyboard entry).

Digital-to-analog converters

Sound effect generators and speech synthesizers are special cases of digital-to-analog converters (DACs), devices which generally perform an operation opposite of that accomplished by analog-to-digital converters (ADCs). The issues raised above about ADC sampling speed, dynamic range, resolution, and signal-to-noise ratio apply also to DACs.

Characteristics. DACs are usually configurations of precision resistors or transistors, the outputs of which can be turned on and off by control bits. These outputs are summed, amplified, low-pass filtered, and amplified again to accomplish some task. Resolution, dynamic range, and signal-to-noise ratio are determined by the number of control bits and the number of resistors or transistors that contribute to the summed signal. One or two channel configurations with 8, 10, 12, or 16 bits of signal control are common. The information presented to a DAC for conversion is a sequence of numbers representing discrete, instantaneous amplitudes and a command which controls the rate at which the sequence of numbers is to be converted. In other words, the input to a DAC is a sampled, discrete-data approximation of a continuous signal.

General purpose DACs can be used to control analog plotters, voltage-controlled analog signal generators, some motors, and a host of other devices. Although general purpose DACs also can be programmed to directly generate tones, tonal patterns, speech, and other complex acoustical signals, dedicated devices based upon DAC technology are inevitable easier to use. Subsystems now available for microcomputers include arbitrary waveform generators, digital oscilloscopes (which obviously include ADCs), and digital function generators capable of producing waves of various shapes (sine, square, triangular, ramps), with or without modulation in the amplitude and frequency domains. Digital function generators offer the advantages of starting and stopping a wave at any point in its cycle and of controlling the duration and/or the number of cycles of an output signal.

Costs. DAC subsystems of more general sensing and control systems are priced starting from a few hundred dollars. Dedicated waveform and function generators start at about a thousand dollars. Prices increase with the number of data control bits and the number of output channels.

IMPLICATIONS FOR COMMUNICATION DISORDERS

This chapter began by describing computers as information processors. What are the implications of contemporary microcomputer hardware for the types and amounts of information and of information processes important to communication disorders?

Computers can store incredible amounts of data, but not infinite amounts. They can process those data with incredible speed, but not if the data fail to conform to some consistent structure. To take advantage of such benefits it is necessary to prioritize information, keeping that which can be used and discarding that which makes no difference. It is necessary to collect and organize information in rigorously consistent ways. It is necessary, also, to become more explicit about the criteria used to classify and categorize behaviors and to better understand the covert reasoning underpinning the best of clinical intuition.

From another perspective, the disciplines of communication disorders have both the expertise and the obligation to generate information about the effectiveness of hardware intended to "listen" or "speak" to people, especially people with communication disorders. For example, what is the effect of hearing impairment upon the receptive intelligibility of synthesized speech? What sort of message designs (controllable events when dealing with computers) can be invoked to improve the effectiveness of communication between machines and hearing-impaired listeners? Between machines operated by nonvocal clients and normal-hearing persons with whom they communicate? Can synthesized speech, with all of its present (but repeatable) flaws, be used to identify or diagnose problems of auditory perception? What are the effects of the quality of synthetic speech upon the affective and attributional responses of those who communicate with VOCA users? VOCAs have a clear impact on the amount and rates of language use, but what effect (if any) do they have on the syntactic, semantic, and lexical development of the people who use them? In one sense, these are issues of communication engineering; in another, they are issues of rehabilitation engineering. Speech-language pathology and audiology should have interests in both areas. These issues will become relevant as computer technology becomes more and more a part of daily life.

THE MARKETPLACE AND THE COSTS OF PROGRAMS

Microcomputer technology has developed as it has for two compelling reasons: (1) microcomputers offer better ways of processing certain kinds of information, and (2) translating those benefits into perceived needs, and the needs into products, has been extremely profitable for manufacturers and distributors of hardware and software.

Four firms have dominated sales thus far: IBM, 37% share; Apple, 34%; Radio Shack, 9%; Commodore, 8%; and all others, 12% (*Data Sources*, 1983). In the 6 months ending in July, 1983, the computer industry (overall) consisted of 1893 products marketed by 566 firms. During this interval, the microcomputer market grew by 29.7% (products) and 28.4% (companies), a far faster growth rate than any other segment (*Data Sources*, 1983). Without question, the market will continue to be extremely competitive and extremely dynamic.

An uncomfortable but simple fact of economic life is that communication disorders is a smaller, less affluent profession than medicine, dentistry, business administration, production engineering, accounting, law, or general education. These professionals have been "blessed" by aggressive development efforts in support of both hardware and software. Although it is possible that the entreprenurial spirit may yet smile upon us, it is just as likely that professionals in communication disorders will have to assume the responsibility for reconceptualizing problems in terms of contemporary technology. This will require changes in the knowledge base of the discipline and in the expectations we hold for educational programs (and the professors, clinical supervisors, and students who people those programs), for continuing education programs, and for working practitioners. The technology of microcomputers has come to audiology and speech-language pathology just as it has to the general public. Now we must meet it.

REFERENCE NOTES

Bird, R. (1981). *The computer in experimental psychology.* New York: Academic Press.
Byers, T. (1984). Micro-to-micro communications. *Popular Computing, 3:*4, 113–115, 118–119.
Frenzel, L., Jr. (1983). *Crash course in microcomputers* (2nd ed.). Indianapolis, IN: Sams Publishing Co.
Harris, J. (1979). ?Proem [sic] to a quantum leap in audiometric data collection and management. *Journal of Auditory Research, 20,* 1–29.
Leibson, S. (1982). The input/output primer, part 5: Character codes. *Byte,* 7:6, 242 and following.
McWhorter, G. (1978). *Understanding digital electronics.* Fort Worth, TX: Radio Shack.
Tyler, R. (1979). Measuring hearing loss in the future. *British Journal of Audiology, 13* (Supplement 2), 29–40.

REFERENCES

Allen, J. (1981). Linguistic-based algorithms offer practical text-to-speech systems. *Speech Technology, 1*:1, 12 ff.
Artwick, B. (1980). *Microcomputer interfacing.* Englewood Cliffs, NJ: Prentice-Hall.
Ashley, R. (1980). *Background math for a computer world: A self-teaching guide* (2nd ed.). New York: Wiley.
Atal, B., & Hanauer, S. (1971). Speech analysis and synthesis by linear predictive coding of the speech wave. *Journal of the Acoustical Society of America, 50,* 637-655.
Bailey, D. (1980). "Basic black" renascent: A new wardrobe. *Behavior Research Methods & Instrumentation, 12,* 96-102.
Bejar, I. (1982). Videodiscs in education, integrating the computer and communication technologies. *Byte, 7*:6, 78 ff.
Blodgett, A. (1983). Microelectronic packaging. *Scientific American, 249*:1, 86-96.
Borko, H. (Ed.) (1962). *Computer applications in the behavioral sciences.* Englewood Cliffs, NJ: Prentice-Hall.
Bull, G. (1983). Special training for special technology: A curriculum use of microcomputer-based tools in speech-language pathology. *The Computing Teacher,* April, 52-56.
Carter, J. (1983). *Electronically speaking: Computer speech generation.* Indianapolis, IN: Sams Publishing Co.
Ciarcia, S. (1983). Build an RS-232C breakout box. *Byte, 8*:4, 28 ff.
Data Sources. (1983). New York: Ziff-Davis Publishing.
Daynes, R. (1982). The videodisc interfacing primer. *Byte, 7*:6, 48-55, 58-59.
Dillon, R. (1983). Human factors in user-computer interaction: An introduction. *Behavior Research Methods & Instrumentation, 15,* 195-199.
Durham, S. (1983). High IQ modems. *Byte, 8*:9, 51 ff.
Durrett, H., & Zweiner, C. (1981). A microcomputer-based laboratory: Real world experience. *Behavior Research Methods & Instrumentation, 13,* 209-212.
Eggebrecht, L. (1983). *Interfacing to the IBM personal computer.* Indianapolis, IN: Sams Publishing Co.
Elovitz, H., Johnson, R., McHugh, A., & Shore, J. (1976). *Automatic translation of English text to phonetics by means of letter-to-sound rules* (Report No. 7948). Washington, DC: Naval Research Laboratory.
Flanagan, J. (1972). *Speech analysis, synthesis, and perception* (2nd ed.). New York: Springer-Verlag.
Flanagan, J. (1981a). Synthesis and recognition of speech: How computers talk. *Bell Laboratories Record, 59*:4, 123-130.
Flanagan, J. (1981b). Synthesis and recognition of speech: Teaching computers to listen. *Bell Laboratories Record, 59*:5, 146-151.
Flowers, J., & Leger, D. (1982). Personal computers and behavioral observation: An introduction. *Behavior Research Methods & Instrumentation, 14,* 227-230.
Fons, K., & Gargagliano, T. (1981). Articulate automata: An overview of voice synthesis. *Byte, 6*:2, 164 ff.
Garetz, M. (1983). The IEEE standard for the S-100 bus. *Byte, 8*:2, 272 ff.
Goldband, S. (1979). Real-time clocks for microcomputers in behavioral research. *Behavioral Research Methods & Instrumentation, 11,* 111-114.
Goldsbrough, P., Lund, T., & Rayner, J. (1983). *Analog electronics for microcomputer systems.* Indianapolis, IN: Sams Publishing Co.
Gordon, W., Foree, D., & Eckerman, D. (1983). Using an Apple II microcomputer for real-time control in a behavioral laboratory. *Behavior Research Methods & Instrumentation, 15,* 158-166.
Hansen, J. (1982). Micros are sounding good. *Microcomputing, 6*:8, 103-108, 110-113.
Hertz, S. (1982). From text to speech with SRS. *Journal of the Acoustical Society of America, 72,* 1155-1170.
Heywood, S. (1983a). The 8086—An architecture for the future, part 1: Introduction and glossary. *Byte, 8*:6, 450-455.
Heywood, S. (1983b). The 8086—An architecture for the future, part 2: Instruction set. *Byte, 8*:7, 299 ff.
Heywood, S. (1983c). The 8086—An architecture for the future, part 3: Instruction set continued. *Byte, 8*:8, 404 ff.
Hon, D. (1982). Interactive training in cardiopulmonary resuscitation. *Byte, 7*:6, 108 ff.
Houston, J. (1984). Don't bench me in. *Byte, 9*:2, 160-162, 164.
Jarrett, T. (1983). The new microfloppy standards. *Byte, 8*:9, 166 ff.
Kamm, C., Carterette, E., Morgan, D., & Dirks, D. (1980). Use of digitized speech materials in audiological research. *Journal of Speech and Hearing Research, 23,* 709-721.

Kieras, D. (1981). Effective ways to dispose of unwanted time and money with a laboratory computer. *Behavior Research Methods & Instrumentation, 13,* 145-148.
King, T., & Knight, B. (1983). *Programming the M68000.* Reading, MA: Addison-Wesley.
Kolotkin, R., Billingham, K., & Feldman, H. (1981). Computers in biofeedback research and therapy. *Behavior Research Methods & Instrumentation, 13,* 523-542.
Laurie, P. (1983). *The joy of computers.* Boston: Little, Brown.
Leibson, S. (1982a). The input/output primer, part 1: What is I/O? *Byte, 7:*2, 122 ff.
Leibson, S. (1982b). The input/output primer, part 2: Interrupts and direct memory access. *Byte, 7:*3, 126 ff.
Leibson, S. (1982c). The input/output primer, part 3: The parallel and HPIB (IEEE-488) interfaces. *Byte, 7:*4, 186 ff.
Leibson, S. (1982d). The input/output primer, part 4: The BCD and serial interfaces. *Byte, 7:*5, 202 ff.
Leibson, S. (1982e). The input/output primer, part 6: Interrupts, buffers, grounds and signal degradation. *Byte, 7:*7, 34 ff.
Lemmons, P. (1983). Japan and the fifth generation. *Byte, 8:*11, 394-401.
Levinson, S., & Liberman, M. (1981). Speech recognition by computer. *Scientific American, 244:*4, 64-76.
Lowe, D. (1983). A Winchester hard-disk integrated computer-assisted instructional laboratory: Hardware and data management considerations. *Behavior Research Methods & Instrumentation, 15,* 181-182.
Margolis, A. (1983). *Troubleshooting and repairing personal computers.* Blue Ridge Summit, PA: Tab Books.
Mau, E. (1983). *Getting the most from your micro.* Rochelle Park, NJ: Hayden.
Mayer, R. (1981). My mistakes with microcomputers (or four years of fun trying to get my computer to run). *Behavior Research Methods & Instrumentation, 13,* 141-144.
McHugh, A. (1976). *Listener preference and comprehension tests of stress algorithms for a text-to-phonetic speech analysis program* (Report No. 8015). Washington, DC: Naval Research Laboratory.
McWilliams, P. (1983a). Fear of interfacing. *Playboy, 30:*10, 119-120, 204-206.
McWilliams, P. (1983b). Computers: Where the joys are. *Playboy, 30:*11, 107, 176, 179-180.
McWilliams, P. (1983c). Decisions, decisions: A personal computer Christmas. *Playboy, 30:*12, 201, 264, 266-268, 270, 273.
Milich, M. (1982). When Apple speaks, who listens? *Softalk, 2:*5, 149 ff.
Moberg, D., & Laefsky, I. (1982). Videodiscs and optical storage. *Byte, 7:*6, 142 ff.
Monahan, J. (1983). Tight squeeze: The HP Series 200 Model 16. *Byte, 8:*6, 110 ff.
Montague, C., Howse, D., Mikkelsen, B., Rein, D., & Mathews, D. (1983). Technical aspects of IBM PC compatibility. *Byte, 8:*11, 247-252.
Moore, M. (1981). Right on target with Winchester. *Microcomputing, 5:*7, 34-36, 38-39, 41.
Moran, T. (1983). New developments in floppy disks. *Byte, 8:*3, 68 ff.
Munro, A. (1982). An overview of speech synthesizers. *Softalk, 2:*5, 149 ff.
Nakatani, L., & Schaffer, J. (1978). Hearing "words" without words: Prosodic cues for word perception. *Journal of the Acoustical Society of America, 63,* 234-245.
Perera, T. (1982). Buying and maintaining micro-computer systems. *Behavior Research Methods & Instrumentation, 14,* 71-76.
Pierrehumbert, J. (1981). Synthesizing intonation. *Journal of the Acoustical Society of America, 70,* 985-995.
Poltrock, S., & Foltz, G. (1983). An experimental psychology laboratory system for the Apple II microcomputer. *Behavior Research Methods & Instrumentation, 14,* 103-108.
Popelka, G., & Engebretson, A. (1983). A computer-based system for hearing aid assessment. *Hearing Instruments, 34:*7, 6-9, 44.
Powell, D. (1984). Monitor buyer's guide. *Popular Computing, 3:*4, 122 ff.
Rabiner, L., & Schafer, R. (1978). *Digital processing of speech signals.* Englewood Cliffs, NJ: Prentice-Hall.
Raskin, J., & Whitney, T. (1981). Perspectives on personal computing. *IEEE Computer, 14,* 62-73.
Reed, A. (1980). On choosing an inexpensive microcomputer for the experimental psychology laboratory. *Behavior Research Methods & Instrumentation, 12,* 607-613.
Reed, A. (1982). The Radio Shack computer in the experimental psychology laboratory: An evaluation. *Behavior Research Methods & Instrumentation, 14,* 109-112.
Rothchild, E. (1983). Optical-memory media. *Byte, 8:*3, 86 ff.
Sarisky, L. (1983). Will removable hard disks replace the floppy? *Byte, 8:*3, 110 ff.
Schneider, W. (1981). Basic computer troubleshooting and preventative maintenance. *Behavior Research Methods & Instrumentation, 13,* 452-459.

Schwejda, P., & Vanderheiden, G. (1982). Adaptive-firmware card for the Apple II. *Behavior Research Methods & Instrumentation, 7*:9, 276 ff.

Sclater, N. (1983). *Introduction to electronic speech synthesis.* Indianapolis, IN: Sams Publishing Co.

Starnes, T. (1983). Design philosophy behind Motorola's MC68000. *Byte, 8*:4, 70 ff.

Stephenson, J., & Cahill, B. (1983). *How to maintain and service your small computer.* Indianapolis, IN: Sams Publishing Co.

Stilwell, T. (1983). *Periodicals for microcomputers: An annotated bibliography* (International Development Working Paper No. 6). East Lansing, MI: Michigan State University, Department of Agricultural Economics.

Sutton, D. (1983). The challenge of hard-disk portability. *Byte, 8*:9, 127 ff.

The, L. (1984). Hard disk drives: Are they worth the price? *Personal Computing, 7*:1, 80 ff.

Thomas, A. (1981). Communication devices for the nonverbal disabled. *IEEE Computer, 14,* 25-30.

Titus, J., Larsen, D., & Titus, C. (1981). *Apple II interfacing.* Indianapolis, IN: Sams Publishing Co.

Toong, H., & Gupta, A. (1982). Personal computers, *Scientific American, 247*:6, 87-107.

Vanderheiden, G. (1981). Practical application of microcomputers to aid the handicapped. *IEEE Computer 14,* 54-61.

Veit, S. (1981). The ABCs of VDTs. *Personal computing, 5*:6, 39 ff.

Voiers, W. (1983). Evaluating processed speech using the diagnostic rhyme test. *Speech Technology, 1*:4, 30-39.

Walker, R. (1981). *Understanding computer science.* Fort Worth, TX: Radio Shack.

Welch, M. (1983). Expanding on the PC. *Byte, 8*:11, 168-184.

Whitaker, L. (1982). Maintenance alternatives for personal computers. *Byte, 7*:6, 452 ff.

Wicat Systems (1982). Interactive video disc design and production. *Byte, 7*:6, 56-57.

Willis, J., & Miller, M. (1984). *Computers for everybody* (3rd ed.). Beaverton, OR: Dilithium Press.

Witten, I. (1982). *Principles of computer speech.* New York: Academic Press.

Witten, I. (1983). Welcome to the standards jungle. *Byte, 8*:2, 146 ff.

Wolf, C. (1983). *Guidelines for the selection of microcomputer hardware* (International Development Working Paper No. 13.). East Lansing, MI: Michigan State University, Department of Agricultural Economics.

Zinagle, T. (1983). Intel's 80186: A 16-bit computer on a chip. *Byte, 8*:4, 132 ff.

Chapter 6

Evaluating Microcomputer Software

Arthur H. Schwartz

Selecting software for clinical, administrative, instructional, or research applications can be a complex, confusing, and intimidating process. The technological nature of microcomputers combined with new terminology make it embarrassing, at best, although it is typically confusing and frustrating. Potential users have concerns about asking the wrong questions, or of not knowing which questions to ask. Similarly, concerns about purchasing the wrong software or not being able to use a program can cause a prospective user to postpone or abandon the decision to incorporate microcomputers. Software evaluation and selection need not be enigmatic, mystical, or restricted to individuals with degrees in computer science. A systematic comparison of software operation with the needs of the user or organization will enable speech–language pathologists and audiologists to evaluate microcomputer software.

Effective microcomputer software must perform accurately and efficiently, be learnable with reasonable effort, and be simple to use. Complete reference documentation and backing by reputable manufacturers or vendors characterizes competitive software. Given the newness of microcomputer applications to speech–language pathology and audiology, the large number of software programs on the market, the lack of development standards, and the costs for programs specific to communication disorders, a logical and organized approach to software evaluation is necessary. This chapter provides a functional explanation of procedures and criteria that can be utilized in making a decision on the adoption of commercial or customized microcomputer software.

A lack of standards for the development and validation of software necessitates that users systematically define their application needs, screen reports on various products, and evaluate programs before purchase (V.B. Cohen, 1983). To make informed decisions in selecting software, it is essential to:

(1) specify the needs the software will fill;
(2) specify the tasks to be completed;
(3) develop a set of performance criteria to determine if a program fills the needs and does the tasks;
(4) identify software programs that might perform those tasks; and
(5) critically evaluate software operation and accompanying documentation.

©College-Hill Press, Inc. All rights, including that of translation, reserved. No part of this publication may be reproduced without the written permission of the publisher.

Planning, preparation, and study of software saves time, effort, and money once the decision is made to purchase and implement a particular type of software program. To evaluate and select effective software some familiarity with the features of microcomputer software is essential.

FEATURES OF MICROCOMPUTER SOFTWARE

The software package

A software package generally consists of the program and supporting documentation. The program is the set of instructions, written in a language and coded into a form understandable to the microcomputer, that directs the operation of the system. Programs can be on floppy disks, cassettes, hard disks, or in a written form called the source code. The documentation accompanying a program provides information about the purposes of the program, its features, and its operation. Accurate, thorough, and understandable documentation is necessary if the program is to be implemented and used as planned.

Types of software

Systems software

There are two basic types of software that govern the operation of microcomputer systems: systems software and applications software (Graham, 1983; Rodwell, 1983). Systems software regulates the internal operation of the microcomputer, displays screen information, accepts keyboard commands, manages information, coordinates activities of peripheral devices, and performs routine functions basic to the operation of the system. It includes both disk operating systems (DOS) and utilities software. Disk operating systems are special program routines that manage the storage and retrieval of information on disks and the management of information to and from the computer. Utilities software systems are specialized operating systems programs which perform tasks such as loading, copying, or deleting information more efficiently, for use with particular applications software to allow the user to modify system operations.

Applications software

Applications software performs specific functions and is categorized as either general purpose or vertical applications software. General purpose applications include word processing, data base management, records management, mailing lists, spread sheets, report generators, and graphics. For the speech–language pathologist or audiologist, general purpose applications software can be adapted for scheduling, client and student record keeping, clinical report writing, financial management, and reporting in a variety of settings. Vertical applications software, on the other hand, performs a series of particular tasks for an individual purpose in a certain context. It represents modifications or enhancements of the general purpose software for particular professions, organizations, or individuals. Software designed for assessment or clinical management of speech, language, or hearing disorders is regarded as consisting of vertical applications programs. For example, a software program to assist in the selection of hearing aids is considered a vertical applications program since it performs a group of related functions but could not be used for other functions such as scoring articulation tests.

Dimensions of software

In the selection of either general purpose or vertical applications software, reference sources recommend determining what operations are to be performed before choosing software and then selecting hardware (Datapro, 1982b,c; Frankel & Gras, 1983; Graham, 1983; and Poole, McNiff, & Cook, 1981). However, when evaluating vertical applications software in communication disorders, hardware requirements for the operation of the program should be considered at the same time rather than after the software has been selected. Vertical applications software, particularly in the area of communication disorders, may be designed to operate on particular microcomputer systems, with particular kinds of peripheral devices, and are likely to be incompatible with other hardware.

STEPS IN SOFTWARE EVALUATION

Several references are available that provide information on the steps involved in evaluating microcomputer software (V.B. Cohen, 1983; Datapro Research Corporation, 1982b,c; Hannaford & Taber, 1982; Roblyer, 1981; and Taber, 1982). A review and synthesis of this information suggests that there are five steps involved in the evaluation process: (1) determining requirements; (2) screening information for software appearing to fit application needs; (3) evaluating the software package operation; (4) selecting the software that meets specifications most easily and efficiently; and (5) installing the program. Figure 6-1 illustrates the five steps in software evaluation. More experienced microcomputer users may find some steps can be minimized. For less experienced users, following a sequence such as this can increase the probability of selecting the best software to fit the requirements of the individual or organization.

The evaluation of software entails two major dimensions: the *steps* involved in identifying and screening software possibilities; and *criteria* for evaluating and selecting programs. Elsewhere in this volume, C. Cohen (see chap. 2) has recommended that, prior to evaluating software, a thorough analysis of organizational operations (products and procedures) should be performed and needs should be identified. In those instances where there is a need to process information faster, more accurately, in different fashions for particular recipients, or if current procedures are costly, inefficient, and time consuming, microcomputer systems may increase productivity.

Determining requirements

The initial step in the evaluation of software entails analyzing current procedures, resources required to perform the task, products, and time and personnel involved. Following the specification of current procedures, it is advisable to enumerate each of the operations performed and evaluate the adequacy of each. Designation of operations no longer adequate or of new procedures needed can be developed from the list of current operations and applications. The resolution of any discrepancy between current procedures and desired procedures, as described by C. Cohen (1983; chap.2), would indicate that a change in either procedures or approaches may be warranted. A microcomputer system may be an appropriate solution if increased accuracy, faster processing, greater output, or different procedures are needed to accomplish the objectives.

Figure 6-1. Five steps in the evaluation of applications software for microcomputers.

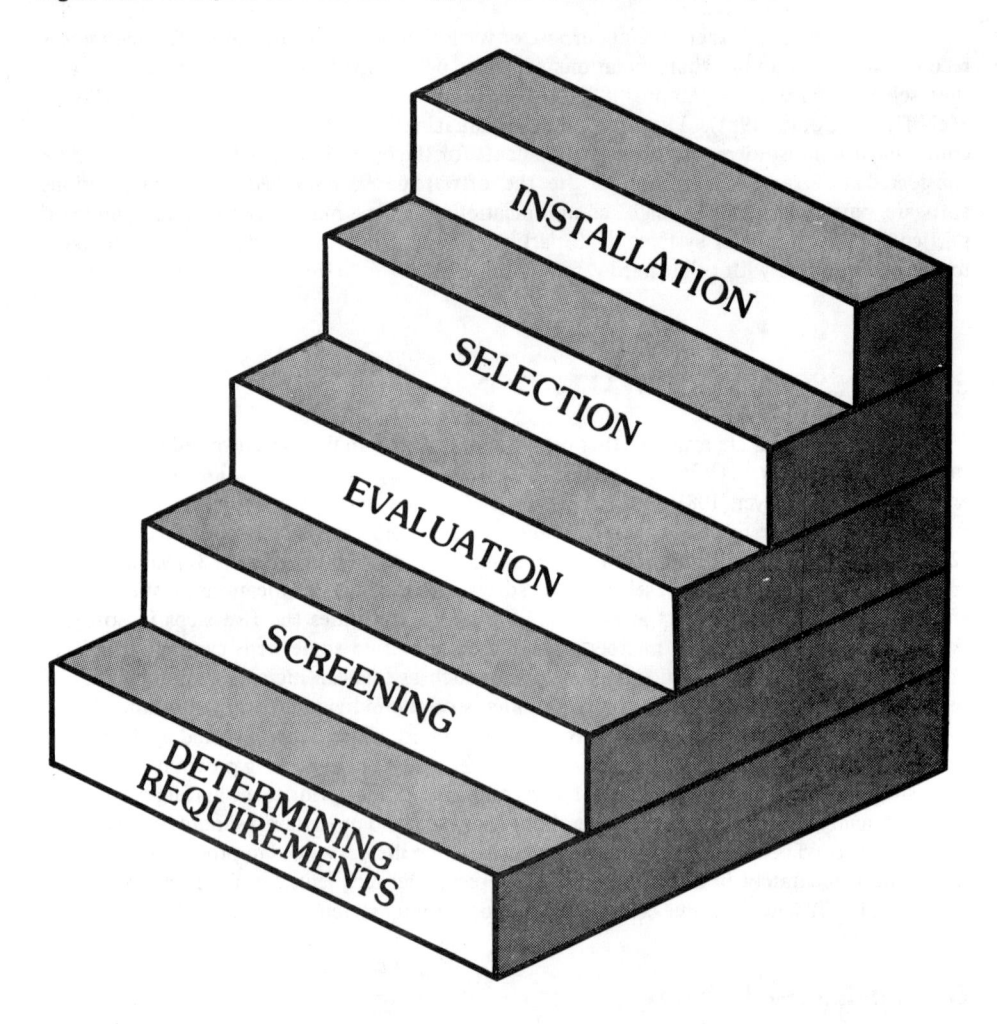

Screening

Screening potential software programs, the second step, is initiated after a needs analysis is completed. Information on applications software can be obtained from published reviews, inquiries to manufacturers and local dealers, specialty shows and conferences, or consultations with other program users (Datapro 1982a; Lathrop, 1982). The purpose of the software screening process is to rule out programs that do not fit the needs of the individual or organization.

Reviews of general purpose software such as word processing, spread sheets, or data based management programs may be found in specialty magazines, software reviews, and technology journals (see Wilkins, chap. 4 in this volume). Reviews of software generally focus on key parameters that make a program efficient to use including performance characteristics, ease of use, documentation, and support. The information in these reviews will be helpful to individuals trying to determine if a particular software program will satisfy certain clinical, administrative, instructional, or research applications.

Because of the individual needs and applications for software, reliance on published reviews seems more appropriate for the screening step of software evaluation than for the more rigorous evaluation step. Surveys of software, particularly in communication disorders, need to be supplemented with information obtained from individuals or agencies who have used those programs. Local computer users' groups can provide an opportunity to contact other users familiar with certain general purpose applications software. The time spent in talking with other program users will help when making a decision regarding software programs to disregard or to pursue for evaluation.

If an organization is large enough or if circumstances preclude systematic evaluation of software packages, an external consultant might be considered. Datapro (1982c) recommends a consultant when time is unavailable for analysis and selection or customized software is needed. In addition, if there are special problems, unique applications, or conflicting information exists, consultants should be able to provide objective advice. Wilkins (see chap. 4) describes resources that can be investigated to locate appropriately qualified consultants.

Evaluation

The third step is the actual evaluation of the software. Software that has been screened is tested to judge if the program meets performance requirements. The evaluation step permits the potential user to verify the adequacy of the software package including accompanying documentation and support. Among the ways to evaluate software operation are to: (1) observe a demonstration; (2) purchase a demonstration disk of the program; and (3) conduct benchmark testing.

Observing demonstrations

Dealers may permit potential users to observe a demonstration of software. This is particularly helpful for individuals with limited experience with microcomputers since the store personnel can show the program's features quickly and efficiently. It may not be possible to obtain a demonstration of each feature since personnel time may be restricted. Another method to observe software operation is at trade shows or conventions. At these meetings, hardware and software manufacturers will be available to demonstrate products. This is particularly relevant in the case of vertical applications software for communication disorders specialists. Much of the application software in speech-language pathology and audiology is not likely to be sold through local vendors. It is published by individuals, companies, or publishers directly concerned with communication disorders. Unless the operation of software can be observed, the user must rely on mail order. Purchasing software without observing its operation is, at best, risky. If the program does not perform as required or the return/refund policy is lacking, the user will be stuck with an inadequate software package.

Demonstration disks

Increasingly, manufacturers of general purpose applications software sell a demonstration disk to assist buyers in determining if the program meets specifications. In a tutorial format, the demonstration disk provides a selection of functions and provides cursory experience with software operation. The cost of the demonstration disk is typically credited to the purchaser's bill if the program is purchased. Accuracy and efficiency of performance, ease of use, and clarity of directions are major factors to consider in a demonstration program. More elaborate information on critiera for software evaluation is provided later in this chapter.

Benchmark testing

The third, and preferable, way to evaluate software is through the use of benchmark tests. Glatzer (1981) has recommended replicating a standard series of steps or operations using the prospective program. Benchmark testing permits comparison of the accuracy, speed, and ease of use of different software. Benchmark testing is a somewhat time-consuming procedure. For general purpose applications software such as for word processing, Datapro (1982b) developed a set of 20 tasks for conducting benchmark tests including a sampling of the types of editing, formatting, storage, and retrieval functions necessary. Benchmark tests are appropriate for other applications software such as that for data management or financial spread sheets. There is need for the development of benchmark tests for vertical applications software in communication disorders.

Conducting benchmark tests with general purpose software for administrative or research applications may be done with a series of tasks that involve data manipulation specific to the user. In its simplest sense, there are three things microcomputers do: (1) receive information from some peripheral device; (2) organize and process information in some manner; and (3) send information to a peripheral device. Speech-language pathologists and audiologists should be able to specify a set of input, processing, and output functions which could comprise a benchmark test in order to evaluate vertical applications software being considered. Due to the limited number of programs, the individualized nature of instructional or clinical applications programs, and the costs involved, special arrangements for benchmark testing may be needed. Either a preview or returns policy should be available.

Concurrent with the software evaluation, all supporting documentation needs to be examined. The accuracy, detail, clarity, and organization of the documentation is as important as the software itself. Specific characteristics and criteria for evaluating documentation are described later in this chapter.

Selection

The fourth step in software evaluation is the selection of the package to fit the needs of the individual or organization. Based on the information from formal and informal reviews, demonstrations, and benchmark testing, the program best suited to perform the desired tasks can be selected. Secondary factors, in addition to performance characteristics and ease of use, can be considered. In the case of both general purpose and vertical applications software, direct and indirect costs become decisive. Direct costs include the programs, documentation, and source code if available. Equipment and supplies not included in the software package, costs for training personnel, and procedures for transferring existing operations onto microcomputers are indirect costs of software. The price of a particular software program may be prohibitive if: (a) extensive modifications in procedures are needed; (b) substantial special hardware is required; (c) additional personnel costs are involved; or (d) the manufacturer of the program fails to provide support. The direct cost of the software package, particularly in the case of vertical applications software in communication disorders, may be secondary to the indirect personnel or instrumentation factors.

Installation

The installation of software is the final step in software selection. After needs have been determined, packages have been screened and evaluated, facilities have been arranged, and staff have been oriented, the software package can be installed (see Cohen, chap. 2). Later in this chapter, ease of installation is discussed as one of the criteria for software selection.

Installation of software should be a relatively straightforward and simple process if appropriate language cards, operating systems, or peripherals for the software are already part of the system. In such a case, the software can be installed by inserting it into the disk drives and turning on the system. In some circumstances, as discussed later in this chapter, minor specifications may be requested when the software is "booted" to configure the program to the particular system. Usable software documentation contains information about the kinds of hardware, operating systems, and configurations needed to install the software and get it operating. Consequently, thorough review of documentation during the evaluation step will identify any additions or modifications needed to make the software operational.

CRITERIA FOR SOFTWARE SELECTION

Perspectives

There has been a proliferation of general purpose applications software which neither performs the functions advertised nor has adequate or complete information about its operation. This trend may be replicated for vertical applications software in communication disorders unless speech-language pathologists and audiologists exercise selectivity in incorporating microcomputers in clinical, administrative, instructional, and research settings. Roblyer (1981) has commented that the lack of standards for software development and validation has placed the user in a "buyer beware" position. It is indispensable that vertical applications software:
 (1) performs the task accurately and appropriately;
 (2) can be previewed or returned if unsatisfactory;
 (3) has documentation that is accurate, readable, and complete;
 (4) permits the user to make or purchase archival copies at a nominal cost; and
 (5) is backed by a service representative who can answer questions about the software.

Additionally, it is convenient if the software can be upgraded as new and more powerful versions become available. Similarly, in the case of vertical applications software, access to the program source code to modify program parameters to accommodate organizational or individual needs is convenient, particularly for clinical programs. While costs may be high, developers still must be held accountable for the quality and accuracy of their products just as they are for services. Until developers, manufacturers, and vendors develop and market software that respects a buyer's rights, pre-purchase benchmark testing is the only protection available to a consumer.

Evaluation protocols

During the software evaluation process, it is advisable to be mindful of several factors. The needs and the applications for both general purpose and vertical applications software vary from organization to organization. It is difficult to state which factors are the most important for evaluating software. Datapro (1982b), Frankel and Gras (1983), Hannaford and Taber (1982), Rushakoff (1982), and Taber (1982) have discussed features that may be grouped into six criteria to be considered when evaluating software: (1) task performance; (2) ease of use; (3) documentation; (4) support; (5) affordability; and (6) ease of installation. Figure 6-2 illustrates these six criteria for consideration. Depending on user needs and experience, certain features may be more important to one individual than another and some may be irrelevant. Each of these six criteria is discussed in the following section.

Figure 6-2. Six criteria to consider in evaluating microcomputer software.

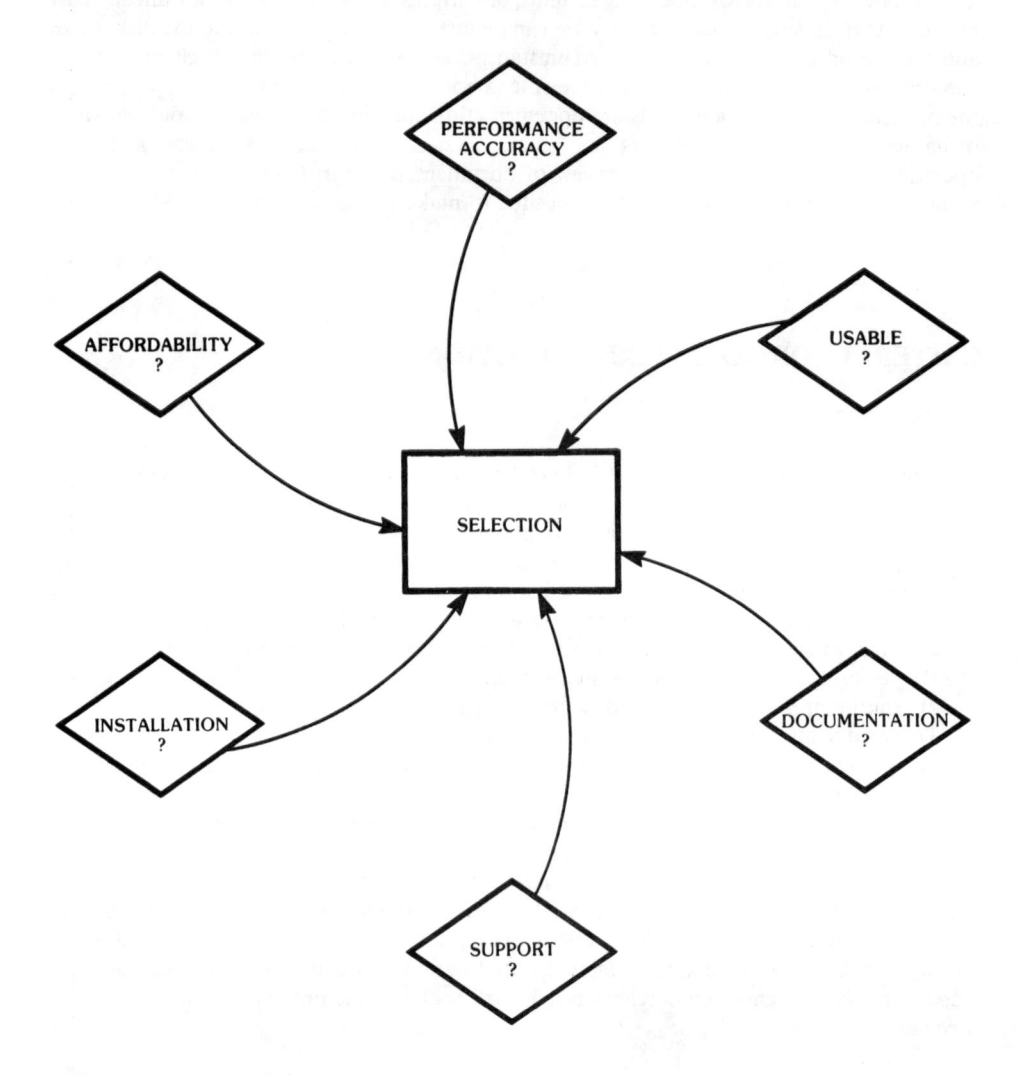

Task performance

The reasons for considering a particular software package include faster, easier, more complete, or less costly processing of information. Within the limits of the system's capacity, software must perform the operations that the buyer is seeking. Unless designed specifically for a user, it is not realistic to expect that software will fit the buyer's requirements exactly. Minor modification in procedures can be anticipated to make software perform to its capacity. Review of documentation and screen menus provides information on all the operations and commands needed to perform software functions. A software program should perform each operation accurately, completely, and in a reasonable time period. Entering, processing, or producing information with as few operations as possible characterizes efficient performance.

Beyond software effectiveness, the remaining criteria to consider have varying degrees of importance relative to specific users. Less experienced users may find that ease of use and documentation are critical for productive applications. Experienced users may be more concerned with affordability than with support. In the case of software in speech-language pathology and audiology that will be used by staff with varying levels of expertise, ease of use may be more important than other factors.

Checklists and rating sheets commonly used for evaluating software programs are informative but may be limited in use. Typically, software rating forms rate a set of features on a numerical scale reflecting the user's judgment. Many of these rating forms are informal in nature and were developed by specific organizations for particular types of software. Systematic studies of reliability and validity of these protocols are lacking. The ratings may be somewhat arbitrary and subjective in nature. This limitation is compounded by the observation that some of the factors identified or the items rated may not necessarily be pertinent to all users or all software. Unquestionably, there is a need for some type of evaluation procedure that accommodates the needs and applications of individual users. Frankel and Gras (1983) have developed a useful approach for the evaluation of general purpose applications software. They differentiate core features such as documentation, user-friendly directions, error prevention and data protection, sorting, and printed output capacities that characterize most software. Within each of these areas, a number of particular features are identified and a short, readable explanation of the feature is provided. The user can select those software features which are essential, optional, or unnecessary for particular purposes. Furthermore, the authors provide elaborate listings of features for categories of general purpose software including word processing, data management, spread sheets, report generators, graphics, and other financial management software. This format might be applicable for software in communication sciences and disorders since it allows the user to select relevant features needed for particular applications.

Using an approach that appears to be an extension of rating scales, Mitchener (1983) reported standards for general purpose software that identify 8 to 10 major categories of features. Rather than rating each feature on a variable scale, a standard, expressed in points, is given for each of these features. In general, the higher the score for a particular software package, the closer the performance to the standards. A standards approach permits the comparison of different software according to some reference. Clearly, some standards for software performance are needed. However, there are certain limitations to the standards approach for rating software. First, no information is provided as to the reliability and validity of the standards. Secondly, the selection of features and the assignment of point values to these features may be subjective in nature. A subjective element cannot be eliminated in the evaluation of software. An evaluation protocol that allows the user to identify relevant features and then rate the importance of each feature to the user's intended application may have the greatest merit.

The rating of vertical applications software in communication disorders is difficult. Because of the limited market, it is unlikely that popular periodicals will conduct such evaluations. While it may be difficult to develop an acceptable set of standards for vertical applications software in speech-language pathology and audiology, professional organizations and special interest groups could take a leadership role in developing review protocols and publishing such information.

Ease of use

User friendliness incorporates several characteristics that pertain to user perception of the ease of getting the program to perform the tasks for which it was designed. Instructions for operating the program, procedures for entering commands, identification of errors that could lead to loss of data, and the ease of starting and terminating operations help users to manage the program productively. User-friendly programs are characterized by instructions that are informative without being technical and intimidating. Directions are short, simple, and clear. A software program may be considered to be user friendly if it can be used on the basis of examination of supporting documentation and tutorials at a reasonable level of proficiency with only a small amount of study and practice. There are numerous general purpose software programs that are powerful and flexible, yet whose operations cannot be mastered through study of the manual and which require special classes or workshops. These may be difficult or discouraging for staff and personnel to learn. Software that has clinical applications must be friendly and easy to use for both the clients and the clinicians.

Command selection

The manner in which operating commands are selected is an important attribute of user friendly software. How users are able to locate the commands to manage program operation determines ease of use. Two major approaches to command selection, menu driven and command driven, can be found in software programs. Menu-driven software displays lists of commands for selecting the function to be performed. In many cases, menu-driven software offers choices that display special screens providing additional explanations of commands or sequences of commands. Menu-driven software is particularly helpful when learning, if a program is used infrequently, or if the user needs a quick means to become familiar with operating commands. On the other hand, software that is command driven relies on user knowledge of specific keys or key combinations rather than screen menus to perform specific functions. Command-driven programs may not seem as friendly as menu-driven software because detailed information is not provided on the screen. Command-driven software tends to be faster. The number of commands, the number of keys or key combinations, and the absence of menus may pose difficulty for users learning a program that is command driven. After the set of fundamental commands has been learned, users typically operate the program quickly and efficiently. With experience and increased proficiency, it is reported that users tend to outgrow the help provided by menus and may even find the menus to be an irritating delay. Some general purpose software offers a combination of menu- and command-driven operations; this allows the novice to obtain the assistance needed as the program is being mastered yet permits the experienced user to bypass menus and execute commands quickly.

Error trapping

Tolerance for errors in operating a software program is a vital component influencing ease of use. Mistakes in entering data, changing intentions, failure to enter operations using commands the program accepts, or even problems in keyboard design can occasionally result in mistakes. Some menu-driven programs may provide a list of choices (i.e., 1 through 4). If a key other than the choices designated on the menu is entered, the program might cease operation. This is termed a "fatal error" since the data would be lost and all information would have to be reentered. Functional software has error-trapping features to minimize the potential for making a fatal error. That is, software programs that are error trapped: (a) will not execute a command unless it is one of the choices presented or (b) will ask for a confirmation from the user before executing a command. For example, in a menu-driven application program, if there are four choices on the screen (i.e., 1 = create a file, 2 = print a file, 3 = delete a file, and 4 = store a file) and the user enters another choice (i.e., "5" or "K"), a program that is error trapped will provide feedback that the character entered is not a legitimate choice. As another example, in word processing programs, if the command to clear the screen of all information is selected, the program will ask for a confirmation and a second command before executing the instruction. This provides an opportunity to confirm an entry before making a fatal error and losing information. If an error is made and the program cannot perform an operation, friendly software should provide feedback as to why the command was rejected. "There is no file by this name" is more informative and less intimidating than computer jargon terms such as "DOS Error."

Operating steps

The number of steps to perform an operation contributes to the perception of ease of use of a program. Information that can be entered, manipulated, or retrieved with one command is simpler to use. Commands that require sequences of key combinations may necessitate frequent referral to a reference card or manual. Software with dedicated keys for specific functions may be simpler to operate than that which necessitates combinations of keys to execute commands. General purpose applications software such as word processing, spread sheet, or data management software frequently has an assortment of commands that perform a diversity of functions. This versatility makes such software powerful. To use powerful programs, particular commands, keys, key combinations, or sequences of commands must be remembered. If a program is not used regularly some of the commands may be forgotten and the user will need to rely on the reference card.

Program entry and exit

Lastly, the manner in which the user can enter the program, change entries, exit a program, or select only part of a program contributes to its ease of use. Many general purpose application programs allow the user to select particular files, operations, or data entry points. Using software that requires a linear progression from the first menu through a series of submenus until the desired submenu is obtained is tedious, cumbersome, and irritating. Rushakoff (1983) has indicated that friendly programs should allow a user to go back and revise a specific entry rather than retrace the entire data entry process if it is discovered that an error has been made. Similarly, simple procedures for exiting a program once the information is obtained or the operation is performed characterize enhanced ease of use.

In summary, ease of use refers to characteristics which provide information and feedback to operate the program. Special menus, designated function keys, error trapping and simplified entry and exit procedures assist in learning how to operate software. Programs which have numerous commands, complicated command combinations or sequences, or rely on the user rather than a menu for command selection may be faster and more powerful, but require more experience and proficiency. Users must decide whether to trade friendliness for power.

Documentation

One of the most important considerations for evaluating software is the acceptability of the documentation. All instructions for the operation of the program including user manuals, reference manuals, reference cards, and program tutorials constitute the documentation. Unless documentation is readable, understandable, and organized—let alone accurate—the program will be difficult to learn and cumbersome to operate (Sohr, 1983).

Comprehensible software documentation has been one of the major problems with some general purpose applications programs. Documentation must furnish information and illustrations to allow the user to accomplish certain tasks with the program. Much of the documentation in the earlier general applications software written for microcomputers was either inaccurate, incomplete, or incomprehensible (Gleason, 1981). Some of the documentation was assembled by programmers or other technical personnel for use by programmers or computer scientists. While appropriate from a technical orientation, it was nonfunctional for users other than programmers or computer scientists. Poor organization, lack of an index, inaccurate tables, illustrations that did not coincide with text, or lack of examples only served to intimidate rather than inform users.

Types of documentation

When evaluating microcomputer software programs, accompanying documentation has to be examined critically. The type and contents of documentation can yield an initial impression about the ease of use of the program. All software should include a manual explaining the purpose of the program, the operations performed, the procedures needed to operate the program, the information the program will process, and the output the program will provide. In addition, the manual should specify the hardware requirements (memory capacity, number of disk drives needed, peripherals required, or special cards or interfaces). It is an admitted challenge for software manufacturers to prepare documentation that is informative and understandable for both inexperienced and experienced users. Increasingly, manufacturers are including tutorials as part of the software package. A tutorial is designed to motivate and teach the novice to use the program. If the program will be used by inexperienced or novice users, it is important that a tutorial program be obtained. Experienced users can bypass the tutorial section and go directly to operating or technical sections of particular interest. The reference manual provides technical information about the program, its structure and organization, and procedures to customize certain operations or products. A reference card, containing the key commands and procedures, is a useful feature. Some recent general purpose software packages include cards or labels to stick to the keyboard for reference purposes. In summary, "good" software programs provide extensive documentation to enable a reader to use the program. Inaccurate, incomplete, or poorly written documentation will necessitate special training.

Organization of documentation

The organization of contents of documentation should also be reviewed. Disorganized documentation makes it difficult to locate information necessary to use the software effectively. One of the major attributes of good documentation, according to Sohr (1983), is organization according to task rather than feature. Manuals organized according to the operations of the program are regarded as task oriented. Users can master contents of task-oriented manuals according to the tasks needing to be performed rather than having to read the whole document in order to use it. Psychologically, it is important for users to be able to locate needed information and get the software operating as quickly as possible.

Unlike task-oriented documentation, feature-oriented manuals present information on the characteristics of the program's organization or capacity rather than the tasks it performs. Feature organization may be of greater interest to the experienced user than the novice. To operate a program that has a feature-oriented manual, nearly the entire document must be read before the program can be used to perform certain functions. This can be frustrating to novice or inexperienced users. The task-oriented manual offers needed information for both the novice and the experienced user.

Editorial highlighting

The organization of documentation can either facilitate or impede mastery of software. Organizers are editorial "highlights" that assist in locating information. Short introductions, margin comments, highlighted section summaries, and synopses by task help the reader recognize key information and serve to integrate a particular topic with broader topics. Examining documentation organizers can enable the reader to determine the effort that was devoted to making the manual instructional. Manuals that have been organized for instructional convenience provide a detailed outline of each chapter at the beginning of the manual and at the beginning of each chapter, as well as an index at the end of the manual. Both indexes and organizers assist in locating information needed to operate the program. Verifying agreement between index pagination and actual appearance of a topic is a way of screening a manual for accuracy and consistency.

Illustrations

Illustrations of commands or operations also promote the understanding of program functions. At least three or four illustrations from a manual should be compared to the surrounding text explanation. Typographical errors and inconsistencies occasionally arise despite the most careful proofreading. It is frustrating and intimidating to study documentation and then find that the outcomes are not the same as shown in the illustration. Users, unfortunately, tend to think that if the command did not work, it was a user error rather than some problem with the manual or the program. Documentation containing inconsistencies and/or errors should be suspect. Before purchase, the buyer should make an extra effort to talk with other users of the program to identify problems.

Support

The fourth criterion for the evaluation of software encompasses manufacturer and dealer support. Manufacturer policies regarding warranty and updating of software need to be examined carefully. In the case of general applications software, some statement of quality assurance should be given in the documentation. Documentation also needs to be scrutinized to determine if the program is being purchased or leased. Careful examination of the documentation may reveal that the software is not being purchased, but rather leased for a one-time fee (Datapro, 1982b). Leased software cannot be copied or modified, as it is the property of the manufacturer. Several prominent software packages assign a serial number to each program leased. Updates, backups, or service to damaged disks are provided only to the leasee of record. Most applications software contains copy protection schemes to prevent unauthorized reproduction. If the program is copied without the permission of the manufacturer, the leasee can be responsible for legal damages. A leased program belongs to the manufacturer and is considered an asset of that company. Should the manufacturer ever encounter financial difficulty, creditors could pursue the assets of the company. A leased program, regarded as an asset of the company, could be seized by the creditors. Users should distinguish between purchase and lease agreements.

Manufacturer support

Manufacturer policies regarding the internal duplication (backup) and replacement of disks are relevant. Piracy, the illegal copying of programs, is a major concern of both general purpose and vertical applications software developers. Obviously, the costs to develop, validate, and market software are defrayed only by the sale of programs. In addition, manufacturers have to spend considerable sums to protect their programs from illegal copying. All of these add to the cost of software programs. The legal, ethical, and economic aspects of this controversy are discussed elsewhere in this volume by Wilson (see chap. 11). However, manufacturers should have policies that permit the purchase of backup or replacement disks in case of loss or damage. Some manufacturers provide an original and a backup copy at the time of purchase. Most manuals recommend that the original program disk should be stored in a safe place and the copy used. Should the copy be damaged, the original can be used and a replacement should be available for purchase at a nominal cost from the manufacturer. Any charge beyond the cost of materials, copying, and postage is unreasonable. Software dealers that charge more than 5% of the cost of the original program in order to obtain an archival copy should be suspect.

Several manufacturers of general purpose applications software provide toll-free numbers to call if there are questions or problems using the program or understanding the documentation. Information about this service can be found in the documentation accompanying the program.

The cost of this service is built into the purchase price. While toll-free numbers may be provided with programs from the larger software manufacturers, this may not be the case for vertical software in communication disorders. Nevertheless, it should be possible to contact the manufacturer directly.

An additional aspect of manufacturer support concerns program updates or upgrades. Periodically, manufacturers may discover and remediate "bugs" in programs, have updates to inform users of those alterations, or produce newer or more powerful versions of the program. If the software is manufactured by a company that also manufactures hardware, new versions of software are produced when new models of microcomputers are introduced. Reputable manufacturers of applications programs may update documentation for registered users periodically. Reduced prices on updated versions may be offered to software owners when newer or enhanced versions of software are marketed. Typically, updated versions are discounted, thereby allowing the user to obtain software that is more powerful and efficient at a nominal cost. Policies on purchase of updates are relevant when considering a software program.

Much of the information about manufacturer support services can be found in the documentation accompanying a software package. If missing, incomplete, or haphazardly assembled, caution should be exercised and perhaps another program should be considered. Vertical applications software in communication disorders is typically marketed by publishers specializing in tests, texts, materials, and journals in the field rather than by the larger manufacturers of general purpose applications software. It should be possible to correspond with publishers of speech-language and hearing references regarding their policies.

Dealer support

The instructional and service capabilities of the dealer must be considered when evaluating software. When considering software, a different kind of support can be expected from a local dealer than from a mail order firm. Local dealers may permit benchmark testing of software. Conducting benchmark tests of software minimizes the need to return programs. Software purchased through mail order vendors may cost less to purchase, but may be difficult to return if problems arise or the program does not perform according to its specifications. If problems are encountered after purchase, a local dealer may be willing to make an exchange for another program of the same make and model. Because of problems with illegal copying of software programs, most dealers cannot be expected to provide refunds. At the time of purchase, it is helpful to inquire as to whether the dealer has backup inventory. If the dealer does not keep an inventory, replacement of the damaged disk will have to be back ordered, resulting in the user being without the program for a period of time. The type of materials and instructional or service support offered by a dealer could be a major consideration for users beginning to implement software programs.

As Wilkins has indicated elsewhere in this volume (chap. 4), mail order houses can save the consumer between 20 and 35% of the costs of hardware and software. For users who know exactly what they want, are able to install the package, and do not need assistance, the mail order dealer is a logical alternative. However, if problems with the product or documentation are encountered, resolution of those problems may become complicated and time consuming. There is no guarantee that local dealers can provide better information or service, however. Knowledgeable staff, selection of hardware and software, reputation, training classes or facilities, and a service department are all features that characterize competent dealers. For users or organizations just implementing microcomputer systems, the convenience of having a local dealer to answer questions, give suggestions, or offer advice on solving problems offsets any price savings available from mail order houses.

Ease of installation

Three factors seem to influence the ease with which a program, general purpose or vertical in nature, is incorporated into daily routines: (1) existing routines and procedures; (2) initial configuration of software; and (3) staff training and supervision.

Existing routines and products
Particularly in the case of clinical or administrative procedures, it is unlikely that existing procedures and products are identical to those of the software programs available. Minor modifications in input, manipulation, and outputting of information are to be expected. The costs of developing software programs that are identical to existing procedures are prohibitive. Some of the more powerful administrative software is flexible enough to accommodate to the unique requirements of many organizations in communication disorders. Similarly, as software that is clinical in nature evolves, the manner in which it is utilized may be more productive than some current procedures.

Software configurations
Before software can be implemented, some attention must be given to any specification of hardware characteristics. That is, some general applications programs such as word processing or spelling checkers will need to be configured prior to actual use. This means that information needs to be entered concerning the brand of microcomputer being used, the make of the printer, the number of disk drives, and so forth. Once configured, the program will "run" on the system without further installation. Other general purpose application programs and most vertical applications software are regarded as "turnkey" programs because immediate utilization without modification of the software is possible; no configuration of the software is needed prior to utilization. If the program is accurate, the documentation is complete and readable, necessary hardware is available, and appropriate language cards are operating, vertical applications in speech-language pathology and audiology are turnkey in installation.

Staff training and supervision
Unless staff are already familiar with the operation of microcomputer software and hardware, some attention must be given to "tooling up." Sturdivant (1983) reported on an inservice project with the Houston Independent School District that was concerned with training personnel to use different software programs. The HISD program is divided into modules of instruction, with each module covering a topic such as authoring languages, word processing, and languages such as BASIC and Pascal. Her findings are of relevance to individuals or organizations needing to know the approximate resources required to get staff to a level of proficiency with different software. On the whole, use of general purpose applications software required approximately 18-22 hours of instruction, practice, and supervision. Proficiency in programming or authoring languages took between 35 and 45 hours of instruction. Unless staff are trained and supervised, neither the hardware nor the software may be used to its fullest potential.

Certain resources must be allocated initially to help personnel learn to use a new software program productively. Release time, incentives, and qualified supervision are helpful both for allaying fears or apprehensions and for enabling employees to operate the program. A transition period of at least 3 months, during which time the new software system is being implemented and the existing system is gradually being phased out, can be anticipated. Until the procedural and personnel factors are resolved, it is wise to have a manual backup system in case the software does not perform as expected. Operating two systems concurrently, therefore, will require additional personnel time and effort, materials, and supplies. After the software has been implemented, personnel trained, and the procedures debugged, the existing procedure can be terminated.

Costs

Costs of acquiring software are a factor in selecting a particular package. Surprisingly, the actual purchase price of software is not necessarily a critical factor. Buyers are prepared for the direct costs of purchasing software. The direct costs cover the software program itself, and all supporting documentation and manuals needed for the program. However, there may be indirect costs in purchasing some software programs that must be investigated before making a decision. Software program literature has to be read carefully to determine if there will be additional hardware or software needed. Special language cards, interfaces, cables, or additional devices add to the cost. If a software program requires a certain type of card or operating system to function, and the user does not have that hardware, the additional cost can come as a rude and unpleasant surprise.

Direct costs
One type of direct cost that should be planned is the purchase of backup or archival copies of software. Several of the manufacturers of general applications software provide backup disks or sell them at nominal costs. Copying of software disks and documentation is subject to the copyright laws governing publications. Backup or archival copies may be made or purchased, but copies cannot be made for distribution. A more detailed discussion of the problems and issues involved in copying software is presented in chap. 11 of this text by Wilson.

Indirect costs
Indirect costs are those expenses not anticipated at the time the software is purchased. One of the major hidden costs of software is the time not only for training but for supervising personnel to use software. Special workshops, tutorials, or release time for classes help personnel develop poficiency in using the program. While it may seem obvious, the amount of time provided to learning a program should be considered in calculating software costs. Small amounts of time provided on a regular basis (1–1½ hours per day over a 2-week span) are more effective than longer segments of time at irregular intervals, such as a half day every 2 weeks. The longer the period between sessions, the more that is forgotten. When the program is used infrequently, the commands and documentation have to be relearned. As with any other foreign language it is less costly to provide regular time for program mastery than to have long intervals between sessions. In the long run, the program will be implemented quicker and more effectively if release time is provided for learning the program.

ADDITIONAL SOFTWARE CONSIDERATIONS

In addition to the criteria described above, consideration must be given to more technical aspects of software. It has been argued that all a user needs to know about software is how to operate it. Like a telephone, an individual does not need to know the technological basis of software operation. This view, while valid in the case of games, is rather simplistic for software to be used for clinical, administrative, instructional, and research applications. A user probably doesn't have to know how to write programs, but does need to know about different languages, versions of programming languages, software compatibility, and other considerations. Unless aware of some of the software and system considerations, the user is in the position of being sold software rather than of buying software. A knowledgeable buyer of software selects software that suits that individual's needs. Lack of awareness of some of the technical aspects can put a user in the position of being sold software that does not do the task completely, cannot be modified, or is not appropriate for intended applications.

One of the first considerations deals with the software system. Software is written to operate on particular hardware systems and will not operate on other microcomputer systems. Between the user and a microcomputer's central processing unit (CPU) are a series of "layers" of software that govern operations. These layers of software act to transform information into content and form that can be understood and executed by the CPU. Closest to the CPU itself is the operating system that governs general operation of the components, communicates with peripheral hardware, and directs other functions of the system. Application programs are based on the operating system formats and requirements and enable the user to perform certain applications functions such as word processing, financial analysis and management, data management, or other specific applications. Several types of general purpose applications software have different versions, each designed to operate with a particular operating system on a particular brand of microcomputer. Care must be taken to verify that a program will operate on the user's microcomputer system.

Programming languages

When software features are being evaluated, consideration needs to be given to three additional factors: (a) the language of the software; (b) hardware considerations; and (c) compatibility with other software. Programming languages differ in characteristics, complexity, and speed of operation. Users need to determine the language a program is written in for the following reasons: (a) to verify that language cards are contained within their system; (b) to estimate the difficulties involved in modifying the program source code to adapt the program if needed, and (c) to ensure that any modifications use the appropriate terms and forms unique to that language.

Programming languages allow the user to write or issue commands in simplified English that can be understood by the computer. The content of the language and the rules for its use reside either within the microcomputer's central processing unit (CPU), on special cards added to the internal circuitry, or in programs stored on disks. Only software written in a language that the computer understands or uses can be operated on a given microcomputer. For example, if the microcomputer lacks the capacity to operate applications software in a certain language (e.g., Pascal), additional circuit boards or language disks will need to be purchased to operate the software.

Program software can be written in any number of languages. Programming languages are classified according to levels. Low-level languages are highly complex languages that allow control of microcomputer operation directly. Ultimately, the only language that a microcomputer acknowledges is machine language. Each instruction in machine language consists of a string of binary digits that designate the operation to be performed and the memory location for that operation. Programs written in machine language are processed quickly. However, writing programs in machine language is complex, tedious, and prone to error, according to Graham (1983), because of the complexities of the coding system.

Assembly language, on the other hand, is also a low-level language that uses codes (mnemonics) to represent operations and memory locations rather than binary strings. As the CPU only accepts commands in machine language, data or commands written in assembly language must be converted. An assembler is a program that translates assembly language into machine language. Because of the type of mnemonic coding of commands, it is simpler for programmers to write or modify programs in assembly language than in machine language. In general, programs written in assembly language or machine language will operate only with specific microprocessors. Consequently, machine language and assembly language programs are machine dependent and are not portable.

Most applications software is written in one of the high-level languages (Graham, 1983). High-level languages use words and terms to designate operations that are meaningful to users rather than letter string codes or strings of binary information. Although there are over 170 higher level languages available, most programs are written in one of about 10 different languages or versions of those languages. Software programs written in high-level languages must be translated into machine language code.

There is a difference between compiler programs and interpreter programs. Interpreters analyze and carry out commands of high-level languages by making an intermediate translation into machine language. Compilers do the actual translation directly. Compilers are software programs which translate high-level languages into machine language for the microcomputer. When using applications programs that involve a compiler, the information is translated and the program is executed in one chunk. Interpreters, on the other hand, translate information from applications programs into machine language on a line-by-line basis (Poole, McNiff, & Cook, 1981). On microcomputers this usually entails rereading the ASCII score every time a line is executed. Software that uses compilers may perform operations more efficiently. Most applications software written in BASIC requires an interpreter program. While easier to modify, software written in BASIC operates slower. Special add-ons are available which compile programs written in BASIC, thereby increasing the speed of operation. The speed of operation may be important for programs that require feedback to the user.

Features of software languages

The ease with which software may be operated or modified, the speed of operation, the amount of memory utilized by the program, and the dependence on a particular microprocessor or operating system are factors to consider in the evaluation of software. Low-level languages and high-level languages are used in each microcomputer system. Low-level languages are considered to be both device and system dependent. Programs written in low-level languages will only operate on systems with a particular microprocessor or operating system. While programs in low-level languages may operate faster and require less memory, their complexity and device dependence restricts them to particular microcomputers.

Most applications programs are written in one of the high-level languages such as BASIC, Pascal, or FORTRAN. Each of the high-level languages has some special characteristic in terms of its lexicon, organizational structure, or memory requirements that make it better for some types of applications than others. Programs written in such high-level languages are simpler to operate and easier to modify than programs written in assembly or machine language. Software programs, particularly those with clinical applications, may need modification for individual clients. While the software may be protected by the manufacturer in order to prevent unauthorized copying, modifiability entails alteration of commands or information so the program operation can be altered.

Table 6-1 presents information about key differences between high- and low-level languages. Eight factors that differentiate the features of the two classes of programming languages are described. Ease of operation, independence, and capability for modifiability are features that characterize high-level languages. Low-level languages tend to require special training, are device

Table 6-1 Features of microcomputer software in different levels of programming languages

	Low level		High level		
	Machine	Assembly	BASIC	Pascal	FORTRAN
General availability	+	+	+	−	+
No special training needed	0	0	0	−	0
Ease of operation	0	0	+	+	+
Speed of operation	+	+	0	+	0
Low memory usage	+	+	0	+	−
System language independence	0	0	+	+	+
Modifiability	0	0	+	+	+
Device independence	0	0	+	+	+

Notes. (+) = Yes, (−) = Qualified yes, (0) = No

and system dependent, and are difficult to modify. Programs written in high-level languages take more memory and may be slower than those written in low-level languages.

SYSTEM CONSIDERATIONS

There is widespread agreement that in the case of general applications software, the selection of software should precede the selection of hardware. However, because of the need for special hardware for clinical and research applications, the needs and constraints of the hardware system must be considered when evaluating vertical applications software in communication disorders. Particularly in the case of software that has clinical applications, hardware characteristics such as memory size and expandability, capacity for peripherals, keyboard characteristics, and the program's language must be evaluated. While the package may include all the necessary software and documentation, there may be additional requirements that would necessitate additional hardware or the modification of existing hardware to operate the program.

Operating system language requirements

Each microcomputer system has its own operating system software. In most cases, an application program is written to be executed in conjunction with a particular operating system (Toong & Gupta, 1982). Software programs written for one operating system may not operate on another without modification of those systems. For example, without a special card or program, software written in Pascal will not operate on many microcomputers. Software specifications and documentation should be scrutinized to determine which language systems are needed.

Memory size

Memory capacity is important for software programs such as word processing, data management systems, or financial spread sheets. Vertical applications software that uses graphics or synthesized speech may require a larger memory component. Toong and Gupta (1982) indicate that the generation of color graphics can raise memory requirements by a factor of 4 or more. When the hardware lacks the memory capacity to operate a software program or if the system cannot be expanded, the program is rendered inoperable. If considerable amounts of the system memory are utilized by graphics, the amount of other data that can be managed concurrently will be restricted. While a minimum of 48K of memory is needed to operate the majority of applications software, at least 64K and preferrably 128K is needed if graphics and animation are involved.

Peripherals and add-ons

Peripherals and add-ons are extra hardware devices that are utilized in the inputting or the outputting of information. Disk drives, speech recognition devices, MODEMs, light pens, digitizer pads, and touch screens are all hardware devices that can be added to the basic microcomputer system. Printers, telecommunication equipment, and speech synthesizers are add-on devices that enable information to be sent in different forms. Each of these peripheral devices expands the efficiency of the microcomputer as a clinical, administrative, teaching, or academic tool. However, the capability of the microcomputer to effectively utilize these add-on devices is dictated by the available software. Special hardware will be of little value if the available software cannot activate those devices. The primary reasons for discussing peripheral and add-on devices in a chapter on software evaluation pertains to the costs that these devices add to the purchase or installation of software. As mentioned elsewhere, special operating systems, cards, or connections may need to be acquired to actualize the capabilities of the software.

Keyboard

The keyboard is the most common way to enter commands and to respond to program requests. The number of keys, the type of keys, the configuration of the keyboard, and the portability of the keyboard may need to be considered when evaluating software. Many microcomputer keyboards have the alphabet and number keys arranged like a typewriter. Special functions such as deletion, control, or cursor movement may have designated or programmable function keys. These extra keys make operations simpler to perform. Designated function keys are particularly helpful for operating more powerful general purpose applications software. However, in the case of programs which involve extensive entry of numerical data, the typewritten arrangement for number keys may be awkward and inefficient. Special numeric keyboards, similar to the number keys on adding machines and calculators, are built onto some keyboards or can be added on with special connectors.

Some additions to a keyboard may be needed for software programs that will be used by children with motor control problems. Large keys or special templates are available for use with children or adults who may lack the coordination to touch a specific key. Several microcomputers have detachable keyboards that are connected to the computer by a cable rather than being built into the unit. The portability of the keyboard may be a factor when considering software programs to be used in a clinical situation where the clinician or client cannot get close enough to the computer to operate a built-in keyboard.

Joysticks, paddles, light pens, a portable "mouse," or touch screens are conveniences to operate some software. These add-on devices may be optional for the clinician, researcher, instructor, or administrator using a microcomputer. However, for motorically impaired clients, these add-on devices are almost necessary for the client to enter information into the computer or operate applications software.

Special cards

Special cards or software programs may be needed to operate peripheral devices or vertical applications software. If the system does not already have these built into the original equipment, they will have to be added at additional cost. Careful screening and evaluation of documentation, together with consultation with other users, should identify which programs will require additional cards.

SUMMARY AND CONCLUSIONS

The evaluation of software is an art rather than a science. At present, criteria and procedures for evaluating software effectiveness are more subjective than objective in nature. The diversity of needs and applications constrains attempts to specify what constitutes effective software. Rather, an enlightened consumer approach to software evaluation is the most productive method for sifting through the maze of applications software. Key factors such as accuracy, ease of use, documentation, support, costs, and installation are all to be considered in selecting software. Analysis of published reviews, consulting with other users, and benchmark testing must be conducted before purchase. In the case of vertical applications software in communication disorders, users should determine the publisher's preview and return policy. Given the cost of software programs, users are as entitled to programs that work accurately, are easy to use, have comprehensive documentation, and have manufacturer or vendor support as the authors are to a profit for their product.

REFERENCES

Cohen, C. (1983, June). *Microcomputer applications: Management, evaluation, and treatment.* Shortcourse presented at the 1983 Director's Conference (American Speech-Language Hearing Association), San Antonio, TX.

Cohen, V. B. (1983). Criteria for the evaluation of microcomputer courseware. *Educational Technology, 23,* 9-14.

Datapro Research Corp (1982a). *User ratings of proprietary software* (MC73-100-101). Delran, NJ: Author.

Datapro Research Corp (1982b). *Perspective: Understanding and evaluating software* (MC13-050-11). Delran, NJ: Author.

Datapro Research Corp. (1982c). *How to select microcomputers for the corporate environment (Appendix A: Selection and evaluation checklist)* (M47-100-217). Delran, NJ: Author.

Frankel, P., & Gras, A. (1983). *The software sifter: An intelligent shopper's guide to buying computer software.* New York: MacMillan.

Glatzer, H. (1981). *Introduction to word processing.* Berkeley, CA: Sybex Publishers.

Gleason, G. (1981). Microcomputers in education. The state of the art. *Educational technology, 21:3,* 7-18.

Graham, N. (1983). *The mind tool: Computers and their impact on society* St. Paul, MN: West Publishing Co. (pp. 73-87).

Hannaford, A., & Taber, F. (1982, October). Microcomputer software for the handicapped: Development and evaluation. *Exceptional Children, 49:2,* 137-141.

Lathrop, A. (1982). Microcomputer software for instructional use: Where are the critical reviews? *The Computer Teacher, 9,* 22-26.

Mitchener, J. (1983). Database standards update. *Peelings II, 4:7,* 39-43.

Poole, l., McNiff, M., & Cook, S. (1981). *Apple II user's guide.* Berkeley, CA: Osborne/McGraw-Hill.

Roblyer, M. D. (1981). When is it "good courseware"? Problems in developing standards for microcomputer courseware. *Educational Technology, 21,* 47-54.

Rodwell, P. (1983). *The personal computer handbook.* Woodbury, NY: Barron's Educational Publishing.
Rushakoff, G. E. (1982, November). *A clinician's beginning model for the review of speech, language, and hearing microcomputer software.* Paper presented at the Annual Convention of the American Speech, Language, and Hearing Association, Toronto, Canada.
Sohr, D. (1983, May). Better software manuals. *Byte,* 286–294.
Sturdivant, P. (1983, Fall-Winter). Technology training: In search of a delivery system. *AEDS Journal, 17:1,* 55–68.
Taber, F. (1982). *Microcomputers in special education.* Reston, VA: Council for Exceptional Children.
Toong, H. D., & Gupta, A. (1982, December). Personal computers. *Scientific American, 247:6,* 86–108.

SECTION III
MICROCOMPUTER APPLICATIONS

Chapter 7

Clinical Applications in Communication Disorders

Gary E. Rushakoff

The microcomputer is a tool which has the capability of serving multiple purposes in the professional field of speech-language pathology and audiology. Speech-language pathologists and audiologists provide assessment, diagnosis, and treatment for the estimated 22 million communicatively impaired individuals in the United States (Wilbur, 1982). The microcomputer has significant potential to serve diagnostic, therapeutic, and administrative functions in areas of clinical rehabilitation.

The microcomputer has the potential to facilitate professional efficiency while at the same time providing for better services in the habilitation and rehabilitation of communicatively impaired populations. Clinically, the microcomputer can administer, score, and profile diagnostic tests; and perform and evaluate certain types of therapy activities, thereby saving the clinician time to concentrate on more complex cases. The microcomputer can save the clinician time in composing and correcting written material, and in maintaining client schedules, records, and therapy data (Rushakoff & Toossi, 1982; Rushakoff, 1983; Hood & Miller, chap. 10). Its data-keeping capabilities allow for ongoing collection of treatment data in addition to collection of data pertinent to planning for projected service needs. Due to the ever-growing availability of microcomputers within elementary schools and clinical rehabilitative services, the microcomputer is no longer an obscure device which has limited clinical utility and accessibility for speech-language pathologists.

RATIONALE

Microcomputer-assisted assessment

There are two basic types of assessment software, (1) microcomputer-administered assessments and (2) analysis programs. Microcomputer-administered assessment programs will present the stimulus item, accept a client response and, when the assessment is completed, provide the clinician with a detailed report of the results. Some programs such as the *Screening Test of Syntactic Abilities* (Quigley, Steinkamp, Power, & Jones, 1982) are solely designed as microcomputer-administered assessment software. However, many therapy programs also provide for baseline scores to be kept (Mills & Thomas, 1982; Wilson & Fox, 1982).

©College-Hill Press, Inc. All rights, including that of translation, reserved. No part of this publication may be reproduced without the written permission of the publisher.

Most of the assessment software available consist of analysis programs which are used by the clinician only after an evaluation. These programs allow the clinician to enter information; the computer then provides a detailed analysis of that information. The two areas where most of the developments have been conducted are phonetic analysis and linguistic analysis.

The two primary advantages of analysis software are that it saves the clinician's time and/or provides more information about the communicatively impaired individual. It is not critical that a program allow the clinician to spend less time working on an evaluation report. If, for example, a clinician normally spends 1 hour doing a linguistic analysis and a computer program also takes 1 hour, it is still of value if the computer program produces *more* information in that 1 hour. The more quality information a clinician has, the more effectively he can make a diagnosis and recommendations and plan for therapy.

There is the potential for some computer assessment software to analyze the information entered and also make suggested recommendations. We all understand that it is not really the computer making the analysis and recommendations, but the speech and hearing professional who designed the program. The computer just asks the questions the professional wants to know and makes decisions based on the instructions from the program designer. The only problem with these "expert programs" is that in the behavioral sciences, it is difficult for a computer program to account for all possible variables in an evaluation. In certain areas, many assessment variables can be taken into account, for example, in recommending possible hearing aids. Programs that present recommendations should be used by the clinician as an additional resource and not a professional dictum.

Microcomputer-assisted therapy

The microcomputer can present a stimulus through any combination of text, graphics (pictures), and speech. It can accept and evaluate a response and then, in some cases, provide a prompt or cue if the response was incorrect. When a response is correct it can also provide feedback and reinforcement. The microcomputer can also change the level of difficulty of the stimuli based upon its evaluation of the responses and also store data on the client's progress. In a very fundamental sense this is the type of task-oriented therapy used in many clinical situations.

The microcomputer with appropriate therapy software can serve as a powerful adjunct to the clinician. It is not clear at this time what percentage of the communicatively impaired population would be able to effectively utilize microcomputer-administered therapy as their primary source of services. Vaughn, Kramer, Ozley, Faucett, and Tidwell (1983) reported progress in Veterans Administration patients who received computer-administered therapy over telephone lines in their homes. Their level of progress as compared to traditional services is still being investigated.

One powerful application of microcomputer-administered therapy is as a supplement to traditional clinical services. Rushakoff and Edwards (1982) reported an improved attitude in a patient when she was able to work with the clinician once a week and several times a week (whenever she wanted) with the microcomputer. The increased time that a clinic patient spends in an interactive learning situation increases the prospect that the problem will be resolved in less time. This in turn may increase the patient's motivation.

Finally, there may be a large segment of the communicatively impaired population who are never seen or are underserviced because there are no professionals in their area or they are unable to regularly schedule direct clinic services. There is great potential for reaching this population through microcomputer-administered therapy or computer-delivered therapy over the telephone (Vaughn et al., 1983).

HISTORICAL DEVELOPMENTS

The multifaceted applications of microcomputers have been discussed in some detail in the educational literature (Allen & McCullough, 1980; Dickerson & Pritchard, 1981; Gleason, 1981; Watts, 1981). Although still in the early stages of development and use in speech-language pathology and audiology, there have been efforts made to use microcomputers for administrative and clinical applications.

Computers have typically been utilized in certain speech and hearing facilities for research activities and for client record maintenance and analysis. However there has been limited application of computers in the areas of assessment and habilitation. The following sections will discuss the use of computers and the early use of microcomputers in client record keeping (Elliott, Vegely, & Falvey, 1971; Harden, Harden, & Norris, 1977; Peterson, 1977; Rushakoff, Vinson, Penner, & Messal, 1979; Rushakoff & Toossi, 1982), assessment (Fields & Renshaw, 1978; Somers, 1979; Telage, 1980; Wilson & Fox, 1981b), and habilitation (Fitch & Terrio, 1975; Nickerson, Kalikow, & Stevens, 1976; Hight, 1981; Macurik, 1981; Mills & Thomas, 1982; Rushakoff & Edwards, 1982; Wilson & Fox, 1982, 1983a).

Record keeping

Elliott et al. (1971), at the Central Institute for the Deaf, developed one of the first programs for computerizing clinical data. The program was designed to serve clinic and research needs based on information from client files. The authors designed computer programs which provided for the updating of client records. Client information, test scores, and audiograms of children enrolled at CID were stored on the computer. This program was used to obtain descriptive analyses of their client populations. In addition, their program had the potential to evaluate the effectiveness of certain clinical procedures.

In the previous study, data were collected on forms and then keypunched for entry into a computer system. Peterson (1977) described an improvement in this data entry process in which the information was filled out by clinic supervisors on custom-designed optical scan forms that could be entered into the computer without keypunching. The major disadvantage of this system was the prohibitive cost of designing a custom form; however, Peterson argued that the cost of the form design was offset by the potential savings on keypunching.

Rushakoff et al. (1979) described a computerized record keeping program on a mainframe computer for a speech and hearing department in a residential facility for the mentally retarded. They collected 50 pieces of information on the 1,100 residents at the facility. The purpose of the project was to provide computerized summary reports on all residents and to plan for projected service needs. For example, from the information compiled from this computerized system, it was determined that 67% of the residents did not or could not communicate through the speech mode. This information was used to determine specific equipment and material needs, necessary areas of specialization for prospective employees, and inservice training needs for speech and hearing clinicians and other staff at the facility. The computerized data also indicated where clinical time could be saved. For example, 98 out of 100 residents who passed an initial hearing screening also later passed a complete audiological evaluation. These data were useful in prioritizing future scheduling for audiologic evaluations.

This project highlighted two major difficulties in maintaining computerized client files. First, it was difficult for the clinicians to agree upon information needed, and how the information could be recorded in a systematic form. Second, because it was necessary to use a computer programmer each time the data were queried and since several days were required to obtain a printout of even one question, the use of the computerized data system was somewhat unattractive to the clinicians on staff.

To maintain expandable therapy data logs, Rushakoff and Toossi (1982) developed a program for maintaining individual client therapy data on a microcomputer system. Its purpose is to allow the clinician to store and update goals and session data. The program continually prompts the user through every stage of data entry and retrieval. First, the program asks for basic identification and demographic information and then prompts the clinician to enter from 1 to 10 therapy goals, to each of which up to 16 updates can be added. The program permits all information to be changed and updated at any time and allows the clinician to sort the records alphabetically by client name. All records, sorted or unsorted, can be viewed on the monitor or printed out.

Maintaining client assessment and habilitation data on the microcomputer is a significant application for speech–language pathologists and audiologists who serve communicatively handicapped populations. This application is becoming increasingly more prevalent as clinicians learn to utilize data base microcomputer programs (Rushakoff, 1983).

Diagnostic and therapeutic applications

It may be difficult to pinpoint the time period when technology first made its appearance in speech pathology and audiology; however, the works by Holland (1960) and Garrett (1968, 1973) are significant in their contributions to the impact of technology in therapy. Holland and Matthews (1963) developed a "program" and a "teaching machine" to study the effectiveness of of self-instruction techniques for teaching speech sound discrimination to children with defective articulation. The purpose of the program was to teach discrimination of the /s/ phoneme to children with misarticulation of /s/. The subject was placed in front of a panel with three large color-coded buttons on it. Prior to the tape recorder playing a stimulus item, the experimenter pressed one of three buttons on a panel hidden in his lap, indicating what the correct response should be. The subject listened to the auditory stimulus from a tape recorder, which then stopped. The subject had to press one of three buttons on a panel in front of him to indicate whether he had heard the /s/ sound. If the button the subject pressed matched the button the experimenter had pressed, the tape recorder went on to produce the next stimulus item. If the subject pressed a different key, the tape recorder rewound and presented the stimulus again. The author felt that the "clatter" caused by the rewinding of the tape recorder qualified as feedback. The program was tested on 27 children with disordered /s/ production. The children who worked with this program showed significant improvements in /s/ discrimination.

One liability of Holland and Matthew's teaching device was the need for the experimenter/clinician to issue the correct answer to the device prior to the subject responding to each stimulus. Garrett improved upon their device in that his Automated Speech Correction program (see Figure 7-1) did not require that the clinician be present during the operation of a program in discrimination training. During the 6 years of the research project the device and its discrimination-training programs were tested on 234 subjects who included college students and public school children with disordered articulation, institutionalized mentally retarded children, adult aphasics, and language-disordered children. Even though the results showed improvements in the subjects, Garrett's primary conclusion was that there were aspects of speech therapy which could be automated!

Although Holland and Garrett both found positive results in some of their subject groups there was a conspicuous non-rush to incorporate this concept of teaching machine/automated therapy further. During the 1970s there was increased use of the computer for clinical assessment purposes (Fields & Renshaw, 1978; Somers, 1979; Telage, 1980), but still very little in the therapeutic area (Boothroyd, Archambault, Adams, & Storm, 1975; Nickerson et al., 1976).

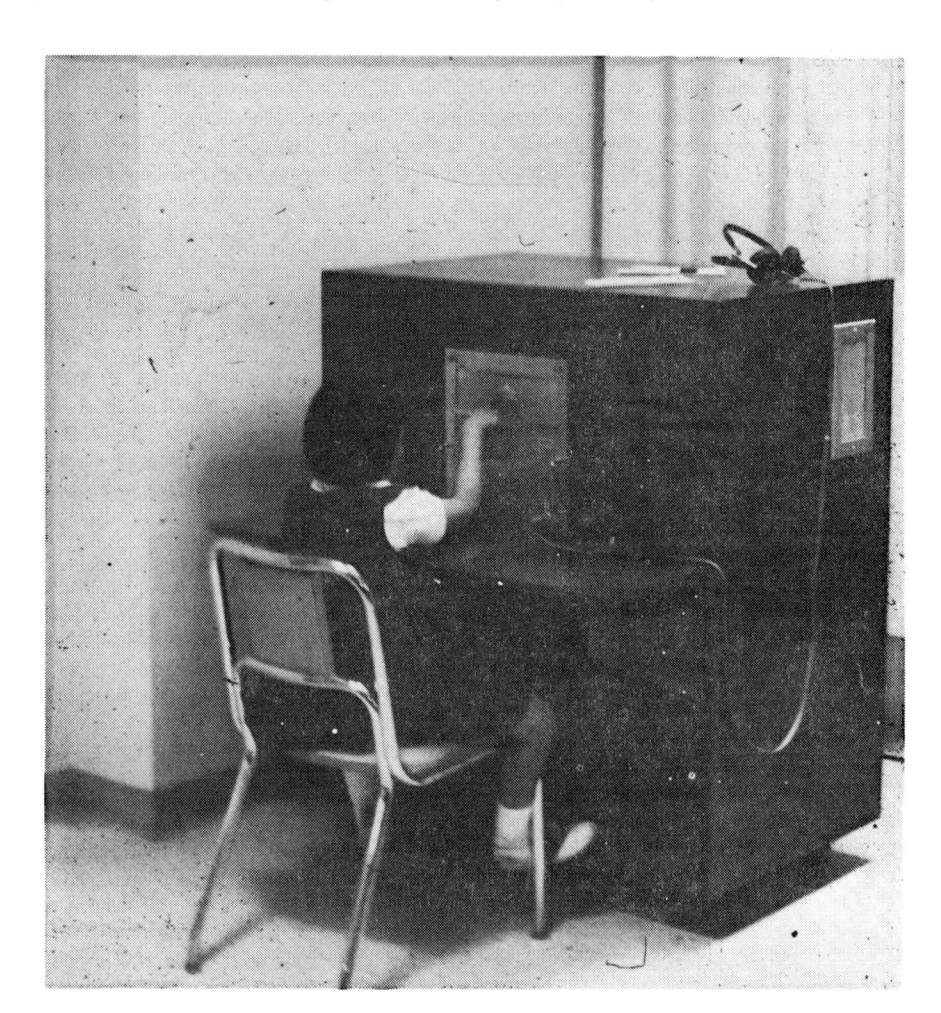

Figure 7-1. Garrett's Automated Speech Correction system (circa 1967).

Fields and Renshaw (1978) used a mainframe computer to analyze the language samples of children to determine if the computer could differentiate between language-disordered children and language-normal children. While the computer was able to discriminate between language-disordered and language-normal children, the investigators found that the computerized procedure was no more time efficient than the traditional manual analysis. They concluded that some of the time involved in the computer process (i.e., typing the transcript) could be delegated to nonprofessionals, thereby freeing the clinician for other clinical activities.

Nickerson et al. (1976) used a computer to help teach articulatory proficiency to 40 deaf and hearing-impaired children at a school for the hearing impaired. They developed several computer programs that provided visual feedback for various phonological components. The computer (DEC PDP-8E) was equipped with a speech recognition unit that analyzed students' verbal responses. The computer monitor provided visual feedback on the children's phonological productions. For example, the Cartoon Face program used an anterior sketch of a head and neck to provide feedback to the student. Voicing was indicated by appearance of an Adam's apple and loudness level was indicated by the size of mouth. The students were able to use the system with teacher assistance or independently. The students did show change in certain phonological skills; however, post-test assessment indicated that overall intelligibility of the test group did not improve significantly.

In a single-subject study, Fitch and Terrio (1975) used a mainframe computer with a voice-operated relay connected to a set of electronic filters to perform articulation therapy with a 6-year-old girl who presented a "functional" /s/ deviation. Stimulus cards were presented to the child by the clinician. The computer was programmed to analyze the child's speech responses and to provide the child with feedback on response accuracy. The computer indicated on the monitor whether the child should move to the next step, return to an easier level, or remain at the same level. The student completed the program in six sessions, a total time of 2 hours. The investigators considered the experiment complete when the subject produced the phoneme correctly and consistently in spontaneous speech. They concluded that the time factor compared favorably with traditional clinical procedures.

Somers (1979) and Telage (1980) have described computer programs to analyze the results of articulation assessment. Somers developed the Computerized Articulation Test to analyze articulation performance data obtained from The Edinburgh Articulation Test (Anthony, Bogle, Ingram, and McIsaac, 1971). He reported that one of the limitations of his program is that it was limited to analyzing data from one articulation test. Once the data are entered into the computer, the program provides seven tables of analyses, for example, an item-by-item comparison of test and target data and statistical feature analyses.

Telage (1980) designed a computer program to perform a series of segmental and componential articulation analyses. The objective of the program was to specify the patient's articulatory behaviors that contributed most significantly to the pattern of misarticulation. This program can be utilized after consonant misarticulations are identified and evaluated using the Deep Testing procedure (McDonald, 1964). The contextual sound error data from the Deep Test were entered into the mainframe computer using a keyboard and video screen. Analyses could then be viewed on the video terminal screen prior to printing a hardcopy. These data could then be utilized by the clinician in designing the most appropriate treatment program. Telage argued that computer analyses of misarticulations can significantly simplify the process of determining an individual's underlying patterns of misarticulation because the computer can easily scan and analyze a large representative sample of articulatory patterns in a short period of time.

Hight (1981) developed a microcomputer program for the Apple II microcomputer designed to assist in training the deaf and hearing-impaired in speechreading. The clinician or client types a word or sentence into the microcomputer. The entry is then displayed on the monitor in a series of animated lip movements. The client must determine which sentence was produced by the lip animation from four printed sentences that appear on the monitor. Data from the training sequence are stored on a diskette so that the clinician can determine the client's progress.

Several microcomputer programs were developed to augment instruction in fingerspelling for hearing-impaired individuals. For example, Kihneman and Salathiel's (1981) microcomputer program for the TRS-80 microcomputer is designed to teach fingerspelling by utilizing the graphics capability of the microcomputer. The program stores graphics (computer pictures) of the 26 hand positions for the fingerspelling alphabet. The user types in a series of letters or words, which are then displayed on the monitor. The speed with which the microcomputer produces the fingerspelling can be controlled so that certain commonly occurring groups of letters can be recognized more quickly.

Wilson and Fox (1981a, 1981b) used the microcomputer to assess language comprehension of prepositions in children. They initially designed the program to assess comprehension of three prepositions, "on," "in," and "under." Computer-generated pictures were presented on the monitor and verbal stimuli were presented by the microcomputer through the Supertalker, a speech digitizer. They used 10 of the 15 assessment plates to teach two young, developmentally delayed Franco-American children prepositions. The subjects were taught the propositions they failed with in the initial microcomputer assessment. The microcomputer remediation program was successful for both children.

Seron et al. (1980) used a DEC PDP-10 with a terminal to provide treatment of writing impairments in aphasic individuals. They tested the program on five subjects between the ages of 35 and 53 years. The subjects were required to type words dictated by the clinician. If the correct letter was typed in its correct position it appeared on the monitor. If a letter was incorrect it was not displayed, thereby "avoiding visual reinforcement of false choices" (p. 45). The results showed a reduction in the number of misspelled words.

Katz and Nagy (1982) reported the results of a microcomputer program to test and treat reading ability in aphasic individuals. The *Computerized Aphasia Treatment System* consists of a diagnostic reading test, five reading treatment tasks, and one math task. Five subjects utilized the program with minimal clinician involvement. One subject had dropped out of the study because he had told the investigators previously of his lack of desire to "work with programmed material or any other activity that did not involve direct and individual interaction with a clinician." Stimulus items were written in a multiple-choice format and presented randomly. Patient data were automatically recorded onto the disk. The results showed varying degrees of improvement.

In a later study, Katz and Nagy (1983) reported the results from five aphasic subjects who utilized a microcomputer program designed to "improve accuracy and recognition time for aphasic patients in reading commonly used words." The program is designed as a drill of sixty-five 1- to 5-letter words. All 13 words in each set are presented on the monitor to familiarize the subject with them. The monitor is cleared and one of the words in large print is displayed on the screen for 0.01 second. Some subjects had to choose the word from a multiple-choice format and others had to type the word from memory. If correct, the next word appears. If incorrect, the item is repeated but appears on the monitor for a longer period of time. The rate is slowed until the subject responds correctly.

With the development of speech recognition devices for the microcomputer several programs have been developed to provide communication habilitation for the deaf and hearing impaired. Macurik (1981) developed a microcomputer program that uses a speech recognition unit. The model of the sound is entered into the microcomputer by the clinician or a tape recording and a visual display of the sound appears on a section of the monitor. The client is required to match the pattern of the model by speaking into the speech recognition unit and compare the visual display produced with the model.

The /s/ Meter (Rushakoff & Edwards, 1982) is an example of a microcomputer program that was successfully completed, but which can no longer be used. It was designed by this author as the result of a clinical experience with a 20-year-old pre-law student who had come to the clinic for an evaluation of a distorted /s/ phoneme due to life-long bilateral hearing loss. She stated that she had received therapy for this problem several times during her life and was concerned that it might affect her career ambitions. At the conclusion of the evaluation it was recommended that she be scheduled for therapy; however, she stated that she had received therapy many times before and had thought there must be something different we could do for her.

The program that was designed used an Apple II microcomputer with the Heuristics Speechlink speech recognition unit (see Figure 7-2) and could discriminate a "target" /s/ phoneme. The program was designed so that it could be used by both children and adults. The client could practice the /s/ in isolation or in the initial position of a syllable or word. The program would judge the sound in one of three levels of production (1) correct, (2) incorrect, but close, and (3) incorrect.

If the phoneme was judged to be wrong (by the designer who programmed that judgment) a green line would appear near the bottom of the screen. At the bottom of the screen would appear the message "Incorrect." If the phoneme was a close approximation the green line would

Figure 7-2. The /s/ Meter as a dedicated device, circa 1964 (top) and microcomputer version with speech recognition unit attached (bottom).

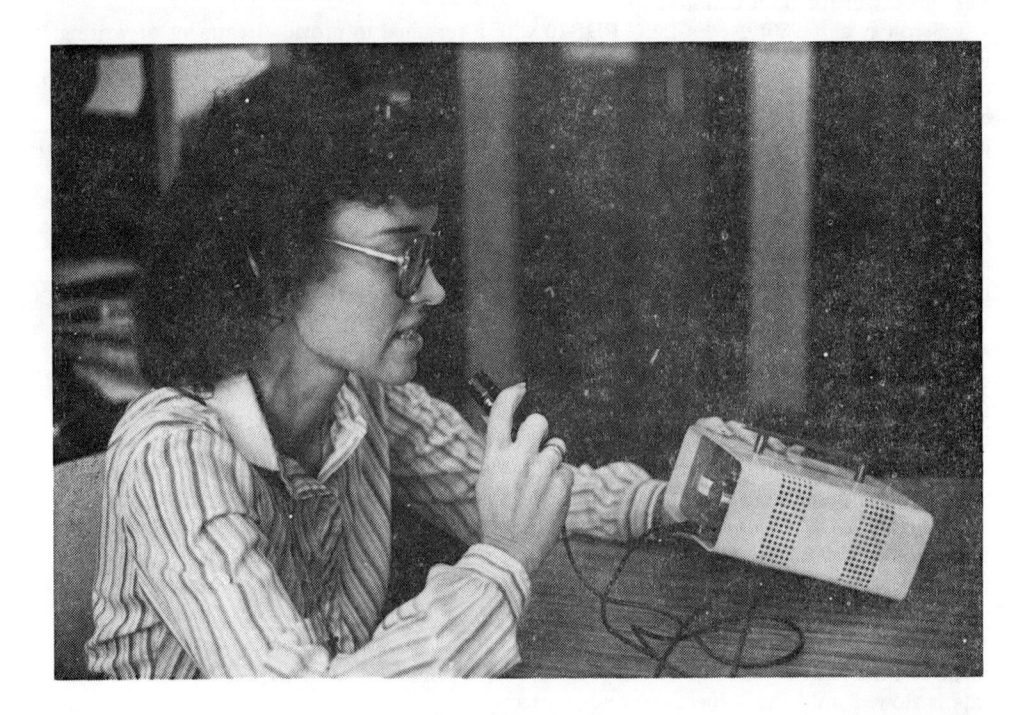

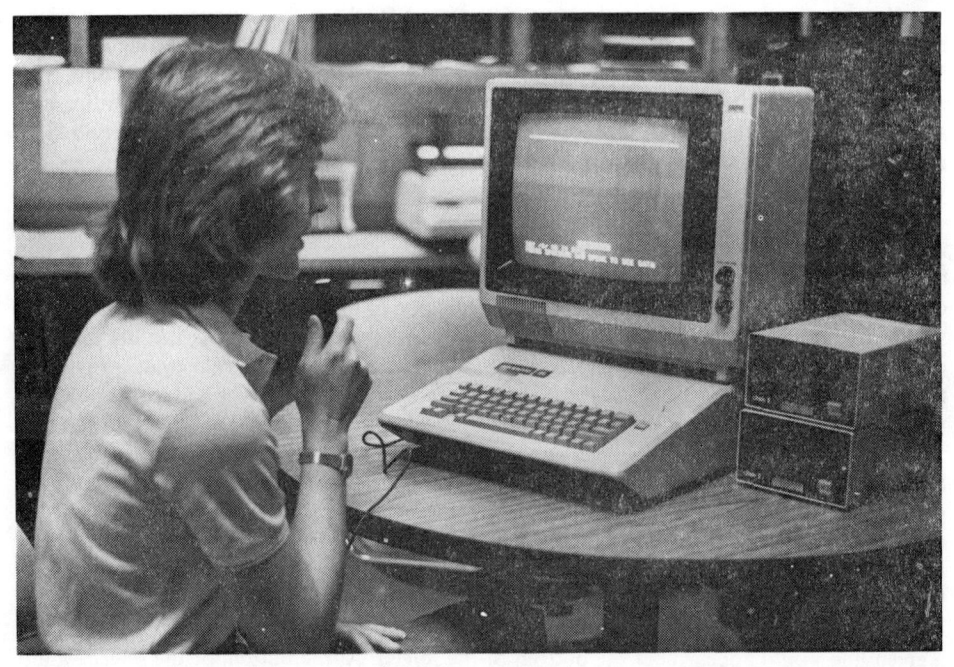

jump to the middle of the screen, paired with an audible "beep" from the microcomputer and the message "Incorrect, but close" would appear at the bottom of the screen. If the /s/ phoneme was correct the green line appeared at the top of the screen, there would be three "beeps" from the microcomputer, and the message "Correct" would appear at the bottom of the screen. Whenever the client wanted to end a session she just had to press any key on the keyboard and the data from that session would be displayed.

When completed, the program was used by another student who had come to the clinic with an /s/ phoneme distortion. She received 4 weeks of traditional therapy and during the fifth week she was shown how to use *The /s/ Meter* on her own. She was very enthusiastic about using the program and signed up to use it three to four times a week for 5- to 10-min segments for the last 2 months of therapy. She stated the microcomputer program increased her motivation because she was able to work on her own and it allowed her to practice more times during the week.

Just as validation studies were being planned for the program, it was learned that Heuristics, the company that manufactured the Speechlink, had gone out of business. This meant the program could only be utilized by those few facilities that had already purchased the device. There will doubtless be more instances in the future where programs are written that utilize certain peripheral devices that may become obsolete.

HARDWARE NEEDS

Main components

The brand of microcomputer and peripherals needed by the speech and hearing clinician are significantly influenced by the microcomputer software developers in our field. If the only application clinicians are interested in is word processing or maintaining client records there are many brands of microcomputers to choose from, since these are "standard" applications. However, if clinicians want to utilize assessment and therapeutic software, they need the Apple II system or a microcomputer which will operate Apple software. The vast majority of the specialty software in communication disorders has been written for the Apple II and fewer programs are available for other brands of microcomputers.

A basic clinical system should consist of the following:
1. Microcomputer with 128K RAM. Due to its relatively low cost, clinicians should purchase the maximum amount of RAM (memory). Several of the programs currently available and others being developed utilize 64K RAM. For an additional cost, the microcomputer can be upgraded to 128K RAM. While clinicians may not need that much memory for assessment and therapy software at this time, it has definite advantages to those maintaining their client records on the system (see Hood & Miller, chap. 10). As stated above, the majority of assessment and therapy software available is written for the Apple II or Apple-compatible microcomputer systems. In most cases, other brands of microcomputers cannot operate Apple II software. There are a few exceptions. For example, with addition of a firmware card the IBM PC can operate most Apple II software. There are disk drives available for the Apple II microcomputer which will permit operation of Apple and some IBM PC software.
2. Dual disk drives. There are a growing number of clinical programs which require two disk drives. Mills and Thomas (1982) utilize the Supertalker speech digitizer which requires two disk drives. Also, some assessment programs such as *Lingquest 2* (Palin & Mordecai, 1982) operate with the program disk in one drive and the data collection disk in a second drive.

3. Monitor. Several therapy programs utilize high-resolution color graphics. A great deal of a program's effectiveness may be lost if the graphics are not used with a color monitor. The problem is that color monitors are not useful for software that utilizes only text. The text on a color monitor lacks sharpness, which if used over long periods of time could be uncomfortable. If the microcomputer is needed for 80-column word processing a color monitor is virtually impossible to use. If one microcomputer must be used both for therapy software with color graphics and with text-only software, it is advisable to purchase a monochrome (e.g., green screen) in addition to the color monitor. It is possible to hook both monitors to the microcomputer at the same time using an inexpensive Y- cord that can be purchased at any local electronics or stereo store. This alleviates the need to constantly connect and disconnect monitor cords. Just turn on whichever monitor is needed. A recent development is a new monitor which can be used as an RGB color, amber, or green monochrome monitor by changing a setting on the monitor's dial.
4. Printer. Several therapy microcomputer programs maintain data on the client's progress. These data can usually then be viewed on the monitor or printed out. Most assessment analysis programs require that a printer be used. It would be a waste of valuable time for the clinician to sit at the monitor and copy down pages of analysis information. Some programs require a specific printer. For example, some phonological analysis software requires dot-matrix printers that are capable of printing phonetic symbols. Since a few printers are available that can be purchased in even the $300–$400 range, this should not be an item that is omitted.

Peripherals

In addition to these basic components, the clinician may find the need for a number of peripheral devices, some of which are currently being used with assessment and therapy software and others which may prove useful in the near future (also see Chial, chap. 5).

Speech recognition

Speech recognition units are devices that allow the microcomputer to "hear" sound. The units available today allow one to "train" the microcomputer to understand a series of words (Gabel, 1982). For example, if a program required the pressing of the return key, in the speech recognition training phase the clinician would type out the word "return," and the microcomputer would then ask her to say that word. It does not care if the word is spoken correctly or with an accent. It just remembers the sound pattern it heard when it asked the clinician to speak the word "return."

Although using this unit as an input device has some interesting applications, its greatest potential would seem to be in its use for speech therapy (Macurik, 1981; Rushakoff & Edwards, 1982). Two of the fundamental aspects of speech therapy are to make qualitative judgments of an acoustic pattern produced by a phonetically disordered individual and then to provide suggestions on what can be done to change that acoustic pattern. Microcomputers with speech recognition units can be programmed to provide a visual representation of a sound. This feature can be especially useful for clients who would like to practice their sound production on their own. There are two severe limitations to this approach. One is that the speech recognition unit can only operate on a sound in isolation (or possibly as the first sound of an utterance). Also, at this time it is doubtful that, based on sound analysis alone, the microcomputer would be able to provide specific, effective recommendations for changing the sound pattern to the target.

Light pen

The light pen is a relatively inexpensive (starting at $30) and, especially for children, easy-to-use alternative to the keyboard. The "pen" is connected to the computer, which can determine where it is being pointed on the monitor. This may be of value in assessment or therapy programs that use groups of pictures; the child merely has to touch (or for some pens just point to) the picture. While there are no clinical programs available at this time which utilize a light pen, some programs may be modified by someone with programming experience so that a light pen can be used.

Touch screen

An even more interesting alternative to the speech recognition unit and light pen is the touch screen (Figure 7-3). The idea is the same as the light pen; however, in this case the individual merely has to touch the appropriate part of the screen. While some monitors are built specifically (and expensively) as touch screen monitors, there are now devices available that can turn most standard monitors into touch screens. One of these devices is a frame with a series of infrared lights embedded in it and placed over the monitor. When a finger touches the screen it breaks the light beams crossing the front of the screen. These devices could also be used by physically impaired individuals who are using other types of pointers such as a head-stick pointer.

The touch screen/microcomputer system with a video disc was used by Thorkildsen, Allard, and Reid (1983) to teach prepositions to learning-disabled and mentally retarded children. The child responded to the program using the touch screen color monitor. The program used live-action video segments, not static computer-generated graphics. For example, one video segment was of a chair with one hat on the chair and another underneath it. The audio portion instructed the child to touch the hat on the chair. If after a certain length of time the child did not touch the screen, it would show a live action video segment of an adult showing the child, that when asked, he should touch the screen. The video segment of the chair was then replayed. After a set number of incorrect responses, a video segment was automatically played of the instructor touching the hat that is on the chair.

There are a few disadvantages to using a touch screen. After a length of time it may begin to get very tiring lifting one's arm up to touch the screen. A possible solution to this problem is to cut a hole in a table and place the monitor with the screen facing the ceiling but with a slight tilt toward the user. Another problem with the touch screen is that it may be difficult to use if the possible choices are too small or too close together on the screen. This can be solved by making sure the choices are large enough and not too close together. A final annoyance is that after continued use the monitor can become a bit difficult to use if covered with hundreds of fingerprints.

Speech output

A number of microcomputer programs have been developed that utilize speech output. These devices have allowed the microcomputer to be used as an alternative communication device by nonspeaking, severely physically impaired children and adults (Rushakoff & Lombardino, 1983). Nonspeaking, physically impaired individuals can operate the microcomputer through the standard keyboard, an expanded keyboard, or even a single switch. Once they can operate the microcomputer they can communicate using a speech synthesizer.

Speech output devices are also enjoying a growing use in therapy software (Mills & Thomas, 1982; Wilson and Fox, 1983a,b). There are two basic types of speech output: (1) digitized speech and (2) synthesized speech. While these two divisions may not satisfy the more advanced user, they form a good basis for the beginning microcomputer user. The speech digitizer comes with a firmware card, microphone, and speaker. If the clinician would like the program to actually

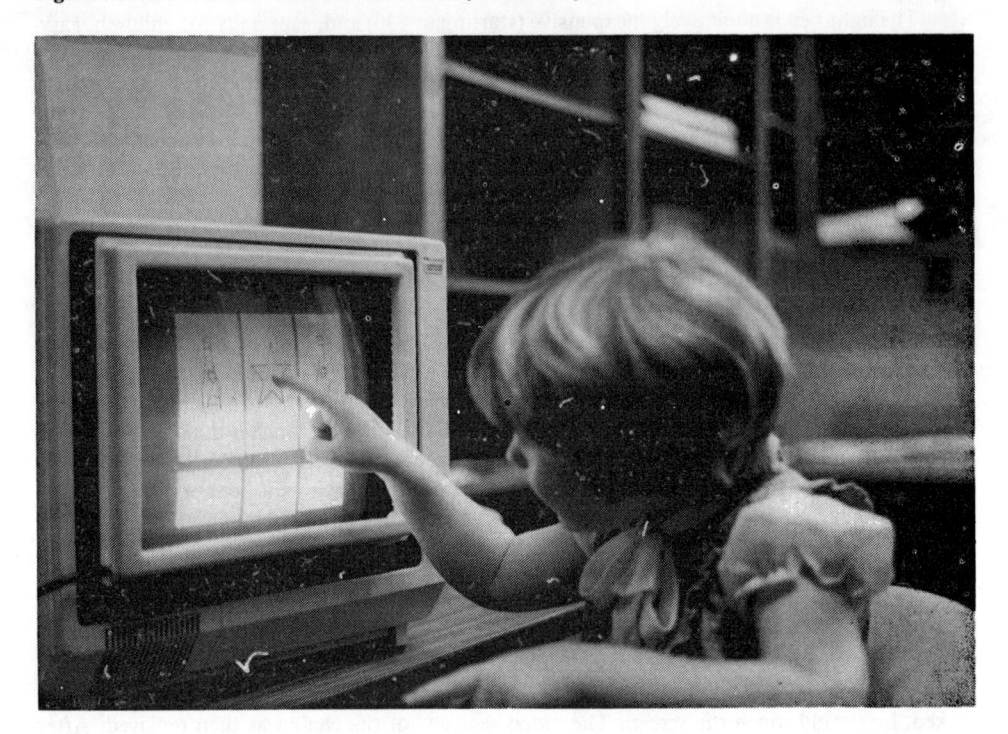

Figure 7-3. Touch screen as an alternative to keyboard entry.

say, "That's correct, keep going," she speaks that utterance into the microphone, which then stores information on how it was spoken on a diskette. When that sentence is reached in the operation of the program, the speech output sounds like that of the individual who spoke it into the microphone. In actual use, most clinicians will be using programs, such as the *Word Recognition Programs* (Mills & Thomas, 1982), where the digitized speech is already included in the software. The advantage of digitized speech is that it sounds "human-like." While the speech sounds "real," the fidelity is not high. The major limitation of this type of speech output is that it requires an enormous amount of space on a diskette. The end result is that a program may utilize only a limited number of utterances. This will change in the future as disk drives become able to hold more data. It can also be expected that there will be improvements in the sound reproduction of speech digitizers.

The other form of speech output is the speech synthesizer, which can range in price from $100 to $600. The phonemes used to generate speech are produced at the factory. These are the synthesizers that even in their improved versions today are occasionally described as having a slight "robot" quality to the speech. The advantage of speech synthesizers is that the program is not limited in the number of different utterances it can speak. One problem is that a program is usually only able to utilize one specific brand of synthesizer. It is likely that in the near future the quality of speech digitizers and synthesizers will improve.

EXISTING CLINICAL APPLICATIONS

In the following section a number of assessment and therapy microcomputer programs are described. The purpose of this section is to document the wide variety of specific clinical applications which have already been addressed by software developers. Their inclusion here cannot atttest to their quality or possible lack thereof but instead to their availability. There is no attempt to turn this section into a "Consumers' Report" of microcomputer software. Clinicians are directed back to the chapter on software evaluation to determine the worthiness of any particular program (see Schwartz, chap. 6). The brief descriptions provided are based upon material supplied by the author/distributor. For a more complete description of a program, clinicians should request information from the author/distributer.

Assessment

Software decision-making guidelines

The first question the clinician must ask is, "Does this program measure what I want measured and/or does it analyze it in the manner in which I want it analyzed?" If an assessment analysis program requires making numerous entries, it should have the capability to easily change, delete, or add an entry. Also, assessment programs should show no analysis information on the monitor that cannot be sent to the printer. It can be very time consuming to have to write down detailed assessment information from the monitor.

Analysis programs

BLACHE phonemic inventory. This program (Blache, 1984) provides information on phonetically delayed or disordered individuals. The following is included in the information summary: an estimate of the first sound system in need of therapy, a listing of defective sounds at each developmental level, a categorization of defective sounds by place and manner of articulation and voicing characteristics of defective sounds, a listing of the distinctive features that need therapy, and a sound substitution analysis program.

Phonological analysis by computer. Responses to 54 items are analyzed from the author's Phonological Process Analysis (Weiner, 1982). Some of the processes analyzed are stopping, prevocalic fronting, velar fronting, denasalization, fricative fronting, gliding of liquids, affrication, velar assimilation, labial assimilation, alveolar assimilation, and deletion of final consonants. The program also provides a process analysis on clusters, inlcuding stop + liquid cluster reduction, fricative + liquid cluster reduction, and /s/ + stop cluster reduction. Finally, a phonetic inventory is computed for each sound in initial and final word positions.

Lingquest 2. This program (Palin & Mordecai, 1982) performs a phonological analysis on a set of phonetically transcribed utterances or the results of formal or informal articulation tests. It analyzes omissions of consonant singletons in the initial, medial and final position of words and also two- and three-element blends in the initial position in words. It also provides a substitution profile, which is based on distinctive feature matrices that collapse the phonemes into their natural classes, presents a ratio of incorrect use for each consonant or vowel in error, and identifies the distinctive feature changes that contribute to a phonemic error. The program also provides a phonological process summary encompassing syllable structure and substitution and assimilation rules. Figure 7-4 shows the Phonologic Process Summary of a child with a phonological delay. It consolidates all of the phonemic substitution and omission analyses. The second column (Total Opps) indicates the total opportunities of occurrence in a speech sample and the first column the total instances of occurrence. The last column provides the total percentage of occurrence.

Distinctive Feature Analysis. Newton's program (1983) can utilize results from an articulation word list or conversational sample to provide a summary of all distinctive features,

Figure 7-4. Phonological Process Summary from Lingquest 2. (From Palin and Mordecai, 1982; reprinted by permission).

Process*	Total Occur	Total Opps	Percent Occur
1. Cluster Reduction	23	29	79%
2. Deletion of Initial Position Singletons	3	53	5%
3. Deletion of Final Position Singletons	35	73	47%
4. Syllable Deletion	3	179	1%
5. Velar Fronting	8	30	26%
6. Depalatalization	2	20	10%
7. Backing	14	240	5%
8. Stopping	25	79	31%
11. Palatalization	1	66	1%
12. Gliding	10	39	25%
14. Vocalization	7	27	25%
15. Labialization	7	97	7%
17. Devoicing of Final Position Singletons	8	40	20%
18. Labial Assimilation	6	88	6%
19. Velar Assimilation	1	97	1%
20. Alveolar Assimilation	8	44	18%
21. Nasal Assimilation	1	89	1%

the percentage of correct and incorrect productions, and a list of phonemes in which the features to be corrected occur.

Lingquest 1. This program (Mordecai, Palin, & Palmer, 1982) provides a grammatical analysis, including grammatical form, grammatical structure, and lexical and verb tense. When provided with contextual cues, an expanded form of the child's utterance can be entered with his actual utterance. The program can then perform a form analysis that includes the number of opportunities for occurrence, the number of correct instances of use, the percentage of correct usage, and the numbers and types of errors for eight form categories. A structure analysis identifies the number of opportunities for occurrence, the number of correct instances of use, and the percentage of correct usage for two phrase types (NP, VP), seven basic (simple) sentence types, eight question forms, and 12 complex sentence types. A detailed lexical analysis (type-token ratio) and a verb tense analysis are provided.

Systematic analysis of language transcripts (SALT). Miller and Chapman's program (1982) provides a detailed interactive analysis of free speech samples from one or two speakers. The program will perform the following measures: mean length of utterance in morphemes and words; distribution of utterances by word and morpheme length; distribution of number of utterances by speaking turn; type–token ratio for words in the first 50 utterances; frequency of occurrence of each word in the sample; bound morpheme frequency table; frequency tables for questions, conjunctions, modal verbs, semiauxiliaries, and negatives; a productivity analysis that determines the grammatical freedom of each different word root in the sample; a summary count of each category previously coded in the transcript; and a search routine to recall and code utterances.

Hearing aid selection. Several programs have been developed to aid the audiologist in selecting hearing aids. The *Computer-Assisted Hearing-Aid Evaluation and Fitting Program* (Popelka, 1983) is designed to assist the audiologist in selecting appropriate hearing aids, evaluating hearing aids, and in making necessary adjustments to the amplification characteristics of hearing aids. *Computerized Hearing Aid Selection* (Fitch, 1983) and the *Berger Hearing Prescription Method* (Berger & Gans, 1983) have also been developed as assessment analysis software to select appropriate hearing aids. The *Computer Assisted Hearing Aid Fitting and Sales Program* (K. Katz, 1984), in addition to suggesting possible aids based on the individual's loss, also suggests the volume the aid should be set at, calculates venting effects on frequency responses, adds in the pinna effect for all in-the-ear aids, and adds in the pinna/concha effect for canal aids.

Computerized assessment of intelligibility of dysarthric speech. This program (Yorkston, Beukelman, & Traynor, 1984) allows the clinician to quantify single-word intelligibility, sentence intelligibility, and speaking rates of adolescent and adult dysarthric speakers. The program randomly selects 50 words and 20 sentences from several hundred possible stimuli. Client responses are tape recorded and judged by another clinician. The scores are entered and the program provides the clinician with an analysis that includes percentage of correct responses, rate of intelligible words per minute, and an efficiency ratio which can be used to rank different dysarthric speakers and monitor change of performance over time.

Frenchay dysarthria assessment: Computer differential analysis. Clinicians can be provided with a precise differential diagnosis of one of five major groups of dysarthria: spastic, mixed, pyramidal, cerebellar, or flaccid (Enderby & Roworth, 1984). The results are based on clinician input of the results of the *Frenchay Dysarthria Assessment* (Enderby, 1983).

Microcomputer-administered software

Screening test of syntactic abilities. This program (Quigley et al., 1982) is based on the screening test of the same name. It provides a profile of a client's strengths and weaknesses in nine basic structures in English, including negation, question formation, relativization, conjunction, verb processes, determiners, pronominalization, and nominalization. The test summary provides percentage correct in each area.

Therapy

Software decision-making guidelines

The software decision-making guidelines which have been discussed previously in this book may sometimes be reduced to a very few major factors. The first is, "What is the objective of the program?" That is the part in the program description where it says, "The purpose of this program is to ..." If you cannot answer this first question, you need more information before purchasing. The second question is, "Is the objective of this program worthwhile?" This may be more appropriately stated as, "Is the objective of this program worthwhile to *me*?" If you

Figure 7-5. Blissymbolics Bliss Drill (From Wertz, Kehrberg, & Wertz, 1983; reprinted by permission).

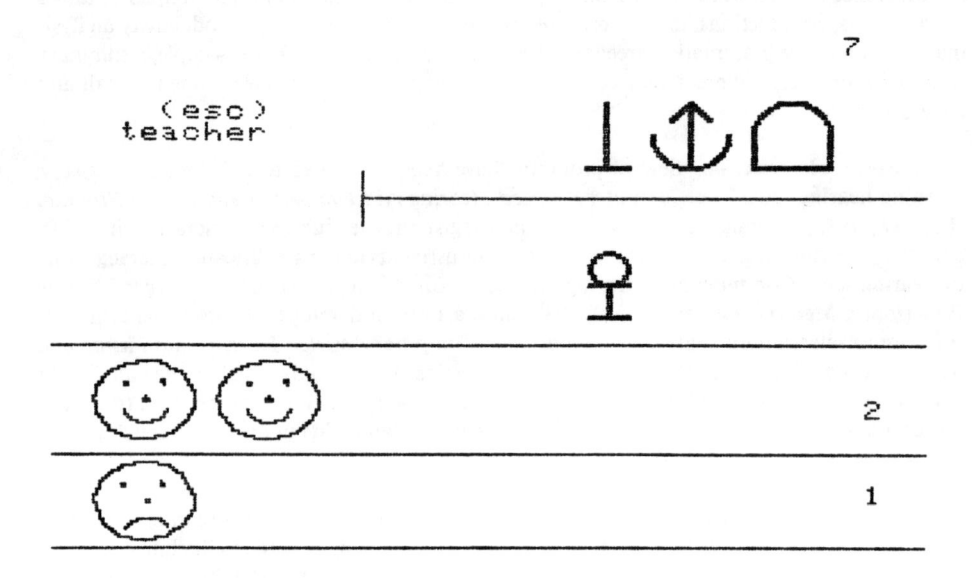

do not have an affirmative response to these two questions, you need to stop and consider whether to purchase the program.

Programs

Blissymbolics Bliss drills. Blissymbols is a symbol system used by many nonspeaking individuals. Wertz, Kehrberg, and Wertz (1983) have designed a program to assist the learning of individual Blissymbols and to distinguish them from others of similar appearance. In the single symbol drill (Figure 7-5), the clinician selects the target symbol and four distractor symbols. The target appears at the top of the screen and the distractors appear one at a time underneath. The child is to press any key (or auxiliary switch) when the matching symbol appears. In the word symbol drill section three target symbols appear at the top of the screen with their associated words just above them. The symbols disappear and soon begin to appear one at a time beneath one of the words. The child is to press a key (or switch) when the correct symbol appears underneath its matching word. These drills can be created and modified by the clinician.

Lessons in syntax. McCarr (1982) designed a computer program to develop the client's skill with eight English structures, including the negative, yes/no questions, Wh-questions, causal clauses (so/because), relative clauses, participles, indirect discourse, and passive voice. The program is recommended for users above the age of 9 with syntactic deficits.

First words. The purpose of this program (Wilson & Fox, 1982) is to train receptive vocabulary, utilizing high-resolution color graphics (Figure 7-6) and speech output with an ECHO II speech synthesizer. It uses 50 nouns that are among the earliest to be understood. There are six instructional levels. The 50 nouns are organized into 10 category sets where two pictures are used to train each word. The child can respond in two ways: either a scanning or direct selection mode. The clinician is able to set the level, category, and parameters of a lesson, including response time and criterion level. A lesson summary is provided at the end of the lesson (Figure 7-7). The level number indicates the instructional level. In this example, level 3 provides instruction, cuing, and feedback. The word category is "nouns" and it is operated

Clinical Applications 163

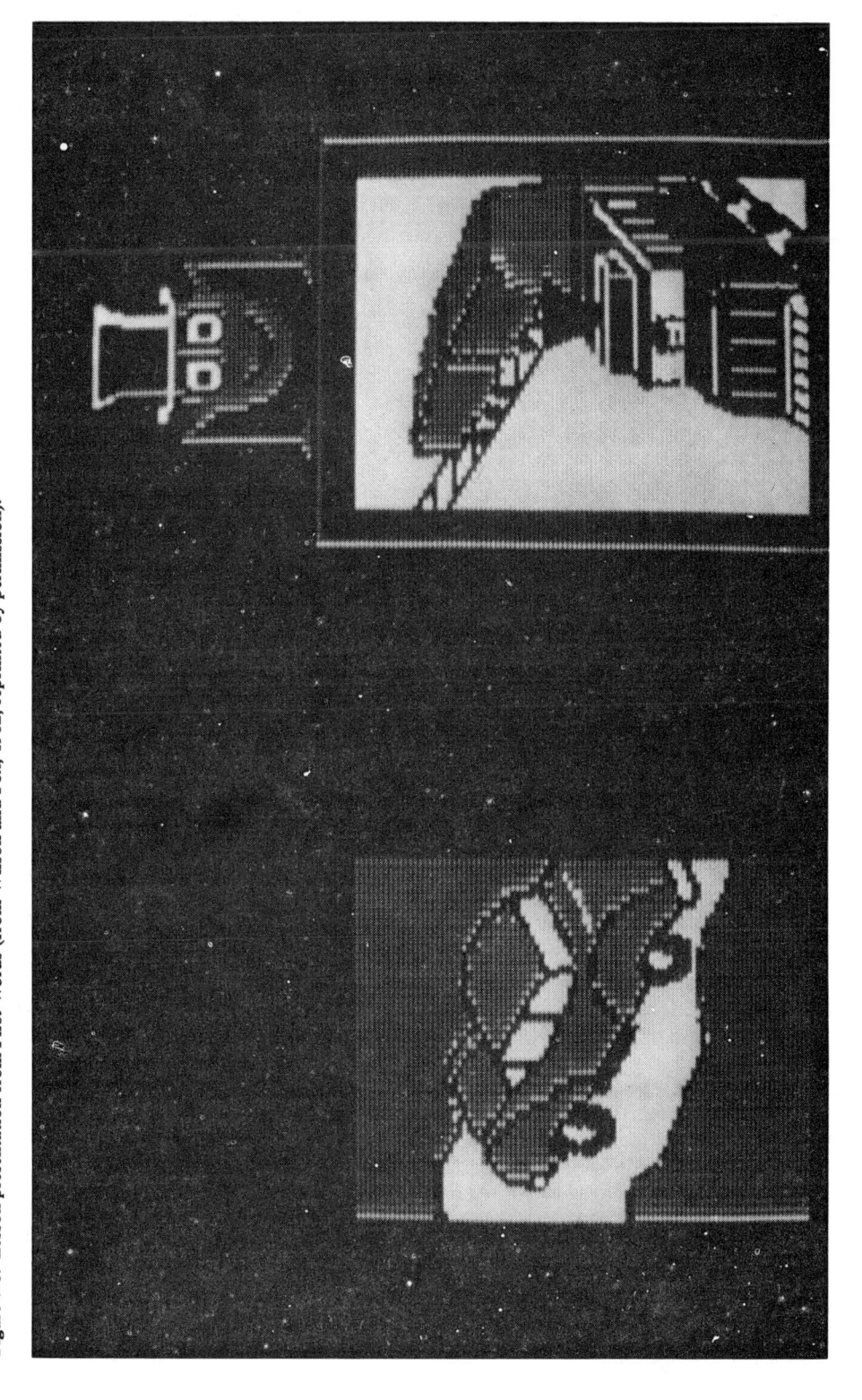

Figure 7-6. Lesson presentation from *First Words* (from Wilson and Fox, 1982; reprinted by permission).

Figure 7-7. Lesson Summary from *First Words*. (from Wilson & Fox, 1982; reprinted by permission).

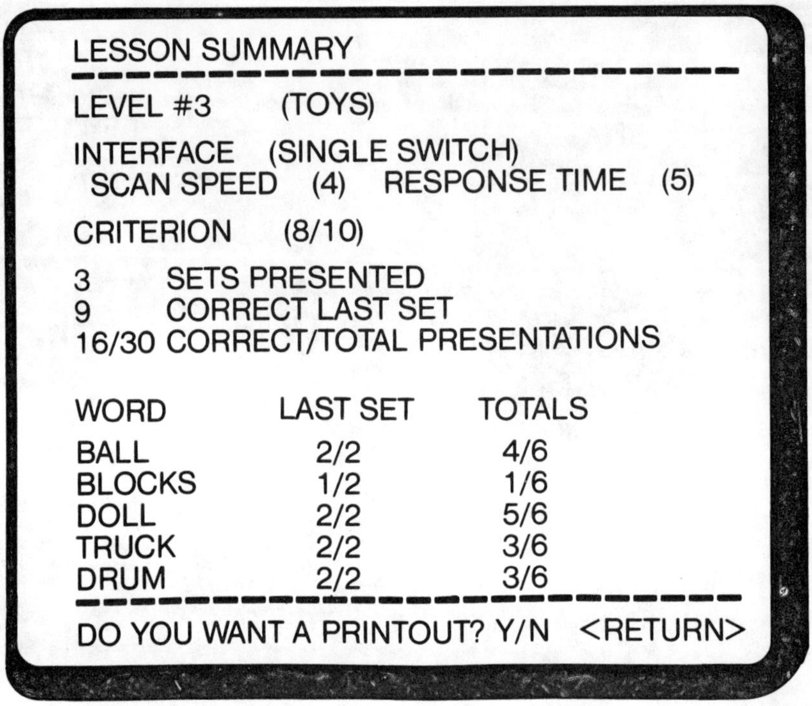

```
LESSON SUMMARY
------------------------------------
LEVEL #3      (TOYS)
INTERFACE   (SINGLE SWITCH)
  SCAN SPEED   (4)   RESPONSE TIME   (5)
CRITERION    (8/10)
3       SETS PRESENTED
9       CORRECT LAST SET
16/30 CORRECT/TOTAL PRESENTATIONS

WORD          LAST SET       TOTALS
BALL            2/2            4/6
BLOCKS          1/2            1/6
DOLL            2/2            5/6
TRUCK           2/2            3/6
DRUM            2/2            3/6
------------------------------------
DO YOU WANT A PRINTOUT? Y/N   <RETURN>
```

by a single switch at a scanning speed of 4 (in a scale of 1-10). The response time indicates how long the program will continue scanning before it moves to the next stimulus item if no response is made. The criterion in this example was set at 8 out of 10. The child went through three lessons, got nine out of 10 correct in the last lesson and 16 out of a total of 30 presented in the three lessons. The remainder of the summary presents data for each of the five words presented in the lesson followed by the scores in the last presentation set and finally the totals for each word from the three lesson presentations.

First categories. This program (Wilson & Fox, 1983a) is also a speech-output program that uses graphics and text to teach six noun categories on three levels of complexity. The program is described as being appropriate for learners at the beginning reading stage and learning-disabled children who have difficulty with categorization.

Micro-LADS. This language therapy program (Wilson & Fox, 1983b), which uses graphics, text, and speech output, is designed to teach the fundamental rules of grammar including verb forms, prepositions, pronouns, negatives, and Wh-questions.

Aphasia I: Noun association. Weiner (1983a) designed a microcomputer-assisted treatment program to help aphasics and others with reading and comprehension problems. This program teaches nouns that are parts of other nouns (foot-toe) and nouns that are associated with other nouns (salt-pepper). There are 20 lessons in this program, designed so that it can be used without the clinician present. The program stores client lesson data which can be printed out.

Aphasia II: Opposites and similarities. This program (Weiner, 1983b) is similar to Aphasia I except that it teaches opposites (hot–cold) and similarities (thin–narrow). The program can store data for up to 28 trials. Data can then be reported in bar graph form.

Minimal contrast therapy. Weiner (1983d) designed a microcomputer-assisted treatment program for children with unintelligible speech. This program utilizes the author's pragmatic approach to phonological disability. The rationale for this approach is described in the program manual. The clinician selects minimal-pairs for the treatment of one process at a time. The goal of this treatment is not correct sound production, but the elimination of the process. For example, if the child pronounced bow and boat the same (deleting the final consonant) any CVC response would be scored as correct and the clinician would act as if she understood the client. The program uses graphics to reinforce the child's correct response.

Word recognition programs. These are a series of programs designed for patients with auditory comprehension and auditory memory impairments (Mills & Thomas, 1982). The stimuli presented in these programs are printed on the monitor and spoken by the microcomputer through the Supertalker speech digitizer. The patient must then choose from one of four high-resolution color pictures on the monitor by entering the number of that picture or using a joystick to position a frame over the picture. The program provides verbal and visual feedback on the patient's response. When the program is completed it provides a data summary of the client's progress.

Understanding questions; Understanding sentences; Understanding stories. These programs (Katz, 1983a,b; Katz & LaPointe, 1983) are reading drills written for the reading-impaired individual (e.g., mildly to moderately impaired aphasic adults). The focus of *Understanding Sentences* is on recognizing and understanding "absurdities" (nonsensical or irrelevant words) in sentences. The program randomly selects 20 out of 40 sentences. The individual is required to read the sentence and indicate the correct answer by pressing 1, 2, or 3 on the keyboard. Performance data are maintained and can be recalled. The *Questions* program focuses on recognizing and understanding "question words" (i.e., who, what, where, why, when, how). The *Stories* program focuses on individuals who need to improve their understanding of simple, short stories.

GENERATING CLINICAL REPORTS

The microcomputer has proven to be equally as valuable to the clinician in nondirect as in direct therapy applications. It has the powerful capability to analyze a clinic population through maintaining client records (Rushakoff, 1983). There are several data base programs available for the microcomputer that allow clinicians to determine what information they want to store on their clients. Information can then be quickly gathered that can be used for administrative reports and in requesting more personnel, equipment, and materials. The information can also be used to pinpoint and provide justification for inservice training needs and, finally, it can be used in supporting documentation for grants.

Microcomputer data base programs which can be used to maintain client records can perform three basic types of processing. The first is *sorting*. With single-level sorting, all of the client records are sorted based on one factor. For example, all of the records can be sorted in alphabetical order or they can all be sorted in chronological order of age or by the date of evaluation. There is also a process called multilevel sort where the records are sorted by two or more factors. For example, they can first be sorted by clients' primary disorder and then, within each primary disorder category, they are sorted in alphabetical order.

Another processing feature of data base programs is sometimes called *frequency of occurrence* or *indexing*. This would answer a question such as, "Of all the clients evaluated during the past 24 months, how many were found to have a hearing loss?"

The most powerful feature in using data base programs to maintain client records is the *multilevel search*. This feature would allow one to give commands such as, "Print out an alphabetized list of male clients between the ages of 6 and 18 who have an articulation deficit, normal hearing, and live within the city limits."

Although microcomputers can maintain client records, they still have their limitations. Even by using every possible precaution and backup, it's still possible to "lose" computer records. It is not advisable at this point for the clinician to replace standard paper records. Also, floppy disks tend to make it a bit unwieldy to maintain large records on a great number of clients. Hard disk drives, although much more expensive, are the most efficient component for maintaining client records.

Word processing may save the clinician time in writing evaluation and progress reports. Some clinics need their reports prepared in a particular format with major headings and subheadings. The "form letter" option of many word processing programs allows the user to type only the body of the various sections and then print out the report with all the appropriate headings and subheadings.

There are a number of programs that allow the clinician to generate IEP reports (Weiner, 1983c; Berryman & Johnson, 1984). And, as has been described earlier in this chapter, there is a program that allows clinicians to maintain therapy data logs.

SOFTWARE AVAILABILITY

One problem that will be with us for a few years has to do with the availability of software. There are a number of reasons why programs which accomplish their objective do not seem to become "available" to other clinicians. One reason is that a number of program authors and developers are making their software available outside of a traditional publishing facility and therefore may not have the means to inform clinicians as to the availability of their software. Some software developers have incorporated, so as to make their software available in a more traditional fashion. These recently developed software publishers actively recruit other authors to submit their material for distribution. The reader may note from reviewing the reference section of this chapter that in 1983 and 1984 a number of publishers and clinical materials producers began marketing a wide range of clinical software.

Another reason for the lack of a wide selection of clinical software may be that some clinical software developers are not able to bring their concepts to fruition. To complete a program a developer must have a useful idea, an appropriate design for the concept, an easy-to-use computer program, clear directions, and, finally, field testing to confirm that all programming and design problems are resolved. Although only a moment of professional insight may be needed to produce the program concept, the other aspects of software development can be very time consuming.

Another problem related to the availability of clinical software is that there are a few facilities which do not recognize the design and development of computer software in the same light of scholarly achievement as a book, test, or journal article. This should change as computer software is reviewed in scholarly journals and is accepted also for distribution by traditional publishing companies.

LIMITATIONS OF CURRENT CLINICAL APPLICATIONS: NEEDS FOR FUTURE APPLICATIONS

Validating assessment software

If an assessment program provides information that a client responded correctly to four out of five tasks we have no difficulty confirming that. However, the myriad of output analyses offered by assessment software compels the working clinician to trust that the designer and the programmer did not make a "slip of the finger" in writing the program, producing an error which might be subtle enough to go unnoticed for a long time. The almost complete faith that computer users put in data printouts should serve to gird the clinician using computer assessments. There is no question about a computer being consistent, but if it is told in the program to divide the wrong numbers, it will do so over and over again with pitiless glee.

The traditional method for confirming that a program is operating appropriately is to compare the results with manual analyses. However, few clinicians would be able to take the time to validate each assessment program they receive. Software developers need to address this issue in their manuals.

Validating therapy software

There may be a tendency to be dazzled by the potential effectiveness of therapy software. Since it is traditional for treatment progams to be scrutinized by the rigors of research, clinicians are entitled to the same information on microcomputer treatment programs. This is a fertile area of research for clinicians. The information they provide would be of value not only to other clinicians but also to software developers, who need this type of rigorous feedback.

One of the significant advantages of computer software is that it can often be updated very quickly with modified versions available to those who purchased previous versions. Clinicians need to be familiar with the traditional system for indicating new versions of a computer program. Textbooks are marked by "edition" and software by "version," sometimes indicated by *Ver.* or simply *V.* The first version of a program will be marked V. 1.0 (or may not be marked at all). If minor changes are made in the program that make it slightly easier to operate or more efficient when running, the decimal number is changed (for example, to Version 1.1). If a substantive change is made which improves upon the objective of the program, then the integer number is changed (for example, Ver. 2.0).

In many cases clinicians may be able to purchase an updated version of their clinical software at a reduced cost. For example, if a clinician has purchased Version 1.0 of a therapy program for $100, she may be able to later purchase the updated version for $25. Clinicians should try to determine company policy on purchasing updated software.

Modifiable software

A future trend will be programs which allow the clinician to make modifications. While writing an entire microcomputer program from scratch may not be a reasonable objective for most clinical microcomputer users, making minor modifications in a program to better suit a particular client is reasonable. The two easiest aspects of a program a clinician can modify are (1) what text appears on the monitor and (2) how the text is arranged (formatted) on the monitor. There may be particular stimulus items that the clinician might think could be stated more effectively or the instructions that often appear on the monitor may not be clear. Changing these PRINT statements in a BASIC program is not difficult. The other problem that is easy to solve is formatting, which is the way text appears on the monitor and on a data printout.

The printout format of analysis software can be changed to make it more understandable to clinicians who have not used that program.

Some developers even advertise that their programs are modifiable. For a program to be modifiable, it must also be "unlocked." It is common to find some developers "locking" their programs. This process is designed to prevent copies from being made by clinicians who did not pay for the rights to use the program. However, locking software also makes it unmodifiable by clinicians who have paid to use it. It is unfortunate that because of the very few professionals who steal software, developers must lock their software, preventing any modification by other users.

Clinician-independent therapy

The potential for clinician-independent therapy and for home therapy is enormous and dazzling to imagine. This potential implies great responsibility for software developers and clinicians who wish to provide their clients with independent interactive therapy activities through the microcomputer. Although it is common for clinicians to assign their clients tasks to perform outside of the therapy session the microcomputer has the capability of providing feedback and modifying the stimuli based on clients' responses. Most of these clinician-independent therapy programs are designed to supplement the client's clinic sessions. The potential dangers may initially make it seem that clinician-independent programs are impossible: (1) prescribing the program to an inappropriate or unprepared client, (2) prescribing an inappropriate program, and (3) prescribing a program which collects data ineffectively. The area of clinician-independent therapy via the microcomputer bestows vast new responsibilities onto the clinician. The effectiveness and potential problems of clinician-independent software need to be rigorously researched.

Vaughn et al. (1983) described a series of computer-assisted therapy programs delivered over the telephone to communicatively impaired individuals in the Veterans Administration (VA) program. The Remote Machined-Assisted Treatment and Evaluation system (REMATE) proved effective with many VA patients who received supplementary treatment at their homes. The system was especially useful in providing certain types of services in areas where speech and hearing personnel were not available and to those who lived in remote areas.

While it is true that a well-designed and -tested microcomputer therapy program can present stimuli, evaluate a response, and provide feedback and reinforcement, it is not capable of responding to the crinkled brow of frustration nor the sparkling eyes of success. Clinicians may remember the introduction of computers in some schools in the 1960s that brought fears of replacing the teacher. It did not take long for everyone to realize that there was more to the learning process than a computer could perform. With an estimated 22 million communicatively handicapped individuals in the country there is no need to worry about the microcomputer assisting in certain therapy procedures.

CLINICIAN MICROCOMPUTER EDUCATION

During the 1960s and 1970s most speech and hearing clinicians who wanted to learn the benefits of computers in communication disorders were sent to the department of computer sciences where they learned how to program in FORTRAN or COBOL. Since few clinicians had access to mainframe computers, for most of them those programming skills proved useless. While some students are now being sent to Departments of Education for coursework, more academic speech and hearing programs are now beginning to offer their own course of instruction in clinical microcomputer applications (Rushakoff & Lombardino, 1984). To be successful clinical microcomputer users, clnicians need to know a relatively limited amount of information about computer programming and hardware. Clinicians who always need to modify commercial software or who desire to develop computer programs need to know more about programming and hardware than most clinicians.

SUMMARY

The microcomputer has been demonstrated to be an effective clinical tool for evaluation and treatment purposes. A primary reason for the initial minimal application of computers in speech and hearing activities has been the price and size of the large mainframe equipment. The recent development and proliferation of economical and small microcomputer systems has enhanced the feasibility of using microcomputers in rehabilitative professions. Although cost may have been the initial reason for the limited application of computers by speech and hearing clinicians, the current problem may be the lack of comprehensive clinical training available to clinicians in the multiple applications of computers.

REFERENCES

Allen, D., & McCullough, L. (1980). Education and technology: The changing basics. *Educational Technology, 20*(1), 47–53.

Anthony, A., Bogle, D., Ingram, T., & McIsaac, M. (1971). *The Edinburgh articulation test.* Edinburgh: Livingstone.

Berryman, J., & Johnson, R. (1984). *Planning individualized speech and language intervention programs: Computer software.* Tucson: Communication Skill Builders.

Blache, S. (1984). *BLACHE phonemic inventory,* San Diego: College-Hill Press.

Boothroyd, A., Archambault, P., Adams, R., & Storm, R. (1975). Use of computer-based system of speech analysis and display in a remedial speech program for deaf children. *Volta Review, 77,* 178–193.

Dickerson, L., & Pritchard, W. (1981). Microcomputers and education: Planning for the coming revolution in the classroom. *Educational Technology, 21*(1), 7–12.

Elliott, L., Vegely, A., & Falvey, N. (1971). Description of a computer-oriented record-keeping system. *Asha, 13*(8), 435–443.

Enderby, P. (1983). *Frenchay dysarthria assessment.* San Diego: College-Hill Press.

Enderby, P., & Roworth, M. (1984). *Frenchay dysarthria assessment: Computer differential analysis.* San Diego: College-Hill Press.

Fitch, J. L. (1983). *Computertized hearing aid selection.* Gulfport, MS: Communicology Associates.

Gabel, D. (1982). Voice command. *Personal Computing, 6*(11).

Garrett, E. R. (1968). *Speech and language therapy under an automated stimulus control system: Final report* (Project Number 3192). Submitted to the US Office of Education.

Garrett, E. R. (1973). Programmed articulation therapy. In W. Wolfe & D. Goulding (Eds.), *Articulation and learning* (pp. 106–138). Springfield, IL: Thomas.

Gleason, G. (1981). Microcomputers in education: The state of the art. *Educational Technology, 21*(3), 7–18.

Harden, R. J., Harden, R. W., & Norris, M. (1977). Computer program for the analysis of clinical enrollment. *Asha, 19*(7), 472–477.

Hight, R. L. (1981). Lip-reader trainer: A computer program for the hearing impaired. In P. Hazan (Ed.), *Proceedings of the Johns Hopkins first national search for applications of personal computing to aid the handicapped* (pp. 4,5). Los Angeles: IEEE Computer Society Press.

Holland, A., & Matthews, J. (1963). Application of teaching machine concepts to speech pathology and audiology. *Asha, 5,* 474–482.

Katz, R. (1983a). *Understanding questions*. Tucson: Communication Skill Builders.
Katz, R. (1983b). *Understanding stories*. Tucson: Communication Skill Builders.
Katz, K. (1984). *Computer assisted hearing aid fitting and sales program*. Tucson: Katz Computer Software.
Katz, R., & LaPointe, L. (1983). *Understanding sentences: Absurdities*. Tucson: Communication Skill Builders.
Katz, R., & Nagy, V. T. (1982). A computerized treatment system for chronic aphasic patients in R. H. Brookshire (Ed.), *Clinical aphasiology: Conference proceedings*. Minneapolis: BRK Publishers.
Katz, R., & Nagy, V. T. (1983). A computerized approach for improving word recognition in chronic aphasic patients. IN R. H. Brookshire (Ed.), *Clinical aphasiology: Conference proceedings*. Minneapolis: BRK Publishers.
Kihneman, K., & Salathiel, R. (1981). Computer fingerspelling. In P. Hazan (Ed.), *Proceedings of the Johns Hopkins first national search for application of personal computing to aid the handicapped* (pp. 33,34). Los Angeles: IEEE Computer Society Press.
Macurik, K. (1981). A vocalization trainer for the hearing impaired. In P. Hazan (Ed.), *Proceedings of the Johns Hopkins first national search for applications of personal computing to aid the handicapped* (pp. 2,3). Los Angeles: IEEE Computer Society Press.
McCarr, J. (1982). *Lessons in syntax*. Beaverton, OR: Dormac, Inc.
McDonald, E. T. (1964). *Articulation testing: A sensory–motor approach*. Pittsburgh: Stanwix House.
Mills, R., & Thomas, R. (1982). *Word recognition programs*. Ann Arbor, MI: Brain-Link Software.
Mordecai, D., Palin, M., & Palmer, C. (1982). *Lingquest 1: Language sample analysis*. Napa, CA: Lingquest Software.
Newton, M. (1983). *Distinctive feature analysis*. Burlington, NC: Southern Micro Systems.
Nickerson, R., Kalikow, C., & Stevens, K. (1976). Computer-aided speech training for the deaf. *Journal of Speech and Hearing Disorders, 41*(1), 120–132.
Palin, M., & Mordecai, D. (1982). *Lingquest 2: Phonological analysis*. Napa, CA: Lingquest Software.
Peterson, H. (1977). More about computer assisted clinical record keeping. *Asha, 19*(9), 617–618.
Popelka, G. R. (1983). *Computer-assisted hearing-aid evaluation and fitting program*. St. Louis: Publications Department of the Central Institute for the Deaf.
Quigley, S., Steinkamp, M., Power, D., & Jones, B. (1982). *Test of syntactic abilities: Screening tests form 1 and 2*. Beaverton, OR: Dormac, Inc.
Rushakoff, G. E., & Lombardino, L. J. (1983). Comprehensive microcomputer applications for non-vocal, severely physically handicapped children. *Teaching Exceptional Children, 16*(1), 18–22.
Rushakoff, G. E., & Lombardino, L. J. (1984). Microcomputer applications. Asha, 26:6, 27, 31.
Rushakoff, G. E., & Toossi, M. (1982). Therapy data collector. In J. Fitch (Ed.), *Software registry number one: Administration and clinical programs*. Mobile: ASHA Committee on Educational Technology.
Seron, X., Deloche, G., Moulard, J., & Rouselle, M. (1980). A computer-based therapy for the treatment of aphasic subjects with writing disorders. *Journal of Speech and Hearing Disorders, 45*, 45–58.
Somers, H. (1979). Using the computer to analyse articulation test data. *British Journal of Disorders of Communication, 14*(3), 231–240.
Telage, K. (1980). A computerized place-manner distinctive feature program for articulation analyses. *Journal of Speech and Hearing Disorders, 45*(4), 481–493.
Watts, N. (1981). A dozen uses for the computer in education. *Educational Technology, 21*(4), 18–22.
Weiner, F. (1982). *Phonological analysis by computer*. Baltimore: University Park Press.
Weiner, F. (1983a). *Aphasia I*. Baltimore: University Park Press.
Weiner, F. (1983b). *Aphasia II*. Baltimore: University Park Press.
Weiner, F. (1983c). *The IEP writer*. Baltimore: University Park Press.
Weiner, F. (1983d). *Minimal contrast therapy*. Baltimore: University Park Press.
Wertz, F., Kehrberg, K., & Wertz, J. (1983). *Blissymbolics Bliss drills*. St. Paul, MN: Minnesota Educational Computing Consortium.
Wilber, L.A. (1982). An open letter to the White House, Congress, executive department, and agency officials. *Asha, 24*(6), 387.
Wilson, M., & Fox, B. (1981a). The bilingual computer: Promise of the eighties. *Asha, 23*(9), 651–652.
Wilson, M., & Fox, B. (1982). *First words*. Burlington, VT: Laureate Learning Systems, Inc.
Wilson, M., & Fox, B. (1983a). *First categories*. Burlington, VT: Laureate Learning Systems, Inc.

Wilson, M., & Fox, B. (1983b). *Microcomputer language assessment and development system (Micro-LADS)*. Burlington, VT: Laureate Learning Systems, Inc.

Yorkston, K., Beukelman, D., & Traynor, C. (1984). *Computerized assessment of intelligibility of dysarthric speech*. Tigard, OR: C.C. Publications.

REFERENCE NOTES

Berger, K., & Gans, D. (1983). *Hearing aid selection by computer*. Paper presented at the American Speech-Language-Hearing Association annual convention, Cincinnati.

Fields, T. A., & Renshaw, S. (1978). *Use of the computer in the diagnosis of language disorders*. Paper presented at the American Speech and Hearing annual convention, San Francisco.

Fitch, J. L., & Terrio, L. M. (1975). *Computer assisted clinical services*. Paper presented at the American Speech and Hearing annual convention, Washington, D.C.

Holland, A. (1960). *The development and evaluation of teaching machine procedures for increasing auditory discrimination skill in children with articulatory disorders*. Unpublished doctoral dissertation, University of Pittsburgh.

Miller, J., & Chapman, R. (1982). *Systematic analysis of language transcripts (SALT)*. Unpublished manuscript, University of Wisconsin—Madison, the Language Analysis Laboratory, Waisman Center of Mental Retardation and Human Development.

Rushakoff, G. E. (1983). *Maintaining client records on the microcomputer: A beginner's guide*. Short course presented at the annual convention of the American Speech-Language-Hearing Association, Cincinnati.

Rushakoff, G. E., & Edwards W. (1982). *The /s/ meter: A beginning for microcomputer assisted articulation therapy*. Paper presented at the American Speech-Language-Hearing Association annual convention, Toronto.

Rushakoff, G. E., Vinson, B. P., Penner, K. A., & Messal, S. A. (1979). *Clinical decision making through electronic information processing*. Presented at the American Speech-Language-Hearing Association annual convention, Atlanta.

Thorkildsen, R., Allard, K., & Reid, B. (1983). *Interactive videodisc for special education technology: Presenting CAI to mentally handicapped students*. Paper presented at the Council for Exceptional Childrens conference on The Use of Microcomputers in Special Education, Hartford.

Vaughn, G. W., Kramer, J. O., Ozley, C. O., Faucett, R. A., & Tidwell, A. A. (1983). *REMATE Computer: Remote machine assisted treatment and evaluation*. Scientific exhibit presented at the annual convention of the American Speech-Language-Hearing Association, Cincinnati.

Wilson, M., & Fox, B. (1981b). *Computer administered bilingual language assessment and intervention: The promise of the eighties*. Paper presented at the Council for Exceptional Children conference, New Orleans.

Chapter 8

Research Applications in Communication Disorders

Robert B. Mahaffey

Microcomputers and their emerging technologies afford challenges and exciting new research opportunities for investigating normal and disordered communication processes, and they provide new measurement techniques and strategies for obtaining information previously viewed as unobtainable. Relative low cost coupled with innovative thinking is opening up possibilities for basic and applied research in sophisticated labs as well as in clinics and schools. The increased availability of microcomputers is nurturing interdisciplinary research that promotes increasingly comprehensive evaluation of communication and rehabilitation problems. Direct patient-computer interfacing provides a much-needed tool for therapy (see Rushakoff, chap. 7), and has the potential for increasing the importance of speech in the early diagnosis of neurological and cardiac disorders (Okada, 1983). Microcomputers have begun a revolution by providing the technology for creative basic and clinical research to those with a bit of ingenuity and a modest equipment budget.

Microcomputers come in many shapes, sizes, and levels of sophistication. The home computer may be designed for recreational purposes rather than laboratory purposes and is thought by many to be a toy. The type of microcomputer discussed in this chapter is the microprocessor-based system with extensive memory, interfacing capabilities, sophisticated operating system, and high-speed processing. These machines have exceeded the capabilities of most minicomputers that are 10 years of age. The term "microcomputer" has become a household word that describes a broad range of systems, but it will be helpful in reading this chapter to think of the "top-of-the-line" microcomputer rather than the recreational systems.

The focuses of this chapter are threefold. First, the impacts that microcomputers are having on research in speech-language pathology and audiology are discussed. Secondly, conceptual considerations for using the microcomputer in a research setting are presented; and finally, techniques are presented that may be helpful in using the microcomputer as both a data gathering device and a stimulus controller.

It is not the purpose of the chapter to suggest research designs, methods, or to review current applications. It is, however, necessary to review the basic terminology of research in order to examine the usefulness of the microcomputer in the process of research.

©College-Hill Press, Inc. All rights, including that of translation, reserved. No part of this publication may be reproduced without the written permission of the publisher.

A RESEARCH FRAMEWORK

Silverman (1977) defines *Research* as the "processes underlying the *asking* and *answering* of questions as well as to the 'answers' that can be abstracted from the observations provided by such processes." He emphasizes a need for reliable *data* obtained through well constructed *systematic observation* in answering questions. The term *data* refers to "numerical and verbal descriptions of attributes of events." *Systematic observation* is a process in which selected attributes of an event are recorded and coded in a manner such that resulting data accurately represent the event. Research methodology is planned with the objective of maximizing reliability and accuracy of observations and their analysis.

The strength of an observation depends upon the accuracy and validity of data collection. Objective data collection categorizes narrowly defined perceptions of attributes descriptive of an event into formats that can be coded as data. For example, a convenient means of researching dialect is to encode speech samples through phonetic transcription. The encoding process depends upon the listener's skills in categorizing ongoing speech into established phonetic categories. When observations are forced into inappropriate categories (e.g., a phonetic category that does not precisely define the proceeded sound), the resulting data are not valid. In the example, once a sound is transcribed as a particular phoneme or allophone its uniqueness is lost, and the encoding does not fully represent the speech sound. Validity of coding depends upon the researcher's knowing precisely what empirical attributes the data represent and what compromises were made during the coding process. Data represent samples of an event and are the products of categorization and integration. As a result, data may not represent all of the attributes and may distort some that they do represent. Coding which relies on human transcription or translation is particularly vulnerable to subjective, categorization errors.

The appropriate use of microcomputers may improve data collection by enabling signals to be directly processed by the system. Direct analysis of responses or other signals may objectify data by eliminating the need for a *subjective* translator or transcriber. However, any researcher using a microcomputer for data collection must be keenly aware that analysis is only as good as the data it massages. It is important not to be misled into thinking that data are absolutely correct and complete because they were collected and stored by a computer.

Even when signals (e.g., speech samples) are processed directly by a computer, there are inherent coding limitations which have the potential for creating validity problems. When analog events (i.e., continually varying), such as speech and other behaviors on a continuum, are directly analyzed, they are coded through an interpolative process which samples the events as a series of sequenced observations rather than as a continuum. Analog signals are continually varying functions; at present, computer technology has not provided a totally adequate means of recording and analyzing them (Witten, 1982). The best, state-of-the-art means of encoding analog signals into the discrete numerical values required for digital processing is by *analog-to-digital* (A/D) *conversion*. The A/D conversion process is a compromise that rapidly samples the voltage of an analog signal at equal intervals and converts the measure to an array of digital values. Because digitized data are handled as strings of numbers, they can be precisely manipulated. However, all intrepretations of these data must be made with the clear understanding that they represent objective samples but not the complete analog signal. To reiterate, it is important not to be misled into thinking that data are correct and complete because they were collected by and stored by a computer.

A/D conversion exemplifies the types of trade-off that must be made for digital analysis of behavioral data. The speed of microcomputers makes A/D conversion an acceptable means of data collection. Even though A/D conversion must be used with some caution, an analog signal that is sampled more than 50,000 times per second is well represented by the resulting data array. Despite their limitations, microcomputers are having significant effects on research because they allow rapid data collection and a means of statistically manipulating samples.

Reliability and validity

Incorporating a microcomputer into a research plan does not guarantee a solid design or worthwhile data. The same fundamental considerations which apply to designs that rely on microcomputers apply to those that do not. Two keys to *reliable* research are the replicability of the experimental conditions and the dependability of measurements. Both keys rely on laboratory tools and the appropriateness of their use. Microcomputers can serve both replicability and dependability by affording precise control of experimental conditions for replicability and precision of data acquisition for dependability of measurements (Silverman, 1977).

The key to *validity* lies with the researcher's choice of problems identified and questions asked. Valid research is a function of the researcher's knowledge of (1) the problem, (2) the effects of environmental factors on the problem, and (3) the limitations of the data collection method. "Askable" research questions depend upon the availability of measurement instruments and the researcher's ingenuity in using them. Computers have had an influence on the types of questions that can be asked by allowing more and different types of data to be collected. Soundness of answers depends on the dependability and validity of the data. Finally, validity is a function of interpretative decisions the researcher makes based upon the information obtained.

Objective measurements

Research tools help code events so they can be conceptualized and quantified, often by indirect measurement. When events are difficult to encode directly (e.g., sound by direct observation), they must be transduced into a manageable medium. Sound must first be interpreted into voltage variations by electroacoustical transducers. For this purpose, microphones produce electrical representations of sound pressure variations. Electricity affords an easily measurable and stable analog coding of sound pressure variations. An oscilloscope provides an analog, graphic representation of waveforms: it also provides a means for measuring magnitude (amplitude) variations as a function of time. Encoding of sound for microcomputer analysis must go an additional step, that of analog to digital (A/D) conversion.

Measurement instruments compare objects or events with standards. For example, a meter stick is used to measure distance by comparing a length to a linear standard (Silverman, 1977). A stop watch measures elapsed time by comparing it to a temporal standard. A sound level meter measures sound pressure indirectly by first transducing the sound into a voltage and then comparing that voltage to an electrical standard. Many noncomputerized clinical tools, such as psychological tests, go one step further and compare behaviors with theoretically constructed standards, such as "intelligence" scales. Measurement tools enable meaningful comparisons of the unknown to standards, and thereby provide for objective quantification of events. Microcomputers enable researchers to develop increasingly complex measurement tools and standards while speeding the measurement process.

It should be noted that computers, in general, do not make measurements; rather, they provide the means for processing measurements and relating them to standards. Their impact on research stems from very rapid and accurate interpretation of basic measurements and from the innovative measurement devices that can be interfaced with them.

The process of measuring magnitude (e.g., amplitude or voltage) takes time. For example, it takes time to use a meter stick to measure the height of a subject. In many instances, the sampling time varies as a function of the required precision. If a subject's height is to be measured, a rough estimate can be obtained quickly, but a precise measurement takes longer. Because magnitude measurements take time, temporal (timing) information in an observation may be sacrificed in exchange for accuracy of magnitude information. The process of A/D conversion is a prime example of a magnitude versus temporal information trade-off. When very rapid sampling of an analog is required, the precision of magnitude information may be sacrificed and vice versa. When an observation contains critical information in dimensions of magnitude as well as of time, as does speech, the researcher must decide where to compromise magnitude for temporal accuracy. If too much emphasis is placed on magnitude information there may be a sacrifice of subtle time-locked information. A significant asset of the microcomputer is that it has drastically reduced the time required for taking and recording magnitude measurements and has helped preserve both temporal and magnitude information in perspective.

With increased use of computers as research tools, scientists should learn about the assets and liabilities of measuring and encoding devices. It is important to know how a sampling device interfaces with the event being measured and to be aware of possible interactions between the device and the event (i.e., artifacts). Considerable effort must be devoted to identifying and controlling possible sources of artifactual and measurement error. It is important to calibrate each sampling device (e.g., microphone, EMG) and data converter (e.g., A/D converters) in the measurement system. Limitations of the measurement system must be identified, and the research design and data interpretation must be modified accordingly. Researchers should be excited and challenged by the new possibilities that microcomputer-based measurements provide.

MICROCOMPUTER IMPACTS ON RESEARCH DIRECTIONS

All too often, technology has dictated the directions of research. Strategies are often based on what can be measured with the research tools at hand, and in the process may ignore attributes of an event that might be critical to a comprehensive answer. Quantitative attributes have been emphasized because these are relatively easy to measure, whereas qualitative attributes are multidimensional, multisensory, and difficult to code objectively.

Research laboratories historically have tooled up to measure specific attributes of events (Flanagan, 1982). Some focused on physiological parameters, others on physical measures, and others on psychological attributes. In part, this division of labor was the result of the high cost of equipping laboratories with sophisticated and highly specialized research instruments. Instrumentation need for physiological measurements is quite different from that used for speech analysis, which again differs from technology needed for language research. Highly sophisticated laboratories were usually dedicated to esoteric research and attracted scholars with compatible interests. In effect, available tools dictated the directions of research efforts and attracted scientists whose interests could be pursued in those facilities. Progress in computer technology has had a significant impact on research. The need for dedicated special-purpose research instrumentation has been minimized and the cost of equipping a laboratory has been drastically reduced. Technology has increased the precision of measurements which can be obtained in the field and has enabled new interactive and artificial intelligence (Frillman, 1982) paradigms that were previously not feasible. The microcomputer is having a singular impact on the scope of research. It extends sophisticated empirical capabilities to remote laboratories and clinical practitioners (Pournelle, 1983). Microcomputer-based research is altering the numbers and academic profiles of those who are regarded as researchers and is stimulating collaborative studies through the use of shared programs and common data bases. Finally, the number of investigative approaches to a given problem that are practical has increased, and innovative and multidisciplinary thinking about solutions to research problems is being stimulated.

As the microcomputer becomes commonplace in the laboratory and in the clinic, the distinction between the two environments is vanishing. If a *researcher* is defined as one who asks and answers meaningful question related to a given problem, it is apparent that the microcomputer is having a favorable impact on the numbers of researchers, who are increasingly including many who are primarily clinicians and secondarily researchers. With this revision, new questions and strategies have emerged. The strategies are often creative and allow new questions to be asked and answered. Creative research thinking has resulted in methods for quantifying behaviors that were previously examined only subjectively (Flowers & Leger, 1982). For example, there are several formal procedures for linguistically analyzing a language sample. Inherent in these systems is a complexity of cumbersome and time-consuming categorizing and tallying procedures. A clinician often opts for a subjective impression of a language sample rather than devoting the time required for the formal analysis, even though the formal analysis may assist in the documentation necessary to support remedial objectives (Mordecai, Palin, & Palmer, 1982). Complex language analysis programs utilize the microprocessor's capability to make systematic decisions according to theoretical models and rules.

As techniques improve for interfacing the speaker and the listener directly to the microcomputer, *real time* processing will become increasingly important. In many mainframe computer operations, most data processing is *batched* for reasons of economy. That is, the user gathers all of the data together and submits it to be processed as a batch—not concurrently with data collection. With microcomputers, concurrent, or *real time* processing is quite practical and economical. Computer logic can process raw data and make decisions about that data in real time. It can process multiple channels of data simultaneously and can make multidimensional decisions (Bird, 1981). For example, a behavioral study may utilize simultaneous data from speech signals, eye blinks, physiological measurements, and numerous other body responses. Response analyses need not be restricted to unidimensional data; a more thorough analysis of communication as a whole-body process has become possible. As a result microcomputers are providing new avenues for behavioral studies and are facilitating the directions of future research.

With creative planning and programming a microcomputer might simulate limited perceptual processes that allow the researcher to examine models of qualitative judgment. This form of artificial intelligence has the potential for simulating normal and disordered communication processes and for changing diagnostic and rehabilitation techniques for sensory and perceptual disorders. Artificial intelligence and perceptual simulation should excite the creative thinking of many researchers. It can provide the means for probing normal differences among perceptual systems and for probing deviations in pathological systems. It may also serve to examine behaviors that were previously studied only by subjective observation.

Given the current, state-of-the-art technology, a bridge is still needed between what the researcher might want the microcomputer to do and what the microcomputer is equipped to handle. Innovative applications of the microcomputer require that the researcher learn something about how the computer "views" data and the rules that it uses to formulate decisions about those data. At present, it is necessary for researchers to bend their thinking to accommodate the conventions of the computer. Such a trend in thinking may provide the researcher with new perspectives on data and concurrently help in adapting the computer to research needs.

Thinking numerically

Digital processing has had an impact on the way in which behavioral measurements must be viewed; computer processing requires the researcher to think numerically. Most audiologists and speech-language pathologists have been taught to think "analog," with oscilloscope tracings indelibly etched in their brains. Tracings accurately represent the analog, or continually varying, nature of speech signals but the are very difficult to record and analyze because of their continuous nature. Computers enable a different conceptual image, that of data arrays in which the amplitudes of the analog signal, at equal intervals, are transformed into a "column" of numbers. It is these numbers that can be stored, retrieved, manipulated, and analyzed. By treating analog behavioral measures as numerical arrays, precise sectioning (i.e., editing), analysis, modification, and recombination of data can be accomplished. For example, a microcomputer with appropriate software and A/D and D/A converters can eliminate the need for tape splicing in the editing of acoustic stimuli. To perform the editing, the acoustic signal is converted to a digitized format and stored in computer memory as a data array. The exact portions of the array that are to be included in the edited version are identified and treated as subarrays. The subarrays (e.g., phoneme segments) can be retrieved and combined with other store segments to reconstruct a new array which is converted from digitized to an analog one, as needed, for output as an acoustic signal. The numerical process of A/D–D/A reconstruction can replace hours of cutting and splicing audio tapes and can increase the precision of the end product. The technique produces a stimulus that is quantifiable and therefore has a positive impact on the validity and the reliability of research.

Numerical thinking affords new insights into analysis techniques. Standard statistical procedures acquire new significance with the microcomputer. For example, the Pearson Product Moment Correlation Coefficient may be used to test relationships between two arrays obtained from concurrent attributes of a given behavior (e.g., neurophysiological measures). It is conceivable that techniques based on the priniciples of factoring may be the key to measuring qualitative attributes which are not directly measurable but which can be factored from multiple channels of physiological and behavioral data. The qualitative notion of "intelligence" is an illusive one, but factoring (i.e., use of factor analysis techniques) can be used to measure it through a series of performance tasks. Factor analysis techniques may have the potential for extracting qualitative measures about communication processes that are not now possible through conventional techniques. Numerical thinking enables the researcher to incorporate probability theory and statistical techniques into routine data acquisition and real time analysis.

Numerical thinking is having a significant impact on systematic analyses of language. Microcomputers simplify the task of phonetic and linguistic analysis by facilitating the task of categorizing, tallying, and analyzing by rules (Telage, 1980). It is feasible to use complex analyses in routine clinical research for investigating language development and the emergence of rules in children's speech (see Rushakoff, chap. 7). Similarly, examining the deterioration of language that occurs with adult aphasia can be facilitated through microcomputers.

Numerical thinking both permits and requires a rigor in examining digitized signals that may not be required in analog thinking. The capability of examining synchronous data points from various sources allows examination of precise, detailed, behavioral responses. Many perceptual and behavioral functions are probabilistic in nature and have been difficult to study with conventional research methodologies (Lutman, 1983; Okada, 1983; Oratio, 1979; Telage, 1980). The microcomputer provides a versatile approach to studying the physiology of speech production (e.g., Keller, 1983) that allows collected data to be analyzed from multiple perspectives. The capability of analyzing multiple channels of data according to perceptual and behavioral models promises to transform the study of normal communication and of disordered communication.

Thinking in patterns and symbols

Numerical thinking is but one example of symbolic logic. The microcomputer is capable of making contingent decisions based on patterns and responding according to rules (i.e., the program) with a prescribed response. In a microcomputer, all numbers and letters are coded as binary patterns. Each number, letter, punctuation mark, or operational key generates a pattern which may be transmitted as electrical pulse patterns. It is fascinating to conceptualize the microcomputer, not as a "number cruncher," but as a "pattern" or "symbol cruncher" because the human nervous system *also* operates as a "pattern" and "symbol" processor. It is even more intriguing to draw parallels between the microcomputer and the pattern-recognition and probabilistic functions of the brain.

Like the brain, a microcomputer operates with patterns of patterns. When the computer handles multidigit numbers, it groups together patterns so that the number "21" would be encoded as "010110010-010110001." Similarly, numerical codes for letters can be combined to encode patterns for words. For example, the word "key" may be subdivided into three letter units, with a code for each unit, or it can be coded as a pattern of patterns (i.e., a pattern of letters, each having its own unique binary pattern). Fortunately, the microcomputer user or programmer rarely deals directly with this coding. It is conceptually important, however, to think of the microcomputer as a symbolic or pattern machine, not a number cruncher when planning a project which uses the microcomputer to interact with the patterns of behavior or the symbols of language.

Perhaps there is a conceptual disadvantage to the term "computer," which implies number processing. It might be more appropriate to think of a microcomputer as a microprocessor which processes logical units rather than simply numbers.

Symbolic thinking can extend well beyond the use of letters and numbers. Movements, sounds, and other responses can be coded as patterns for processing by the computer. Joysticks, A/D converters, graphic tablets, and other devices can be used to convert behavioral responses into symbolically coded data. Creative symbolic coding offers a wealth of opportunities for an innovative researcher.

Psychologists, neurologists, educators, linguists, physiologists, phoneticians, psychoacousticians, and many others study the way in which the human mind and body process patterns. The microcomputer's ability to be programmed to process patterns and to make logical decisions based on those patterns affords the researcher a valuable tool for examining the ways in which the nervous system processes stimuli.

Most numerous of the current symbolic processing applications of the microprocessor are programs which analyze language structure. Speech pattern recognizers, brainstem-evoked response averagers, and computerized audiometric test equipment (Flanagan, 1982; Lutman, 1983) are also becoming commonplace. A significant effect of the microcomputer will be the increased study of patterns and symbols.

Thinking clinically

Microprocessors enable clinical observations that were possible only as clinical judgments 10 years ago. Clinical observations are complex, multifaceted measurements that require decisive processing to be meaningful. Clinical judgments fit many simultaneous, simple measures into diagnostic categories based on probability. Because behavior is multidimensional, the number of measures that must be made and processed simultaneously may be staggering. The microcomputer can provide a handle on complex data gathering and clinical decision analysis.

Clinical thinking presents challenges to the creative researcher. The components and rules of a clinical decision must be defined objectively rather than being based on insights and intuition. Microcomputers offer the potential for clinical measures to be objective samples of physiological and behavioral attributes. Clinical expertise may be transformed into definable rules for interpreting those measures. As a bonus, microcomputers may motivate researchers to convert clinical expertise into rules that intelligent systems can implement.

Interactive research

Learning about the environment and about other individuals occurs through interaction; some of the process is through speech, but much of it occurs through nonverbal interactions. Stimuli are tossed out to see how the environment and other people react to them. People stimulate and observe, alter stimuli accordingly, and observe again. Learning is a very interactive process.

The microprocessor is capable of making high-speed decisions based on multiple data acquisitions and established rules. It may be programmed to follow a mode of operation contingent upon decisions made. High-speed decision functions allow for interactive research in which the "intelligence" or contingency of the program alters the course of data gathering according to the subject's responses. Interactive processing enables a *stimulus–response* research paradigm for pursuing the most direct path (critical path) to an answer. For example, a computerized audiometer can be programmed to employ conventional audiometric paradigms to interact with a patient in establishing a hearing threshold. The psychometric process is interactive because the system varies its subsequent presentation according to the patient's responses. It is a critical path strategy because it does not test *all* stimulus possibilities but tests only those that are necessary for making an efficient decision about the threshold. Interactive systems can emulate the stimulus–response procedures which animals use to learn about their environment and to communicate with other animals.

Interactive processing and critical path analysis coupled with artificial intelligence may facilitate the probing and modification of behaviors that are intuitively obvious but are difficult to objectively quantify. A prime example of interactive probing is critical path diagnosis in which a program probes the patient's symptoms, "learns" from the responses, and alters its probing accordingly. At its command are banks of data about symptoms, probabilities, courses of pathologies, and other epidemiological data. By comparing the patient's responses to stored data and pursuing the most direct path of data acquisition, the program gathers critical diagnostic information. An example of interactive behavior modification is computer-assisted instruction (CAI) in which the student interacts with the computer to be "taught" information (see Shearer, chap. 9). The microcomputer presents information and the student responds. The processor evaluates the response and varies its course accordingly. By interacting with the student, the computer and its program establish a critical path of stimulation to facilitate learning. The same interactive strategies have been applied to other types of behavior modification. In research, interactive probing and modifying can provide valuable information about behavioral mechanisms and how they function.

Answering research questions

Microcomputers often help the researchers ask and answer new questions because of the system's flexibility and versatility in measuring responses and in analyzing data. Their speed and multiple task capabilities can generate stimuli and measure multiple channels of response data. Many stimulus signals may be directly generated; others may be generated by instruments under computer control.

STRATEGIES FOR RESEARCH APPLICATIONS

In research, stimuli are carefully controlled to optimally test a system or hypothesis. By comparing the output of a system to a known input, the operations of the system can be assessed. Discrepancies between input and output are clues to the rules of its operation or behavior. In a complex system, rules are typically not simple, so that a given stimulus many cause a response with many attributes. To answer a question thoroughly, a researcher must account for as many of those attributes as possible. The microcomputer is a suitable research tool because it can generate tightly controlled stimuli and can sample multiple simultaneous responses. It can also store data as a function of their time of occurrence to facilitate a direct linkage between stimulus and response. In effect, the microcomputer serves as an integrated *input* source and an *output* analyzer, capable of answering increasingly complex research questions.

Expanded response data collection enables the testing of complex models of behavior. The ideal model would be one which accepted multitudes of data, processed them, and responded to them as a human would. Such a model is well beyond the capabilities of state-of-the-art microcomputers; however, preliminary applications of artificial intelligence (Pournelle, 1983) have laid the groundwork, and increased memory and processing capabilities will facilitate the process.

Artificial intelligence (Hirsch, 1984) utilized the computer's logical capabilities to make decisions based on complex sets of rules and multitudes of input data. The program then modifies its course or "behavior" based on these decisions. The use of artificial intelligence *(AI)* will enable researchers to ask new kinds of questions that probe the dynamics of perception, cognition, and communication. Effective use of AI programming depends upon sophisticated interfacing between the person and the computer.

Interfacing responses

Digital interfacing is the process of logically linking one piece of equipment or one person to another. The most obvious interfaces on a microprocessor are the keyboard and the CRT screen. The keyboard allows the user to enter information, and the CRT allows the user to obtain it; these are the primary input and output (I/O) channels (see Chial, chap. 5). Both of these are high-level I/O channels requiring extensive coding on the part of the user. To generate simple stimuli and to sample simple responses and attributes, other types of interfacing are required.

Numerous devices are used by speech-pathologists and audiologists to measure the attributes of the speaker, the listener, and the communication process. Many of these serve to transduce analog responses into electrical signals. Examples of these devices are microphones, EMG recorders, simple switches, and air flow meters. Each device interacts with an attribute of the speaker, listener, or acoustic signal to create an electrical signal that correlates with the event. To some extent, a researcher's ability to use microprocessors for communications research depends on clearly defining those attributes which are to be measured, to interface measuring devices to those attributes, and to interface the devices to the computer. To a greater extent, the researcher's success depends on the logical processes that the computer performs on the data and the interpretations placed on those results.

Successful interfacing depends upon an understanding of the microcomputer system and the system (person) being interfaced with the computer. Typically, the process is best carried out by a team consisting of an electronics technician and the researcher who understands the behaviors that are to be measured. It is not a requirement that the researcher become an expert in microcomputers, but that the investigator communicate with the technician about interfacing needs. However, an increasing number of researchers are taking the time to learn skills of hardware interfacing through instructions available in recent publications.

As discussed above, microcomputers are logic machines that process information as patterns of binary states. The patterns are routed along *data buses*, are processed by binary logic processors, and are the sole basis for a computer's operational flow. The user has access to data buses through a series of *ports*. One or more of the I/O ports are usually dedicated to a keyboard, a printer, and a CRT. But there are usually others which are available for special-purpose interfacing. It helps to view I/O ports as arrays of switches that can be turned "on" or "off" individually.

A researcher must be creative to interface measurable attributes of behaviors with the array of "switches" that are available. It requires careful assessment of which attributes are to be encoded and the precision (i.e., amount of information) with which they are to be encoded.

Despite their speed and power, microcomputers have finite processing capabilities. It is critical to encode enough but not too much information. If too little information about a response is encoded, necessary data are lost; if too much is encoded, the system may become overtaxed with unnecessary processing. For example, if the response to be encoded is the prosody of a speech signal, relevant information may be lost if a voice-operated relay is used to detect only the presence or absence of sound. On the other hand, if a simple push-button response is all that is required, a complex procedure for encoding amounts of finger pressure during the pressing of the button would provide too much information and would unnecessarily tax the processor and program.

Simple switches

Any response that can be measured with a simple switch can be fed into a microcomputer as binary information. The response may be a depressed key, a loudness detector coupled with a microphone, or a physiological sensor detecting EMG activity. Binary information is fed from a switch to the microcomputer as a voltage level which switches on and off as the response exists or does not exist. Data ports receive binary information according to their operating characteristics. Data port inputs are of two basic types: *level detectors* and *event detectors*. Level detectors are switched on only so long as a given condition exists. For instance, a level detector switch can be rigged to be "on" so long as an acoustic signal exceeds a given level. When the signal drops below the specified level the switch turns "off." Level detectors are useful in providing input information to the computer about the current state of a parameter. Event detectors, as the name implies, detect that an event has occurred. Unlike level detectors, these remain turned on until switched off by the computer or external device. They do not represent the current state of a parameter but rather a record of the occurrence of an event. Each application dictates which type of detector is most applicable, and the research design should specify which type is to be used.

Simple switches used with computers are usually of the SPDT (single-pole, double-terminal) type. When the switch is in one position the line going to the computer data port is held to ground (0 V); when it is in the other position, the line is held to a given voltage (e.g., +3 V). The computer interprets the 0 V as "off" and the +3 volts as "on."

The simple switch can be the most efficient and easily managed measuring device for a speech–language pathologist or audiologist. It can be used to code simple conditioned responses, as in the case of an audiological test; and it can be used by neurologically and motorically handicapped persons to encode bodily movements that are not conventionally used for communication.

In many instances it is useful to encode more than an "on–off" response to the pressing of a switch. Coded switches are used to inform the processor which response was made when a key on a computer's keyboard is depressed; a binary pattern is generated which indicates which specific key or switch is depressed. A numerical keypad can be a convenient means of encoding nominal data into a computer. The system is programmed to recognize each of these codes as the letter or number it represents. It is feasible, however, to use the keys on a keyboard for more than one purpose by programming the microcomputer to recognize the codes differently for specific applications. For example, if a researcher wanted to provide phonemic transcriptions of speech samples, each of the keys on the keyboard could be assigned to one phoneme. The program would then recognize the codes from the keyboard as phonemes rather than as letters and numbers. Recall that the computer is a pattern recognizer, and that the program dictates how each pattern is processed.

Interfacing analog signals

Each researcher must make an important decision when planning to encode analog information for a computer. How much information is to be encoded and what it represents must be determined prior to planning an interface. It must be decided whether the entire signal should be digitized and fed into the computer or if an extract from that analog signal might be more appropriate.

Schmitt triggers

Although A/D conversion provides the maximum precision in coding information from an analog signal, it may in some instances be "overkill" to use it. A Schmitt trigger is a useful analog/digital measuring device which functions as a threshold detector. When an analog signal exceeds a predetermined and specified threshold the trigger's binary output is on; when the signal drops below that threshold, the output is off. As in the case of a simple switch, it forces a logic line to 0 V or +3 V to indicate the analog signal's level relative to threshold. The Schmitt trigger can be interfaced as an event detector or as a level detector to provide the computer with a binary decision about the intensity level of an analog signal.

The Schmitt trigger is different from an A/D converter and derives less information from the analog signal than does the converter. The trigger forces magnitude information into one of two binary categories (i.e., it exceeds or doesn't exceed threshold) whereas the converter codes the analog magnitude into a range of categories that depict the actual magnitude of the signal. The Schmitt trigger exemplifies efficient use of digital processing when only threshold-related information is needed. It is an example of delegating decisions about stimuli to peripheral devices to ease the load on the computer.

In research designs that require a procedure to begin after an event (e.g., phonation) has begun, the Schmitt trigger is useful and efficient as an event detector. The program "watches" for the trigger and alters its course when the event occurs. Because it can be set to trigger at a wide range of voltage levels, Schmitt triggers are useful as signal overload detectors and can function much like the "peak level" detector on a VU meter. If an analog signal is to be digitized by an A/D converter for computer processing, it may be convenient to couple a Schmitt trigger to the same analog signal with threshold set at that point where the signal just about overloads the converter. The trigger can be used to send a signal to the computer as a warning that the signal is about to be distorted.

Analog to digital converters

The A/D converter is used throughout this chapter to illustrate points about data collection because it is so well suited to speech–language pathology and audiology. The A/D converter is the most direct means of encoding *interval* scale data about an analog signal (e.g., speech) to the microcomputer. It is a powerful device, but it must be used carefully and with an awareness of its assets and its limitations. Some of the basic considerations the researcher should bear in mind are (1) the precision of the converter, (2) the sampling speed used by the converter, (3) the consistency of the interval between samples, (4) the manner in which it is interfaced with the computer, and (5) the load that it places on the processor. Chapter 5 discusses the specifications of A/D hardware and should be used as a co-reference for this chapter.

Precision. The *precision* of the converter refers to the number of units in its amplitude scale. For example, a 12-bit converter uses 4096 steps to encode amplitude so that the most negative voltage in a signal may be encoded as −2048 and the most positive voltage encoded as +2048, with the midpoint being zero. This range may seem adequate for encoding any analog signal, but it may in fact be inadequate for the nuances of music or the information of speech that is carried in the very low magnitude energies of consonants. A 16-bit converter provides a resolution of over 64,000 steps and provides significantly better resolution for most microprocessors because it affords high resolution and it can be stored in 2 bytes (8-bit units) of memory. There are also A/D converters of greater precision which may be needed for certain projects. The greater the precision (over 16 bits) the more difficult it is for a microcomputer to store and manage the data. The technology associated with A/D converters is changing so rapidly that it is wise to consult with knowledgeable vendors and engineers when selecting these devices.

Sampling rate. The second consideration is that of A/D sampling rate. The Nyquist rule of thumb (Witten, 1982) states that sampling rates should be at least double the highest frequency to be sampled. If a research design calls for the analysis of a signal with meaningful components up to 10,000 Hz, the sampling rate should be at least 20,000 samples per second. If an inadequate sampling rate is used, alias properties may appear in the data. These alias properties are artifacts of the sample rate and appear to represent waveform traits that are not present in the original signal (see chap. 5). Digital recording engineers indicate that a sampling rate of five times the highest frequency is needed for low-noise, high-fidelity conversion. If the audible range of hearing is to be faithfully digitized, a sampling rate of 100,000 conversions per second is required. Converters which sample up to 200,000 samples per second are currently available, but most contemporary microcomputers are not capable of processing input at these rates.

The sampling rate of an A/D converter is controlled by a clock which is located either within or peripheral to the computer. It is this clock which provides the researcher with a very high degree of temporal accuracy in the analysis and generation of signals. The user should verify that it initiates each sample at equal intervals and at the prescribed speed regardless of the other tasks being performed by the computer. The advantage of using a peripheral clock directly interfaced to the A/D converter is that it operates independent of the system's other tasks and therefore may be more reliable than the microcomputer-driven converter.

The instruction to a peripheral clock and A/D converter might be, to paraphrase, "sample the analog voltage every 2 μs." The peripheral device then functions independently until instructed to stop. A converter that relies on the computer for timing must be instructed to begin each sample. If the CPU is also engaged in other tasks, there will probably be times when the instructions to begin samples are slightly delayed. The effect is an irregular A/D sample rate and erroneous data.

High-speed A/D converters generate data at rates greater than most microcomputers can process them. There are several options for overcoming this problem: (1) a sophisticated, high-speed CPU, (2) direct memory access (DMA), (3) an external microprocessor with its own buffered memory, and (4) modification of the research design.

A researcher should consider, when purchasing a microprocessor, the maximum rate at which data need be processed and the maximum amount of data which must be readily accessible to the processor. Most microcomputers are not designed for speed data processing. If a low capacity microcomputer is purchased, the researcher can generally expect to pay more for peripheral A/D equipment with external clock and buffer. Sophisticated laboratory microprocessors typically have CPU speeds which exceed those of most "personal computers" and can accommodate high-speed data input and bulk storage which are adequate for A/D conversions. A "laboratory microcomputer" (probably classed as a minicomputer rather than as a micro) is designed for ease of data input and rapid data routing and storage.

Laboratory microcomputers often have the capability for a peripheral device to access RAM (memory) directly without having to obligate the CPU to process each piece of data that is stored. Direct memory access (DMA) permits a peripheral A/D, clock, and controller to sample and store data directly in the computer's memory. Detailed programming tracks which piece of data is where and which sample in time it represents. DMA, in conjunction with A/D, requires special programming that can allow it to serve as a general data collector for various analysis programs (see Figure 8-2).

The third option for adapting a high-speed A/D converter to a slower microcomputer delegates almost all A/D-related processing to a peripheral device that interfaces with the microcomputer. Several commercial products are on the market that perform the A/D data conversion, peripheral memory (buffer) storage, and retrieval with a small microprocessor built into the device. The computer's microprocessor communicates with the peripheral device's microprocessor in a master-slave relationship. The device makes the A/D measurements; it stores the digital data in a temporary buffer and transfers it to the computer upon demand. The system performs its functions and then interfaces with the host computer via a logic card that plugs into the host. Special purpose software provides a turnkey system that is available for specific applications with a minimal amount of user programming. The turnkey programs are packaged software programs that allow the researcher to specify the parameters of data collection and manipulation with little or no knowledge of programming (see Schwartz, chap. 6).

One example of such a system, as shown in Figure 8-3, equips a low-cost microcomputer for measuring brainstem-evoked response potentials. The device performs the sampling and buffering at a very rapid A/D sample rate. The system interacts with the clinician or researcher and the peripheral device to set the parameters of the data acquisition and analysis, to store needed data, and to communicate the results to the user through graphic and tabular representations. The system is a compromise between dedicated hardware and a general purpose computer and has the advantages of both. An advantage of microprocessor-based systems is that with programming changes, their functions can be modified to meet specific needs at a minimal cost.

The fourth option for adapting a research need for A/D conversion to a slow microcomputer is to modify the research methodology. Of the four options, this requires the most thorough knowledge of laboratory instrumentation and the greatest amount of creative thinking. The problem of getting A/D information into a microcomputer is one worthy of careful consideration, and the researcher must decide which information is most critical to the study and how best to get it into the computer.

If the available microcomputer will accept output from an A/D converter but not at an adequate rate of speed, the analog signal must be slowed down to acquire the necessary number of samples per waveform. Tape recorded analog information can be stretched by replaying the tape at half speed. This effectively doubles the A/D sampling rate. If the analog recording equipment is of high quality the signal can be rerecorded at half speed and replayed at quarter speed with an effective factor-of-four increase in the A/D sampling rate.

The minimum rate for A/D conversion sampling is dictated by the amount of information to be extracted. If not all the information in an analog signal is needed for an analysis, the A/D process may be simplified by preceding it with an electronic circuit (e.g., fundamental frequency extractor, filter integrator) which extracts from the analog signal only the needed parameters. For example, if a researcher needs information about the amplitude envelope of a speech signal rather than the entire waveform, an inexpensive integrator circuit can serve to derive the envelope information. The derived information, rather than the whole signal, can be entered into the microcomputer via the slow A/D converter.

If a study specifies only information about the fundamental frequency of a signal, analog bandpass filtering of the signal prior to A/D conversion will minimize the amount of information to be extracted and allow for a slower sampling rate.

As a last resort, the experimental design may be altered to use analog measuring devices with the readings being directly or manually transferred into the microcomputer. Many new clinical and laboratory instruments are equipped with RS-232 connectors (see Chial, chap. 5), which allow for direct communication between the instrument and the microcomputer. The connection permits a two-way exchange of information between the microcomputer and the instrument. It provides a means of control over the device and of entering data directly. Manual

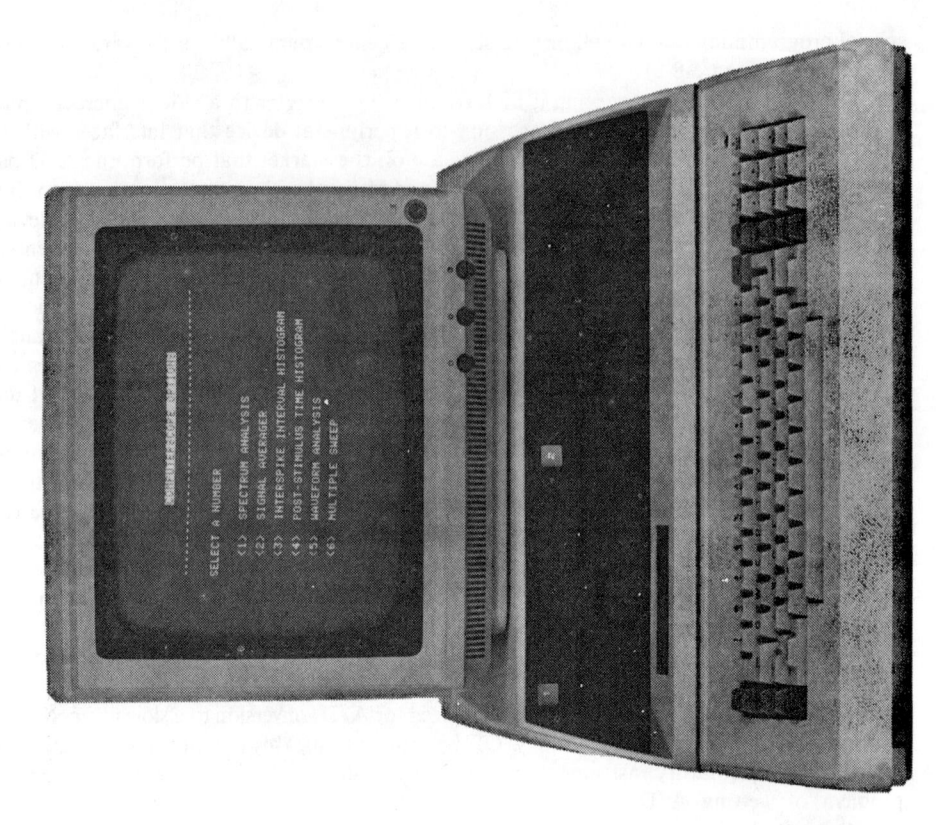

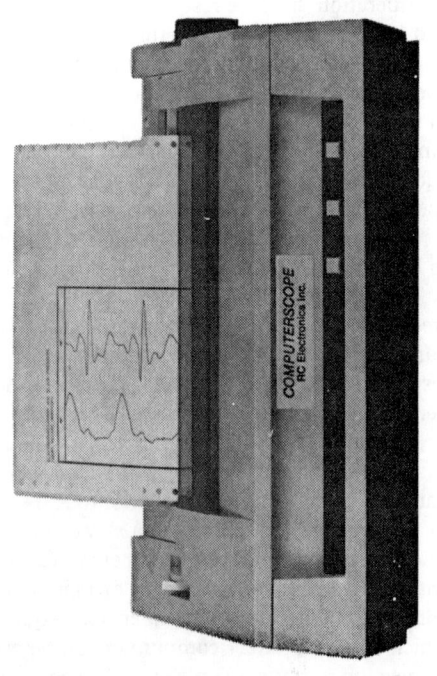

Figure 8-1. Microcomputer and dedicated hardware that can be utilized for research applications (courtesy RC Electronics).

Figure 8-2. Logic board for microcomputer.

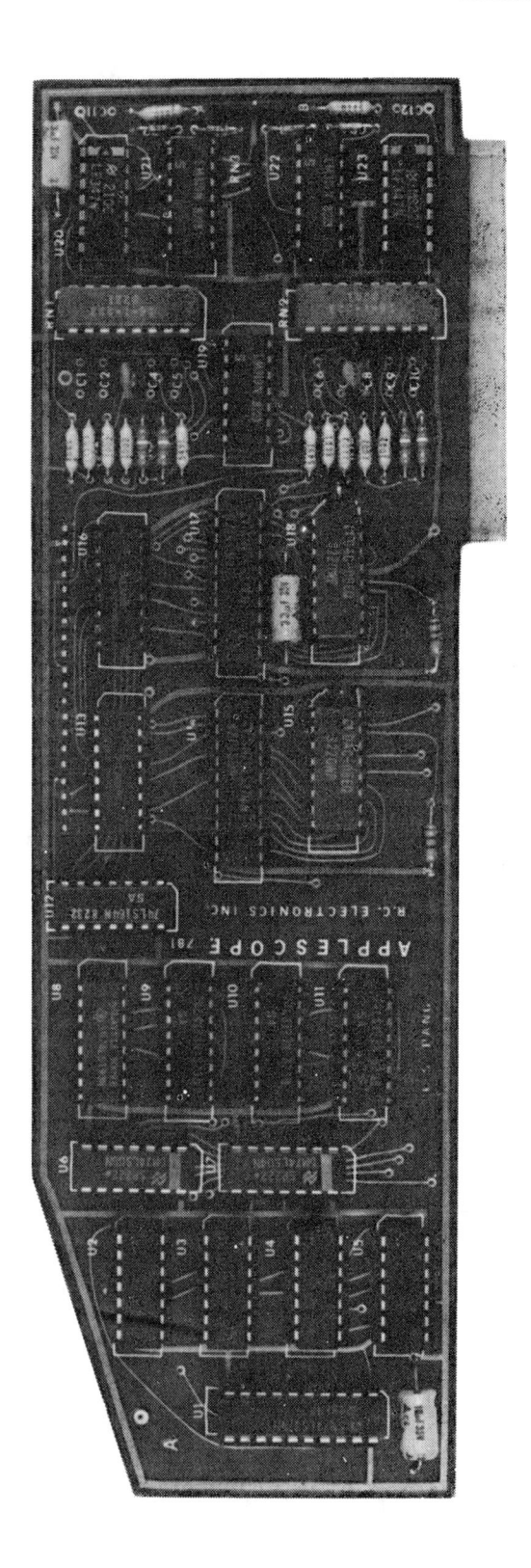

entry can be cumbersome, but when extensive processing of the results is required it may be worth the effort. For example, if a study is to compare the spectra of many phonemes using a spectrum analyzer, the analyzer can do most of the data reduction so that only spectral information need be keyed into the microcomputer. This greatly reduces the amount of information that must be entered. In this example, if for each phoneme to be compared, a 200-ms analog signal is to be analyzed at a 50,000 sample per second rate, 10,000 A/D conversions must be made and fed into the microcomputer. If a spectrum analyzer is used and only the spectrum is fed in, possibly 50 data points need be entered. Thus, by using a peripheral analyzer, the amount of data that must be entered into the microcomputer is reduced from 10,000 to 50 data points per phoneme. In the example, the microcomputer serves the role of comparing spectra among the phonemes, and the spectrum analyzer serves the role of analog data reduction and analysis. Such a division of labor optimizes the use of each piece of equipment.

Digital to analog converters

The reciprocal of A/D conversion is D/A conversion (see Chial, chap. 5). The D/A process is useful for controlling and synthesizing stimuli from a digital array. Analog signal generation is particularly useful when a research design specifies an auditory stimulus that is not found in nature or that is not easily managed with analog devices. When an optimal system is available, analog signals can be computed as data arrays which can be converted to an analog format for use as an audio signal. As with high-speed A/D this requires a sophisticated computer and a high-speed D/A converter. In most instances microcomputers are not well suited to such tasks but some laboratory microcomputers are. When such capabilities are not available, the researcher must be resourceful and delegate tasks to microcomputer-controlled peripheral devices as with A/D input.

Many of the same considerations that apply to A/D conversion apply to D/A conversion. Whereas A/D is the extraction of information samples from an analog sample, signals generated by D/A conversion are produced from representative data points and not from a comprehensive array. When a signal is synthesized through D/A conversion, there are artifacts (noise and higher harmonics) that must be accounted for. Typically these are well above the frequency response that is intended and are often above the D/A conversion frequency. For instance, if the intended signal is to be a 5000-Hz sine wave and the D/A conversion rate is 10,000 conversions per second, it is likely that there will be harmonics of the 10,000 Hz generated in the process. Filtering can minimize these artifacts, but it must be used with caution and with the understanding that filtering can alter the phase relationships within a signal.

Just because a researcher has acquired a microcomputer, trusted analog equipment that has been acquired through the years should not be discarded. In many instances, the laboratory that combines analog and digital instrumentation is the most versatile. The D/A converter can be a useful device for indirectly generating stimuli. With the aid of peripheral instruments, the microcomputer can effectively control frequencies and amplitudes of pure tones through D/A converters. The output of a D/A converter is a voltage that can be precisely controlled. The D/A voltage can be used to control the parameters of waveform generators to produced desired tonal stimuli at a moderate cost. Certain types of waveform generators have the capability of being controlled by input voltages. Voltage controlled amplitude (VCA) waveform generators accept an input dc voltage and vary the amplitude of the signal it produces accordingly. Through this system, the output of the computer can modulate the amplitude of a waveform. Voltage controlled generators (VCG) waveform generators vary their output frequency according to the voltage in. With two D/A converters and voltage controlled functions, a microcomputer can vary the amplitude and the frequency of a pure tone as needed for a research procedure.

The output from a D/A converter can also be used to control instruments which accept analog voltage control. There are other devices which produce analog output without using the D/A converter. Waveform generators which are capable of accepting digital information directly can be programmed through a data link to produce a given frequency, a given waveform, or a given sequence of analog variations.

One of the most exciting potentials of the microcomputer for perceptual research is its capability of generating tightly controlled auditory stimuli that are not derived from pure tones. There is a huge gap in our research on perception. On one side of the gap is pure tone research and its many significant findings. On the other side of the gap is a very impressive collection of phonological and linguistic research which examines complex auditory perception that has linguistic attributes. In between is a vast absence of research that examines perception of the basic acoustic events that carry the information of speech. There is little research that examines the perception of transients, independent of phonology, and there is little that examines the clinical perceptual changes that occur with hearing loss. There is little research that examines the basic auditory differences between a person who can easily extract a signal from noise and a person who cannot. There is a need for studies that explore auditorily evoked potentials to determine what types of acoustic patterns pass the basal ganglia and reach the cortex and which do not.

The computer's capacity to generate hybrid acoustic stimuli that are sculptured according to design and are not dependent upon pure tones and waveform generators should excite basic researchers and clinicians alike. A researcher should think carefully of the possible applications that might be made of microcomputers before selecting a specific system. As Cohen (see chap. 2) notes, it can be a frustrating experience to invest equipment money only to find that the hardware that was purchased does not have the capability to meet future needs.

Joysticks and other devices. As described by Chial (chap. 5), a joystick is a mechanical device, familiar to all video arcade fanatics, that encodes two-dimensional movements for computer input. The paddle and the roller ball also encode movements into computer-compatible formats. Although these devices are typically thought of as recreational tools, they should also be regarded as research tools. Each one is capable of sensing and encoding the dynamics of movement. Motor control for speech is a whole-body process, and dynamics of hand movements during speech are integrated facets of the communication process. Developmental researchers might examine models of learning through perceptual-motor skills, with the joystick being the sensor of these skills. Clinical researchers should be observant of the entire person as a communicator and should consider all movements as possible sources of data that might lead to a better understanding of the communication process.

Graphic displays. An advantage that a microcomputer has over mainframe, multiuser systems is that the microcomputer is practical for generating colorful and animated graphics. Easy-to-use software packages enable relatively inexperienced programmers to develop displays for depicting research results in graphic form, and for creating complicated perceptual-motor stimuli and motivating illustrations for computer-assisted instruction (CAI) teaching modules.

Graphics software packages are available for most microcomputers that display data as bar graphs, as pie charts, or as line graphs. They allow the researcher to display the results of data analysis in several forms and can ease the task of data interpretation. Graphics packages, in conjunction with high-density graphics printers, can prepare camera-ready illustrations for publication.

Microprocessors can serve as digital storage oscilloscopes for displaying speech or other transient waveforms as well as for displaying the results of a spectral analysis or brainstem-evoked response analysis. It is capable of displaying two-dimensional figures and of three-dimensional displays with color as the third dimension.

Computer graphics are powerful research tools in that they can create dynamic visual stimuli for perceptual and conceptual studies. Computer graphics afford the same degree of control over visual stimuli that D/A converters provide for auditory stimuli. Images can be generated according to rules and prescription, and they can be varied as functions of the viewer's responses. Interactive graphics can be generated readily with most "personal" types of microcomputers and afford the perceptual-motor scientist a means of examining interactions between the hand and the eye. A visit to the showroom of perceptual-motor devices (the video arcade) will provide many practical strategies for the innovative researcher.

The interactive graphic capabilities of microcomputers are well-suited to the study of biofeedback. With appropriate biological sensors interfaced to the computer, flexible response analysis programs, and graphics routines, the researcher has an extremely versatile tool for exploring biofeedback possiblilities. These potentials exist for all areas of human response, including biofeedback control of voluntary motor functions, autonomic functions, and psychological behaviors (Kolotkin, Billingham, & Feldman, 1981; Zicker, Tompkins, Rudow, & Abbs, 1980). Most biofeedback studies have dealt with single modalities; the computer provides a tool for multimodality biofeedback studies. Artificial intelligence coupled with biofeedback procedures has the potential for conditioning the nervous system to perform highly specialized perceptual-motor tasks. Knowledge from these studies may provide exciting breakthroughs for rehabilitation of patients with communication disorders. These applications may contribute to new ways of creative thinking about diagnosis and therapy.

ADMINISTRATIVE APPLICATIONS IN RESEARCH

It is estimated (Pournelle, 1983) that more microcomputer time is devoted to administrative applications than to all other applications combined. Word processing is the most used of these applications with spreadsheets taking second place. These applications can assume important roles in a research facility because of their time-saving features. These and other administrative applications are discussed by Hood and Miller (chap. 10) of this handbook.

Two specific applications of word processing for research purposes are (1) proposal writing, and (2) report writing. Manuscripts that concern a given project or group of projects typically share key content sections. These may be philosophies, review of literature, or bibliographies that will be used in several manuscripts with minor modifications. Word processing saves time and effort by enabling text to be stored, retrieved, and modified for the various forms it must take. The review of literature that appears in a research proposal will probably be appropriate, with modifications, in interim or final research reports. The stored text from the proposal can be retrieved and edited for the report as needed.

Word processing can be used with bibliographical retreival systems to generate bibliographies directly from a master information data base, such as MEDLINE, ERIC, and other commercial services (see Wilkins, chap. 4). The user must have a telephone MODEM to access networked data retrieval systems. Through the microcomputer and the network, the user communicates with a mainframe system to search for references that are relevant to the research. The data base system downloads the bibliographic references through the network to the user's microcomputer. The computer builds data sets from these references that can then be edited for the user's specific needs.

Word processing programs are also useful for less conventional applications. The editing and character string search functions of word processors can be used for compiling lists, maintaining files, and organizing data. Spreadsheet programs can also be used for nonconventional applications. They provide a means for organizing data (see chap. 10), revealing trends, and summarizing results.

Smooth administration in a research setting can mean the difference between an efficient study and a sloppy study. Hood and Miller in chap. 10 elaborate on other applications that should be considered.

The research potential of the microcomputer must be emphasized by training programs. Realization of this potential depends upon special technology and the widespread understanding and use of that technology (Bull, 1983). The computer is a useful device for instruction (see Shearer, chap. 9), and will be useful in teaching students about its own capabilities as a research tool. Collective efforts are needed to develop instructional packages that will convey a general understanding of the computer and its potential in research and as a clinical tool.

SUMMARY

The purpose of this chapter has been to stimulate thought about the research applications that can be made with microcomputers. New approaches to problems and creative solutions are possible with microcomputers, and the research scenario is changing as a result. A review of published research applications indicates that the potential has barely been tapped and that there are many possibilities that have not even been tried.

REFERENCES

Bird, R. (1981). *The computer in experimental psychology*. New York: Academic Press.

Bull, G. (1983). Special training for special technology: A curriculum use of microcomputer-based tools in speech–language pathology. *The Computing Teacher*, April, 52–56.

Flanagan, J. L. (1982). Talking with computers: Synthesis and recognition of speech by machine. *IEEE Transactions on Biomedical Engineering*, April, 29(4), 223–232.

Flowers, J., & Leger, D. (1982). Personal computers and behavioral observation: An introduction. *Behavior Research Methods and Instrumentation*, 14, 227–238.

Frillman, L. W. (1982). The development of your programs for the microcomputer—a process approach. *American Annals of the Deaf*, 127(5), 591–601.

Hirsch, A. (1984). Artificial intelligence comes of age. *Computers and Electronics*, March, 63–67, 93–95.

Keller, E. (1983). Computerized measurements of tongue dorsum movements with pulsed-echo ultrasound. *Journal of the Acoustical Society of America*, April, 73(4), 1309–1315.

Kolotkin, R., Billingham, K., & Feldman, W. (1981). Computers in biofeedback research and therapy. *Behavior Research Methods and Instrumentation*, 13, 523.

Lutman, M. E. (1983). Microcomputer-controlled psychoacoustics in clinical audiology. *British Journal of Audiology*, May 17(2), 109–114.

Mordecai, D., Palin, M. W., & Palmer, C. B. (1982). *LINGQUEST 1 (Manual and Program)*. Napa, CA: Lingquest Software, Inc.

Okada, M. (1983). Measurement of speech patterns in neurological disease. *Medical and Biological Engineering and Computing*. March, 21(2), 145–148.

Oratio, A. R. (1979). Computer assisted interactio analysis in speech–language pathology and audiology. *ASHA*, March, 21(3), 179–184.

Pournelle, J. (1983). The next five years in microcomputers. *Byte*, 8(9), 233–250.

Silverman, F. H. (1977). *Research design in speech pathology and audiology*. Englewood Cliffs, NJ: Prentice-Hall.

Telage, K. M. (1980). A computerized place-manner distinctive feature program for articulation analysis. *Journal of Speech and Hearing Disorders*, November, 45(4), 481–494.

Witten, I. (1982). *Principles of computer speech*. New York: Academic Press.

Zicker, J. E., Tompkins, W. J., Rudow, R. T., & Abbs, J. H. (1980). A portable microcomputer-based biofeedback training device. *IEEE Transactions on Biomedical Engineering*, April, 2(2), 97–107.

Chapter 9

Academic and Instructional Applications for Microcomputers

William M. Shearer

THE MICROCOMPUTER AS INSTRUCTOR CONCEPT

Introduction

The most obvious application for microcomputers in the area of instruction is, of course, "computer-aided instruction," commonly called "CAI." Variations of this term include MCAI, "microcomputer-aided instruction" and ICAI, "intelligent computer-aided instruction." The latter term refers to the application of instructional programs using languages that have the capability to interact in a conversational or intelligent manner with the student. The CAI assumes the role of an individual tutor who not only presents new material to be learned and administers tests, but who also conveys a rather friendly, positive, and perhaps even charitable attitude toward the learner. Although the issue of exactly what circumstances are best or least suited for CAI application has not been clearly resolved, it is generally agreed that the academic CAI is not really intended as a substitute for the teacher or instructor, but is most effectively used in conjunction with a more traditional type of instruction. Furthermore, the computer is most realistically viewed simply as one of many effective teaching media and techniques at the teacher's disposal (O'Shea & Self, 1983). The "real teacher" is still absolutely essential to assist, evaluate, and organize the learning process. By allocating some of the more routine aspects of teaching to the microcomputer, the instructor can be more effective in teaching a course with greater depth, and enrichment, and can reach more students or provide more individual attention where greater personal contact is essential. The microcomputer can provide information and evaluate responses rapidly and efficiently but it cannot understand the student's needs, confusions, and other obstacles to the learning process; this requires the presence of a live, experienced teacher (Scanland & Slattery, 1983).

From the student's point of view one of the main advantages in using CAI is that one may learn new material or take a quiz to check one's comprehension level at a convenient time and as often as necessary in order to progress at one's own pace of learning. In some university computer-oriented study programs the student may even have the convenience of using the CAI in his/her own dormitory room from a personal computer or terminal access to the large central mainframe computer system. The implications of this type of learning system implemented on a widespread basis can literally stagger the imagination; however, the actual benefits and

---

©College-Hill Press, Inc. All rights, including that of translation, reserved. No part of this publication may be reproduced without the written permission of the publisher.

other aspects of the learning experience are yet to be evaluated on a systematic and reliable basis (Dence, 1980).

Microcomputer–teacher function

From one point of view the model of computer-aided instruction is the teacher him/herself, in that the computer is to explain the topic (or refer to textbook information), show the student what is to be learned and how to learn it, give a test over the designated information, and finally give the student a test score and/or evaluation of progress (Orwig, 1983). The CAI is less threatening than the teacher, however, in that in most cases the students' progress is tested only for their own information and can be treated as an informal learning exercise. In this sense, the test grade is not "real" and a poor score on the display screen is definitely more tolerable than a poor score in the grade book.

In the role of tutor, the CAI program is often provided with a personality, and treats the student with kindness and good humor. In some cases the computer's personality might be considered even too jocular to suit the learning situation and could possibly engender some reaction of disdain on the part of the learner if it were to appear too "cute" for an adult level program. Ideally, the program should display a sense of encouragement, reward for achievement, and a specific, but tolerant, accounting of errors and incorrect answers.

General outline of the CAI program

Most CAI programs have a somewhat standard format (Gagne, Wagner, & Rojas, 1981) that may include the following:

1. Introduction and instructions. This explains the purpose of the program, and informs the user about keys to be pressed and operational procedures of the instructional program that must be followed. It usually sets a user-friendly tone to the learning situation by greeting the student by name and inviting him/her to participate.

2. Informational contents. Information for the learning situation may be included in a written paragraph, an illustration shown on the display screen, or a reference to outside readings or lecture material.

3. Questions. Questions must be objective in nature—true–false, multiple choice, or matching. Other possibilities in the nature of problem-solving strategies may eventually be utilized more routinely with more advanced CAIs, but the present methodology requires that the CAI program must be able to match the student's answer precisely with the correct answer stored in the program.

4. Feedback. Evaluation of the user's answer as being right or wrong. This may include a message of encouragement and/or penalty and would usually also include a subroutine to tally the scores. Some CAIs do not proceed to the next question until the user finally gets the correct answer. More elaborate CAIs also give a hint following an incorrect answer or explain why an answer is wrong.

5. Tally. A final tally is displayed on the screen after the last test item. It may be a raw score or a percentage score. In some cases the score may be even further evaluated, as to whether it is average, below average, or excellent, to let the student know how s/he might compare with others in the class. In some types of CAI the program also keeps a check of each student's record so that the instructor can see who is and is not doing the homework.

6. Scores. Display of the test score is usually followed by a choice either to quit, to take the test again, or to go on to another test.

7. At the termination of the program the computer informs the student that the session is over, and might also add a cordial good-bye.

Uses for CAIs

Nearly all computer-assisted learning programs in use today fall into three major categories. Beginning with the area of most usage, these are (1) microcomputer programs for learning about BASIC language and the nature of computers themselves. These are produced mainly by the microcomputer manufacturer and are often included as standard equipment delivered with the new microcomputer; (2) programs for the teaching of new courses. Many of these fall into what is commonly called the "adult education" categories such as how to play bridge, how to speak a foreign language, or how to understand the stock market. One widely circulated program in the area of communicative disorders is a package for the learning of fingerspelling. It is written in BASIC and portrays the finger letters in surprisingly clear graphics; (3) remedial class material. These are mainly children's programs including areas such as math, science, biology, and English. Of particular interest in the speech–language category are quite a few programs in remedial language. These consist mostly of vocabulary, understanding of nouns and verbs, and other linguistic concepts. They tend to be very colorful, using good graphics and animation and sometimes sound. Most are inclined to present very limited material at a very primary level. Nevertheless, these represent a substantial beginning of incorporating language concepts within the motivational features of the microcomputer and will no doubt serve as the practical base for more advanced and more useful programs that can be tailored to serve the needs of specific professionals in the language development field.

In the classroom situation the CAI is usually employed in a role similar to that of an adjunct teaching experience, as part of the class course requirements, or as an optional self-help opportunity for the individual who needs some additional study of the regular class material.

As a part of the class organization the material is assigned as a type of laboratory learning experience to be completed by all members of the class. The advantage is that the instructor may use the CAI to teach the fundamentals of objective material, while using the classroom situation itself to pursue more advanced or more creative types of information. A common complaint of some instructors is that when a class consists of students from too many divergent levels or backgrounds the course must be geared to the slower student while the more advanced students are bored and ready for a higher level of instruction. CAI can be used to make sure that the class can start as a more homogeneous unit from a reliable base and that all members have the necessary vocabulary to follow the advanced lectures, readings, and discussions.

The second use of the CAI could be considered remedial in nature. Intended literally as a tutor for the student who is experiencing particular difficulty in preparing for classroom participation and tests, the CAI in this situation is set up principally as a series of review exercises.

The third use for the CAI is in the form of self-study programs in which an individual wishes to learn a topic simply on the basis of his/her own interest. These are currently available in the form of self-instruction in learning how to use a microcomputer itself and are designed mainly for children although some are available for all ages. They are often produced by the microcomputer manufacturer and may come as standard software with each new system. These are in the form of cassettes, disks, or other cartridges in which the user who has just purchased a microcomputer can insert a disk or tape and be guided through a series of steps illustrating use of the commands. Unfortunately, some of these self-learning programs appear to be hastily compiled and are often composed by professional programmers or engineers who do not always have an accurate feeling for the needs of the beginner.

Instructional applications in speech–language pathology and audiology

The workshops available in instruction in computer literacy for speech–language–hearing professionals are sometimes quite poor, being taught by personnel who have little or no concept of the needs in the area of communicative disorders. Fortunately, however, the quality of these offerings is improving steadily, as specific needs become better defined. The field is currently wide open in terms of potential software. At this writing most contributors in the field of computer-assisted instruction agree that much of the currently available software is inadequate, primitive in its content, and unimaginative in its mode of presentation. This deficiency, however, is sure to be short-lived because of the overall dynamic nature of the microcomputer technology field (Kurshan, 1981).

On the other hand, the availability of adequate hardware is already quite good and continues to get better each year (see Chial, chap. 5). Small microcomputer systems (including computer board, cassette storage, and TV screen hookup) may be purchased for even as little as $1000 at this writing. For the more professional user, the entire package (including board, screen, two-disk storage, phone MODEM, printer, and word processing software) is available in the $3000 range. Hardware also includes relatively inexpensive speech synthesizers that can make some learning programs available to preschool children and other nonreader participants (Trachtman, 1984). Needs for instructional applications are currently in the following areas:

1. Software programs for many of the standardized texts that are most widely used. These CAIs will have best application in areas that deal mainly with objective—as opposed to discussion—types of material. Some of the more obvious areas include anatomy, audiology, acoustics, neurophysiology, language development, and speech science. However, some of the broader discussion-type areas might also be utilized through the use of true–false questions dealing with the views of various authorities, uses of selected diagnostic methods, or pros and cons of certain arguments within the field. More advanced types of programs can also deal with discussion material, but these are considerably more difficult to prepare.
2. Graphics programs for the learning of anatomy need to be extended. A good start in this direction has already been achieved by Rushakoff (1984), who has combined text and color graphics to teach many of the primary aspects of speech and hearing anatomy. Sophisticated graphics programs tend to be beyond the capability of most amateur programmers and will probably have to be made primarily by professionals with course instructors as consultants. The use of graphics for interest and motivation in all learning programs is recommended but is not critical except for use with small children. Many graphics software packages also tend to require more RAM storage than is contained within the least expensive microcomputers. This may inhibit the development of instructional graphics for the time being, but will not be a problem for the newer models of microcomputers that will probably contain a minimum of 65K to 128K as standard storage capacity.
3. Case study programs should be designed to show the student how to think through evaluations of various communicative disorders. These should include decision-making simulation problems for students both in speech pathology and audiology, involving the diagnostic procedures that must be included in the test battery for each type of patient.
4. Hearing aid evaluation programs should be available in order to give the student a comparison of his/her choice of recommended aid compared with the one chosen by the microcomputer program.
5. Simulation programs for student familiarity with the variables involved in private practice, such as time schedules, fees, personnel, payroll, overhead, taxes, and legal regulations.

6. Collections of simple software programs to be used for teaching microcomputer literacy to students and for inservice training of professionals in the field. These should consist of word games, elementary graphics exercises, and number games that can be easily programmed and activated in a short period of time.
7. Research problems to be designed, in which the student selects the experimental procedures, the population, the controls, and the statistical treatments. The microcomputer could "run the study" and present the strengths and weaknesses of the results.

It would appear that the ingredients needed for CAI development are physically possible at the present time including technology, expertise, and reasonable cost. The only obvious limiting factor is time; professionals in the field have not had the opportunity to learn microcomputer programming languages nor to begin assembling the software that will fit their needs adequately. The current surge of interest in CAI implementation and computer literacy in general should change this picture in a positive direction within a few short years. The use of microcomputers is relatively self-proliferating, in that the more common their use becomes, the more other uses can be envisioned and subsequently developed (Grossnichle, 1983).

Summary

Computer-aided instruction (CAI) can be a great aid to (but not a replacement for) the instructor. As a supplement to the classroom experience the CAI can offer the student extra materials or special tutoring arranged at the student's convenience, complete with text, graphics, and sound, as needed to motivate and to highlight the material. Most CAI programs even project a friendly and encouraging personality to the student. Programs can be either simple or very complicated but all have much the same essentials, in that they present material to be learned, test the student, and evaluate the student's achievement. CAI programs are most easily applied to objective material, such as anatomy and speech and hearing science; but virtually every phase of speech, language, and hearing can be reached through appropriately designed programs. The technology is still very new and unfamiliar, but professionals in the field are catching up rapidly.

APPLYING MICROCOMPUTER INSTRUCTION

Advantages and disadvantages of the CAI

In considering the positive and negative features of computer-assisted instruction, a reader is led into the areas of realism and perhaps also of philosophy. The age of computer-assisted instruction is definitely here; how much can and will be taken advantage of it is still a matter of consideration (Scandland & Slattery, 1983). Teachers are sometimes skeptical of having their role delegated to a machine, which lacks the human factor of personal interaction. They are inclined to view this new gadget as being "good" or "bad," and thus to jump on the bandwagon or to resist it with passionate belligerence.

Taking a detached view, it is of course neither good nor bad, nor is it always helpful or advantageous. Some of the strengths/advantages and weaknesses/disadvantages are listed below.

Strengths/advantages
1. Students can use the CAI program at any time to fit their schedules. Labs are usually open all day and may also be open in the evening or even all night.

2. Students can progress at their own rate. This allows the plodding learner to proceed at a deliberate rate while the very fast learner can advance through the program swiftly.
3. In classes where some basic concepts are essential to comprehension of the lectures, the CAI program can be mastered by all of the class members on their own time to ensure a good understanding of some fundamental information by everyone. The class may then proceed from the same uniform base of knowledge. In some respects this may serve as a short course for prerequisite material that would otherwise have to be treated as review preparation before the course could really get underway.
4. The few students who tend to seek a disproportionate amount of classroom time would be able to utilize the computer learning situation and thus allow the instructor to use his/her time more effectively.
5. The experience of being pretested by the microcomputer would help uncertain or inexperienced students to know whether or not they were actually ready for the "real" examination to be held in the classroom, and to be more realistic about classroom preparation.

Weaknesses/disadvantages
1. The more inexperienced students tend to be confused by the computer hardware and software and to call upon the instructor for continual assistance. This situation is not always the fault of the student; some microcomputers and programs are temperamental and somewhat unfriendly to the naive user. Hopefully, this will become less of a problem as students enter the educational situation with greater computer literacy.
2. Some students who are actually unqualified to proceed in a certain major area—such as communication disorders—tend to persist doggedly through remedial or tutorial efforts to the point where an unrealistic passing grade is obtained in some of the basic courses. In these cases it is often argued that a student who will be unable to pass advanced courses should get a realistic appraisal of his/her academic capacity in the earlier stages of the curriculum, rather than to discover at a later stage that it is really too difficult. The unlimited tutoring aspect of the CAI may thus give some students a false assurance of their ability to learn difficult material in order to be competitive in the advanced courses of the major curriculum.
3. A major weakness in the ability to produce good instructional programs may persist for quite some time because of the obstacles in combining computer programming skills with expertise in curricular subject matter. At this moment, few instructors in the speech and hearing sciences have programming skills or the time to learn them well enough to set up original CAIs in their areas of interest. Through the availability of additional workshops and other in-service training efforts, however, this deficit should gradually diminish.

Instruction for young children

Both parents and preschool program personnel are increasingly interested in the age at which children might first become familiar with the microcomputer. Although this aspect of instruction is entirely new, some firsthand accounts have suggested that one may begin at any early age in which a child expresses an interest in the events appearing on the screen and has developed the eye–hand coordination to manipulate the keyboard. At the beginning of this kind of endeavor one should expect the child to want to press all the keys at once and to push at the keyboard with the whole hand. This is not only normal but should be expected and encouraged at this preliminary stage. Of course, the keyboard can't stand up under full-force pounding but the child will naturally begin by pressing and poking at everything to see if anything happens. This is the way the child will be trying to understand this strange new object—to see how it feels— and to see if the picture on the screen changes as a result of these actions. The child, in other words, learns by handling, and so handling should be used as the preliminary computer-readiness stage of initial progress. Some have suggested using a membrane-type keyboard for young children at first because of their tendency to have food and sticky hands that could damage the keys. The membrane-type board does not have individual moving keys, and can be wiped clean easily.

The second point to keep in mind is that the young child will be most responsive with familiar objects and pictures, such as pets, foods, clothes, and various favorite personal possessions. These should be used where possible in the early graphics or speech responses from the microcomputer.

Matching activities, primarily with graphics, should be the first formal microcomputer activity for the young child. Fortunately, quite a bit of colorful animated software based on matching has begun to appear on the market and some of these packages are even reviewed in parent's and in children's magazines. Word building and other simple language programs are a good place to start. As the child matures (the next level should not be rushed) s/he may be led into the concept of computer programming itself through play at making lists of events in their proper chronological order. These may include sequences such as "How do I get dressed in the morning," "How I get to school from my house," or "How I play with my toys." In these serial games, which can be drawn first on paper and then put on the microcomputer display screen with the help of simple graphics and simple key words, the series must include each detail in logical order, so as to make an appropriate learning activity for the sequences used even in the most simple computer programs. An adult version of these children's programs may be made up to illustrate the fundamentals of series program:

1. Get up
2. Eat breakfast
3. Call in sick? (Y/N)
4. If "Y" go back to bed
5. Go to work
6. Work one hour
7. Coffee break? (Y/N)
8. If "Y" go for coffee

For young children, LOGO can work well at ages as young as 5 or 6 years with those who are relatively mature for their chronolgocial age, but as a general rule this language is perhaps more reliable for beginners in the 8- or 9-year category. LOGO, although considered perhaps the simplest of all languages to learn, nevertheless requires about 30 hours of actual instruction in order to be learned to a functional level. Unfortunately, the research into its effectiveness in terms of related areas of development has not been well documented. Most reports of its benefits are in terms of anecdotal accounts or of surveys of general impressions of its value. The literature is slowly beginning to show that simple computer skills, particularly in the use of LOGO, have produced observable gains in language and fine motor skills—both in learning disabled and gifted learners. One of the tangible advantages of the computer display screen is that it eliminates the messy papers typical of the early ages, with multiple erasures and rewrites over the same sheet of paper. The printer produces a fairly neat final page regardless of how much rewriting the child may do on the viewing screen. Teachers also report that the inherent motivating power of the microcomputer is particularly advantageous among children who do not ordinarily respond well to school work. The microcomputer is a symbol of status and importance in modern society and the child has some extra sense of purpose upon realizing that s/he can actually control the complicated electronic device.

The microcomputer has also been reported as effective with hyperactive children; the fast responses of CAI programs appeal to those with impatience and short attention spans. Some teachers have reported that hyperactive students tend to complete about twice as many math problems or similar exercises on the computer than they do with the more tedious pencil-and-paper tasks. Even drill exercises are reported to be definitely more motivating for hyperactive as well as normal children when performed on the computer.

Teachers in nearly every imaginable area of special education have reported in one way or another that the microcomputer is well adapted to the needs of children with special types of educational problems (Ryder, Cox, & Tilley, 1983). These have included slow learners, deaf, blind, cerebral palsied, and even autistic children. The children respond well to the novelty of the device, to the feeling that they are doing something in the nature of an adult skill, because the computer teaches the concept of structured activity, and because the final result on the screen or printer gives the child a sense of pride and accomplishment because of its neatly printed format.

A rather universally observed advantage of computer-assisted education for children is that the child finds him/herself in charge of the situation and literally in charge of the microcomputer. This is especially true if the computer language is a child's language, such as LOGO. The computer has the capacity not only to convey information but also to challenge children at their own level and ultimately therefore to teach the children to think as well as to learn information (Trachtman, 1984).

Critics of CAI—who are fewer and fewer as computer literacy increases—say that the human element is missing in this kind of instruction, or that the technology-dependent child may draw away from other people and become introverted as the microcomputer is substituted for real companionship. Experience, however, does not bear out this prediction—in fact, the microcomputer tends to foster conversation and to bring about social interaction of mutual interest among computer users. Although many parents have reported that their child can scarcely leave the computer alone for the first few weeks, or even months, it eventually comes to be treated as any other useful instrument in the household, such as the family telephone or the television.

Meeting the instructional demands

Within any instructional setting, such as a school district or university department, a definite plan is necessary to get faculty and student involvement in microcomputer instruction (see Cohen, chap. 2). Ultimately, microcomputer literacy must precede instructional application. Simply buying a microcomputer for the department does not accomplish the goal.

The initial cost of the computer, with the necessary disk drive, software, monitor screen, and printer, will probably average out at approximately $3000 to $5000 at current rates. However, educational discounts on some machines, such as Apple, Acron, and IBM, would substantially change the price estimates. At least 64K and CP/M capacity are recommended in order to accommodate some of the graphic oriented instructional programs, and to take advantage of the variety of programs designed to run on CP/M BASIC language. As newer hardware packages emerge, they will be designed in both directions of cost; more rugged equipment containing extra features and designed for heavy use will probably approach the $5000 level or higher. At the opposite extreme, the more popular home computer producers will probably strive toward turning out cheaper models designed for personal light use, offering a practical setup in the $1000 category.

Most writers of the instructional software agree that, aside from the actual purchase of the microcomputer, the most critical aspect of getting an instructional program underway is the designation of one specific person to develop and coordinate the applications program within the group or department. In some cases, this may entail sending the coordinator to some workshops or night school courses to learn the elements of BASIC and the ins and outs of microcomputers and their peripheral equipment and to be responsible for setting up workable materials, reference manuals, sample programs, and maintaining an up-to-date knowledge of the rapid developments in the field. Adjustments in the resource person's working schedule or some release time is highly recommended to compensate for the extreme drain of time spent in initiating the total venture if success is to be assured (Cohen, chap. 2).

Inservice workshops, individual tutoring and consulting, and provision of sample software to be arranged by the computer coordinator represents the next step in spreading computer literacy into the potential areas of computer instruction.

In a computer literacy program designed for the staff or faculty in any training or clinical facility, the best computer consultant is not necessarily the one who knows the most about microcomputers and programming. Some organizations have reported that the expert is sometimes too formidable a person to interact with the beginners and that a better choice is someone with a generally sound knowledge of the topic. The effective resource person has a warm, friendly, interactive personality and will not intimidate the hesitant beginners or point out their mistakes too forcefully. They should be persuasive and patient in their consulting role.

The main thrust of the program at this point is to train the rest of the staff to be able to select and operate commercially available instructional programs. Ideally, however, most educators agree that a few instructors should develop some programming ability of their own in order to tailor certain programs to be more effective in specific and unique types of learning situations.

The inservice training workshops and similar presentations have been found to be most effective if they are designed for the special interests of the audience. In other words, they are minimally effective when taught as a general introduction to microcomputers or microcomputer programming. For optimum benefit from the experience, the courses should be presented as "Computer Use in Audiology," "Instructional Programming for Speech and Hearing," and so forth. The course content itself should be carefully reviewed. Some earlier professionally sponsored workshops were given attractively appropriate titles but the contents were disappointingly geared toward computer electronics or professional programming.

For the training of elementary BASIC microcomputer literacy, most reports recommend that "whole program" learning is likely to produce better results than "single command" learning. In other words, the trainees should be given small programs to work with right from the beginning instead of tediously going over all the commands in the computer language followed by instructions on how to put them together into a program. This is sometimes also referred to as "project-oriented" learning, as opposed to "vocabulary-oriented" learning.

Long- and short-range implications of the instructional development efforts should be kept in mind and evaluated periodically. The instructional staff showing the most aptitude toward computerized teaching techniques should be encouraged and given opportunities to upgrade their expertise in keeping up with developments in the field. The instructional effort should not be left to plod along with older and less efficient techniques and materials. The goal of the instructional programs themselves should evolve from mastery of the rudimentary systems of matching lists and simple multiple choice formats into use of more advanced and thought-provoking teaching techniques where the students must think through solutions to problems (see Mullendore, chap. 12). These latter techniques have been found to instill a higher quality of learning from the instructional experience and also to enable clinicians to incorporate the full capabilities of the computer.

Eventually, the use of CAIs must be put to the test of accountability (Steinberg, 1983). Research in various model programs of computer-assisted instruction should be carried out to determine which features of this methodology pay off in greatest learning advances and which features are inefficient, disadvantageous, or even detrimental to the learning process (Steffin, 1983). Cost effectiveness should also be taken into account by comparing more expensive with less expensive products and procedures for programmed materials; cost effectiveness should also be included in the year-end report.

A MICROCOMPUTER INSTRUCTIONAL PROGRAM

Functional aspects of the CAI program

Viewing the computer-assisted program from the perspective of the programmer, most instructive models are set up according to the following outline:
1. Display introduction.
2. Display information or reference to readings or lecture material.
3. Display question No. 1 of the test, and wait for response.
4. Judge or grade the response to question No. 1.
5. If the answer is right, say "good" and go to the next question. If the answer is wrong, tally the error, say "try again" and repeat the question.
6. As an optional step, stop the test if the student is making too many errors.
7. After the last question, say "Test is complete," and display the student's score.
8. Ask the student whether s/he wants to continue on to the next test, repeat the present test, or quit. Depending upon the student's response, the computer program should jump ahead to the next section, go back to an earlier line number, or go to the next line and say "good-bye."

Diagram of the CAI

Once the programmer has the general sequence of the program in mind, it is customarily set up as a series of subroutines, or building blocks, to make the total program, as shown in Figure 9-1. These are arranged in boxes, each representing a subroutine, laid out in sequence much like the diagrams used to show the arrangement of laboratory equipment.

A short version of a working CAI program for anatomy of the ear follows. This program repeats the question until the student gets the correct answer, then goes to the next question. At the end, the student's tally of total incorrect answers is displayed and the student is given the choice of stopping or taking the test again. The full microcomputer program looks like that displayed in Figure 9-2.

Expanded CAI program features

Although the outline shown in Figure 9-2 is simple in its most elementary form, a great many extra features can be added to enhance CAI attractiveness and effectiveness. For example, the amount of time that the informational material remains on the screen can be controlled to introduce a certain speed factor into the learning situation. The time allowed for the student's answer can also be controlled or prodding messages can be inserted to speed the test along such as, "Please hurry—my circuits are heating up." In the commercial CAIs graphics play a major role in presenting the stimulus material in an animated display, in rewarding correct answers, or in congratulating a high level of achievement. This latter display, for example, might show a clown doing somersaults on the screen or other exuberant displays such as those that sometimes appear on athletic scoreboards following a home run or touchdown.

Advanced instructional materials have included a more subjective or thought-provoking format such as the presentation of a diagnostic case study followed by a series of questions concerning the recommendations, referral, therapy plan, prognosis, and related considerations about the disposition of the patient. This mode of CAI is not always scored but may rather be printed out and used for class discussion. It could be analyzed, of course, based on the student's ability to solve the problem by the most efficient means. This would involve the amount

Figure 9-1. Diagram of computer assisted instruction.

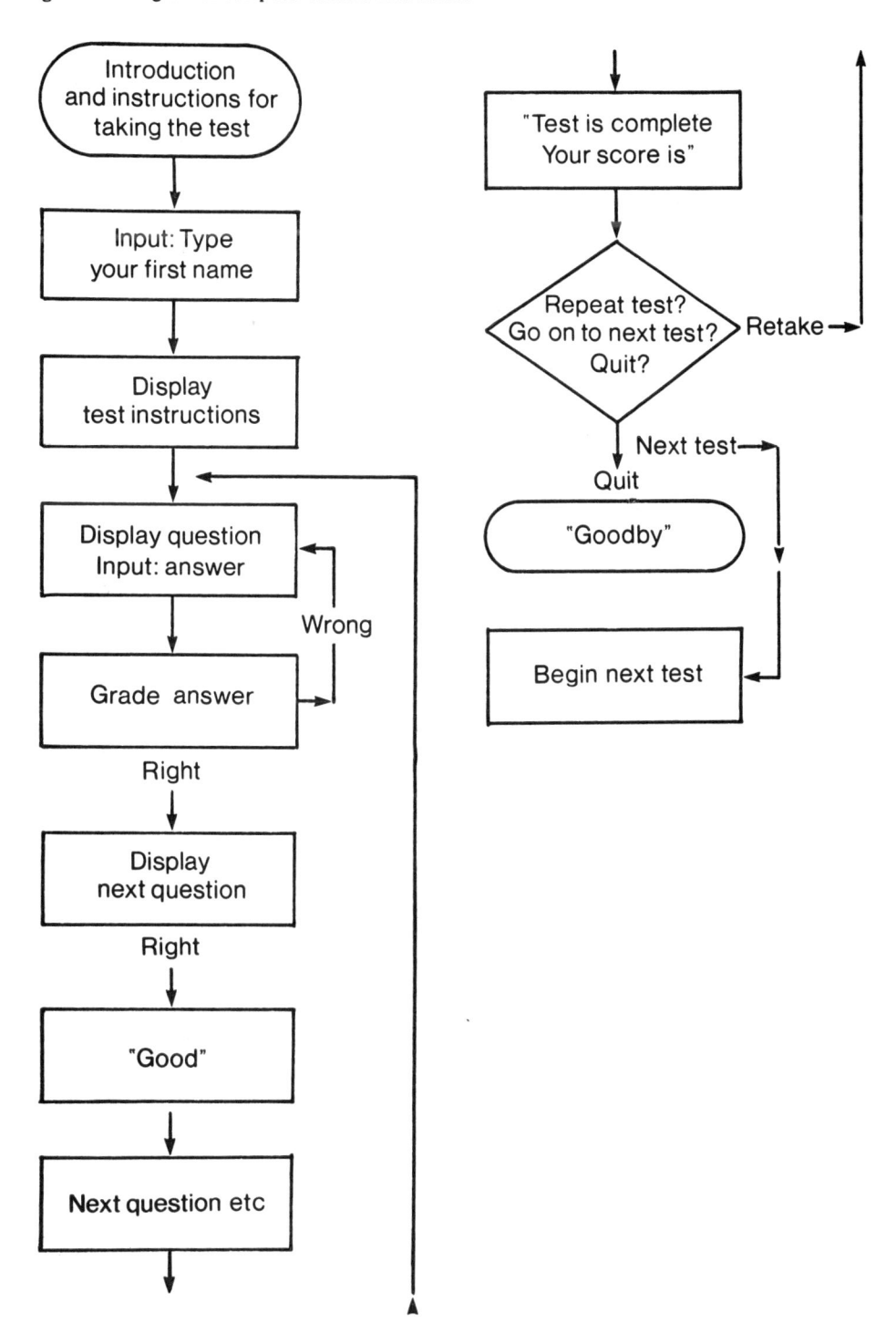

Figure 9-2. CAI program listing for anatomy of the ear.

```
10   PRINT   "WELCOME TO COMPUTER ASSISTED INSTRUCTION ON THE"
20   PRINT   "HEARING MECHANISM."
30   PRINT   "PLEASE TYPE YOUR FIRST NAME, AND PRESS THE 'RETURN' KEY."
40   PRINT   INPUT   X$
50   PRINT   "THAT'S FINE, "X$
60   PRINT   "NOW READ THE FOLLOWING PARAGRAPH:"
70   PRINT   "THE RIM ON THE TOP OF THE EAR IS THE HELIX,  AND THE"
80   PRINT   "HOLLOW IN THE CENTER OF THE EAR IS THE CONCHA, AND THE"
90   PRINT   "FLAP ANTERIOR TO THE OPENING OF THE EAR CANAL IS"
100  PRINT   "CALLED THE TRAGUS.  THE EAR CANAL IS ABOUT 25 MM. LONG, "
110  PRINT   "AND CONTAINS WAX CALLED 'CERUMEN'."
120  PRINT
130  PRINT   "ENTER ANY LETTER TO CONTINUE (AND PRESS RETURN)."
140  INPUT   Z$
150  FOR     C=1 TO 30
160  PRINT
170  NEXT    C
180  PRINT   "WHAT IS THE ANTERIOR FLAP BY THE EAR CANAL?"
190  PRINT   "A=CERUMEN, B=HELIX, C=TRAGUS, D=CONCHA"
200  INPUT   R$
210  IF R$ = "B" GOTO 260
220  N=N+1
230  PRINT   "SORRY," X$
240  PRINT   "WRONG ANSWER; TRY AGAIN."
250  GOTO    180
260  PRINT   "RIGHT !  HERE IS THE NEXT QUESTION."
270  PRINT
280  PRINT   "WHAT IS THE APPROXIMATE LENGTH OF THE EAR CANAL?"
290  PRINT   "A=5MM, B=15MM, C=25MM, D=CONCHA"
300  INPUT   S$
310  IF S$="C" GOTO 340
320  PRINT   "WRONG ANSWER.  TRY AGAIN," X$
330  GOTO    270
340  PRINT "YOU GOT THIS ONE RIGHT, TOO," X$
350  REM...PAUSE...
360  FOR P = 1 TO 1200
370  NEXT P
380  REM ...CLEAR SCREEN ...
390  FOR C=1 TO 30
400  PRINT
410  NEXT C
420  PRINT   "THIS COMPLETES THE QUIZ," X$
430  PRINT   "THE NUMBER OF INCORRECT ANSWERS WAS " N
440  PRINT   "DO YOU WISH TO TAKE THE TEST AGAIN?"
450  INPUT   "Y OR N"; S$
460  IF S$ = "Y" GOTO 70
470  PRINT
480  PRINT   "GOODBY,"X$
490  PRINT   "SEE YOU AGAIN SOMETIME."
500  END
```

of time required to solve the diagnostic question or the number of steps used in arriving at the solution. More imaginative applications of CAIs have seen little use so far except perhaps in finance and some areas of business (Herschler, 1983) or administration in which strategy is part of the activity. Using a game format, the student must follow certain ground rules and plays to "win" by using a problem-solving approach to the task presented.

Simulation problems

The advanced types of instruction, sometimes called "simulation problems," are designed according to the following format:

1. The overview of the problem is presented to the student, who is to arrive at the solution in the most effective means possible. The problem should be realistic in nature, challenging, and should contain a certain amount of unusual or attention-getting material. It should require some thought.

2. It should contain a problem that has features actually encountered in the field (Herschler, 1983). Possible simulation problems might include scheduling a typical group of children from five elementary schools, writing individualized education programs (IEPs) for several types of children, determining a malingerer in a hearing test, conducting a complete speech evaluation for one or more types of clients, or running a clinical enterprise, such as a clinic, hospital department, agency, or private practice function.

3. The student can call upon all the types of information that might reasonably be available, such as interview material, medical reports, observations, and test results.

4. As part of the instruction plan, there is a limit to the amount of information that can be accumulated by the player. This might be limited by the client's fatigue, availability of the clinic facilities, or the clinician's time, or by the expense of client's travel to the clinic.

5. When the student arrives at the solution to the clinical problem his/her answers are scored on the basis of (A) whether or not the answer agreed with the recommended solution, and (B) how efficiently the students used the cumulative clues as the problem was being solved. Sometimes the simulated information is weighted according to how important or superfluous it was in getting to the heart of the problem.

6. As with other games, the task may be repeated in order to achieve a better score.

Annotated CAI outline

1. Display the title of the learning program, the author, and other similar designations.

2. Give instructions to the student about the function of the program and the use of the computer keyboard in making responses to the test items and in controlling the progress of the program itself.

    THIS PROGRAM IS TO TEST YOUR COMPREHENSION OF THE ANATOMY OF THE EAR.

3. Present the informative material or refer to the assigned reading or lecture used as the basis of the test. Perhaps for the purist, the CAI should be entirely self-contained, including the content material to be learned. However, realistically, the CAI information should be presented through whatever medium is the most appropriate for the content and the learning situation. More often in the future the information content is likely to be displayed by taped video picture in the display screen, in the form of lectures, graphics, and laboratory demonstrations. For the time being, however, the simplest way to display the information is through the text paragraph on the display screen:

    THE OUTER EAR IS CALLED THE PINNA, WHICH CONSISTS OF SEVERAL IMPORTANT SUBSTRUCTURES THAT MAY AID SLIGHTLY IN HEARING OR IN THE

PROTECTION OF THE EAR ITSELF. THESE INCLUDE THE HELIX, OR UPPER RIM, THE TRAGUS OR ANTERIOR FLAP, AND THE CONCHA OR CENTRAL BOWL.

4. Display the test question. Of necessity, all questions must be objective because the program has no capacity to grade other types of questions. Ideally, there should be no room for interpretation of the wording as having more than a specific single meaning. The choices of answers to the questions are nearly always presented in the form that can be answered by a single letter or number. Whole-word answers can be handled by the computer but any variation in spelling or even in upper and lower case will be interpreted as an incorrect answer.

WHAT IS THE NAME OF THE UPPER RIM OF THE OUTER EAR?
A = PINNA   B = HELIX   C = LOBE

The first few questions often include a reminder to press the RETURN key to enter the answer.

5. Check the answer. Following the student's response to each quiz question, the CAI program matches the student's answer with the correct answer stored in the program. If it is a perfect match, the screen typically displays a message of reinforcement, such as "THAT'S RIGHT!" and then goes on to display the next question. If the answer is incorrect, some programs are made merely to ask the student to try again. Others go into elaborate branching routines to correct areas of misinformation. However, this part of the CAI tends to be gauged to fit the tolerance level of the students. Some simply ignore the error and say "TRY AGAIN" while others may be a bit more pointed, as in "SORRY, BILL, THAT'S WRONG. TRY AGAIN."

As an additional feature, some CAIs are designed with a built-in progress report that counts the number of errors part way into the test and may ask the student if s/he wishes to go back to an earlier learning step. At a more stern or pedantic level, some CAIs simply inform the student that s/he has missed too many items and is not prepared for the test. It is therefore terminated at that point.

"YOU HAVE MISSED 10 ITEMS UP TO THIS POINT; THE TEST IS NOW TERMINATED. REREAD YOUR TEXT AND TRY AGAIN."

6. After the last question, the program informs the student that the test has been completed and the test score is displayed. Sometimes an evaluation of the score is also included.

THIS COMPLETES THE TEST. YOUR TOTAL NUMBER OF ERRORS IS 3.
YOUR SCORE IS VERY GOOD, BILL.

7. At the end of the CAI program the student is asked whether to (A) terminate this program, (B) take the same test again, or (C)—if the CAI is fairly long and divided into sections—to continue on to the next section.

Making a sample CAI program

The outline shown in Figure 9-3 may be used directly as is, for a model CAI program, simply by copying the program word-for-word and filling in the blanks. The program is written in BASIC and is designed to run on Apple, Commodore, and NEC, but should also run on nearly all other microcomputers. However, all makes of microcomputers have small idiosyncracies and small modifications of BASIC language that will cause error messages to appear on the screen at various stages of the program. Therefore, small adjustments may have to be made for use of this program on certain computer models. With experience using this CAI template, a "programmer" may then want to experiment with different messages to the student and expand or modify the program to fit individual teaching and learning situations more closely.

Figure 9-3. CAI template outline.

```
10      PRINT TAB(15) "WELCOME TO COMPUTER AIDED INSTRUCTION."
20      PRINT
30      PRINT "THE TOPIC IS . . . . . . . . . . . . . . . ."
40      PRINT
50      PRINT "INSTRUCTIONS:"
60      PRINT "YOU WILL BE PRESENTED A PARAGRAPH TO READ."
70      PRINT "PLEASE READ IT CAREFULLY, UNTIL YOU COMPREHEND "
80      PRINT "IT COMPLETELY AND ARE READY FOR THE QUIZ QUESTIONS."
90      PRINT "AFTER EACH QUESTION, TYPE IN YOUR ANSWER "
100     PRINT "AND PRESS THE KEY MARKED 'RETURN'. "
110     PRINT "WHEN YOU ARE READY FOR QUESTION #1 TYPE THE "
120     PRINT "LETTER 'R' AND PRESS THE 'RETURN' KEY."
130     INPUT R$
140     FOR C=1 TO 30
150     PRINT
160     NEXT C
165     REM . . . TYPE IN YOUR PARAGRAPH . . .
170     PRINT " . . . . . . . . . . . . . . . . . . . . . . . ."
180     PRINT " . . . . . . . . . . . . . . . . . . . . . . . ."
190     PRINT " . . . . . . . . . . . . . . . . . . . . . . . ."
200     PRINT " . . . . . . . . . . . . . . . . . . . . . . . ."
210     PRINT
220     PRINT "PLEASE PRESS THE LETTER 'C' AND 'RETURN' TO CONTINUE."
225     REM . . . CLEAR SCREEN . . .
230     FOR C=1 TO 30
240     PRINT
250     NEXT C
252     REM . . . TYPE IN THE QUESTION . . .
255     PRINT " . . . . . . . . . . . . . . . . . . . . . . . ."
260     PRINT "TYPE IN THE CORRECT ANSWER AND PRESS 'RETURN'."
270     PRINT "A= . . . . . . . . . .        B= . . . . . . . . . . ."
280     PRINT "C= . . . . . . . . . .        D= . . . . . . . . . . ."
290     PRINT
300     INPUT "ANSWER";A$
310     IF A$="." GOTO ???
315     REM . . . T = TALLY . . .
320     T=T+1
330     PRINT " . . . . . . . . . . . . . . . . . . . . . . . ."
340     PRINT "SORRY, TRY AGAIN, "N$
350     GOTO 170
360     PRINT "THAT'S RIGHT, "N$
370     PRINT "PRESS 'C' (AND 'RETURN') TO CONTINUE"
380     INPUT I$
385     FOR C=1 TO 30
390     PRINT
400     NEXT C
410     PRINT "THE NEXT QUESTION IS:"
420     PRINT " . . . . . . . . . . . . . . . . . . . . . . . ."
430     PRINT "A = . . . . . . . . . .      B = . . . . . . . . . . ."
432     PRINT "C = . . . . . . . . . .      D = . . . . . . . . . . ."
440     INPUT B$
450     IF B$="." GOTO ???
460     T=T+1
470     PRINT "SORRY, TRY AGAIN, "N$
480     GOTO 420
490     PRINT "RIGHT AGAIN, "N$
500     INPUT "ENTER C";I$
```

Figure 9-3. CAI template outline. (Continued)

```
505    REM . . . CLEAR SCREEN . . .
510    FOR C=1 TO 30
520    PRINT
530    NEXT C
540    REM . . . ADD MORE PARAGRAPHS AND MORE QUESTIONS, FOLLOWING THE
550    REM . . . SAME PATTERN SHOWN ABOVE, UNTIL THE TEST IS COMPLETE. . .
1000   PRINT "THIS CONCLUDES THE TEST, "N$
1010   PRINT "WOULD YOU LIKE TO STOP NOW, TAKE THE TEST AGAIN,"
1020   PRINT "OR GO ON TO THE NEXT TEST?"
1030   INPUT "S, A, OR G";R$
1040   IF R$="A" GOTO 30
1050   IF R$="G" GOTO 1080
1060   PRINT "GOODBYE FOR NOW, "N$
1080   PRINT "HERE IS THE NEXT TEST, "N$
```

INSTRUCTIONAL LANGUAGES FOR CAI

Microcomputer language

The "real" language of the microcomputer is the language of binary numbers—a symbolic system made up exclusively from the group of numbers with digits that consist only of 0 and 1. From this base it is relatively easy to function in the languages of mathematics using the symbols found in arithmetic, algebra, trigonometry, and so on. Most humans, however, must communicate in their own language system consisting of words, phrases, and sentences. These are easy for humans to manage but are slow, clumsy, and very awkward for computers. Therefore, any communications between humans and computers are always some form of compromise between our two divergent native languages. A relatively simple compromise can be made by using a language based mainly on single words instead of mathematical symbols. These are found in common command statements such as RUN, LIST, and PRINT. Other mutually understood parts of the language consist of the most common mathematical symbols, such as those used to indicate addition (+), subtraction (−), multiplication (*), and division (/). In the future evolution of CAI design it is essential that the computer interact in a "user-friendly" manner with the student, and also that the computer be able to accept programs made by non-computer specialists, that is, by specialists in non-computer fields.

As professional applications become more advanced, microcomputers will undoubtedly be able to communicate in a more conversational manner. Learners, in turn, will become more sophisticated and tolerant of the microcomputer's native tongue. By far, the greatest contributions in CAIs are being made in BASIC. This is the language of the "amateur" programmer and yet is robust enough to handle rather long and complicated programs. It is also fairly easy to learn and comparatively easy to debug—that is, to correct errors in the program. "Easy to learn," however, realistically implies about 6 months of spare time practice as an average period for learning the language well enough to set up a one-page program and make it do the task for which it was intended. The advertisements that suggest writing one's own programs within a few hours after the computer is unpacked from the box are highly misleading; the beginner's exercises are a far cry from programs that will serve a practical and useful purpose.

Two other relatively simple languages for the noncommercial programmer are LOGO and PILOT. These are gaining in popularity rapidly, and will soon become as common as BASIC. LOGO is perhaps already the most common computer language among children and preschool educators. PILOT will perhaps also surpass BASIC among educational users, because of its CAI applications, relative ease of learning, and low cost of software. Pascal and C have also demonstrated promise as all-purpose languages with better efficiency than BASIC for CAI applications. Both of these, however, are definitely harder to learn than BASIC. Both languages are nevertheless available as options in most microcomputers.

Artificial intelligence languages

A newer class of languages that will find perhaps more use in the future in instructional programs are sometimes called the "artificial intelligence" languages (O'Shea & Self, 1983; Roberts & Park, 1983). They are so named because they can be programmed in somewhat less specific terms and they have the capacity to carry out commands in a rather general way that need not be clearly specified by the human programmer. The simplest of these is LOGO but the more advanced types include Smalltalk, FORTH, and LISP. These latter languages are considered to be difficult for the casual user to master but the future is likely to produce languages that are easier to use and many will probably be in the nature of "broad concept languages." With increased computer literacy among the next generation of humans to match the increasingly human-like capacities of the next generation of computers the end result will clearly be much better effectiveness.

In the future, moreover, as the CAI concept evolves in the direction of learning through problem-solving strategy, some of the artificial intelligence languages will find greater employment in the medium of games that teach users to think through problems more effectively (Roberts & Park, 1983). The characteristic of these languages that makes them suitable for artificial intelligence functions is that they have the capacity to adapt to a situation by changing their own commands slightly as the program develops (O'Shea & Self, 1983). In other words, the programmer inserts the concept of the task and the program calculates the way the command should be carried out. As a result, the student has more of a sensation of interacting with another imaginative being rather than with a simplistic machine.

BASIC

BASIC stands for "beginner's all purpose symbolic instruction code." This has become almost the universal language of the microcomputer but it has many dialects that prevent its use from being completely standardized. Fortunately, most of these variations are not within the main body of the average program but are related to operating systems of different makes of microcomputers or to certain makes of printers and other peripheral devices. Therefore, a program written in BASIC will more or less run on all microcomputers (and many large mainframe computers) except for minor commands, such as clearing the screen or activating the printer. Some of these variations or dialects in the language are MBASIC, CP/M BASIC, Applesoft BASIC, NBASIC, SBASIC, and integer BASIC.

CP/M BASIC is a version of BASIC which has many universal types of software. Most microcomputers have either a built-in CP/M chip or provision for adding CP/M (control program for microprocessors) at extra cost. For the serious programmer, and particularly in dealing with instructional software, the capacity to develop and run programs on CP/M BASIC is essential if the resulting software is intended to have a universal acceptance.

BASIC is about the simplest language for most people to learn. It can produce elaborate and lengthy programs as well as simple exercises for the beginner. It is, however, an inefficient, bulky, and clumsy language for the computer to run and is even a bit tiresome for the skilled programmer. If computers had the capacity to become bored they would definitely react to BASIC in this manner. There have been no studies to show that BASIC is in fact a better all-purpose language for beginners than are any of the other microcomputer languages such as Pascal or Ada, for example. In fact, both LOGO and PILOT are probably better for educational purposes. However, BASIC has a considerable head start over any other language as many microcomputers have used it as their main language. Eventually, Ada, or perhaps Pascal, might become the main built-in language for the microcomputer but so far neither of these has seemed to catch on. This is especially surprising in the case of Ada, because it was developed specifically as an all-purpose standard and was field-tested to reduce programmer errors.

LOGO

The most elementary example of general concept language is LOGO. It is particularly well suited for use by children, having been designed at Massachusetts Institute of Technology by Papert (1980) specifically to teach children the essentials of computer programming through the medium of graphics. LOGO accepts commands that are very close to conversational speech and much of its function is based upon moving color graphics. This aspect of LOGO is called "turtle graphics" because it is controlled by moving a small triangle—called a turtle—around on the screen. The turtle moves any commanded distance in any direction toward which it is pointed and is used to set up lines and other figures that can be programmed almost instantly to move or expand on their own. By this extremely simple and rapid technique, the user can make up a working game in full color, complete with space ship figures and laser gunfire in a matter of minutes. The commands are actually so simple and obvious that the inexperienced programmer can often guess the correct terminology. This feature of the language is called "intuitive vocabulary." An advantage of LOGO for beginners is that it treats mistakes by the user not as mistakes but rather as a novel type of programming; it tries to make something out of a strange command instead of simply printing an error message (McDougal et al., 1983). Vague "error messages," common to other languages, are often quite intimidating to the new user of the language. For example, if the student were to type in an incorrect command, such as JUMP, LOGO would simply answer, "I can't jump." Other languages would respond with "INVALID COMMAND" or "SYNTAX ERROR."

For more sophisticated purposes, however, LOGO has the capability to learn new vocabulary as it is programmed, and its workings become fascinating in this respect. If, for example, the user makes a wave form on the screen and inserts the word "wave," "to wave" then becomes a verb in LOGO's vocabulary. From then on, "to wave" is accepted as a regular command to draw a wave on the screen. This process encourages children to develop new words. It is also adapted to children with physical or learning disabilities because it will function even with the child's newly invented commands. By analogy, the same types of controls that perform the graphic presentations on the display screen are also capable of making similar compositions in a sound system using musical notes. Musical patterns can be composed and put together in unlimited combinations to make tunes or rhythmic patterns. The music function, however, is a comparatively recent development of LOGO and its effectiveness and usefulness have yet to be evaluated.

LOGO first appeared in the 1960s as a system for the fast arrangement of graphics, and has since developed into a delightful children's game language. It is now available to be run on most of the common brands of computers. For all its flexibility and simplicity, LOGO has many very significant limitations.

1. It does not have the structure and uniformity needed for general purpose programming, as is found in BASIC. In other words, it could not be used very well to make the tightly organized question-and-answer types of CAI. It is also too slow for the types of programs that are intended to have a practical use with larger amounts of data to be handled with timely efficiency.
2. It works better in more sophisticated hardware, preferably with a 16-bit rather than an 8-bit system, and it needs a large storage system, in excess of 64K, if it is to be operated with its full options. A RAM storage capacity of 64K will accept a rather large software package, but will leave little room for the user to build the program.

3. A high-quality screen makes a big difference in displaying the color graphics at their intended level of clarity and effectiveness.
4. Finally, the serious user who intends to purchase LOGO for educational purposes should be aware of the many versions of LOGO that are available. The less expensive versions are not likely to contain the capability of the full language package. Although all versions contain turtle graphics, the more complete sets include additional functions, such as list processing and other data handling routines.

PILOT

"Programmed inquiry learning or teaching" makes the acronym PILOT. This language was designed specifically to help teachers make instructional training programs. In its high degree of organization, PILOT is closely akin to Pascal. It has been considerably expanded since its development and is now available in a form called "SUPERPILOT." It is designed to incorporate color graphics and sound effects into the CAI, in addition to the regular written text. PILOT is in the category of "authoring languages"; that is, it can be used by a teacher to write a teaching program, wherein the clinician does not need to know much about computer programming per se. All that is needed is to fill out the form, so to speak, and PILOT will present the information to the student in the form of a test, complete with interaction instruction (Hazen, 1982). An especially attractive feature of PILOT is that it gives messages to the student in the form of conversational sentences. It is best suited for making games and similar learning activities that are much like many of our familiar word games.

It is also easily programmed for drill exercises, comes in several versions, and is priced quite reasonably. A distinctive part about the workings of PILOT is that it can scan the student's answers for key words much as an instructor might grade an essay test, checking to see whether the main concepts were included in the writing. This scanning procedure takes slightly longer than does the checking of an objective test but the end result is much more interactive for the student. In addition, PILOT includes a graphics function that is similar to LOGO. It is easily programmable for charts, graphics, and abstract designs that can be interspersed with written test. Designed exclusively as an instructional language, PILOT does not work very well for general programming of a noninstructional nature.

Pascal

This language is usually considered to be one step more advanced than BASIC. It is slightly more structured than BASIC and, therefore, employs a few more rules of form that must be followed by the programmer (Price, 1983). Once learned it can be programmed faster than BASIC on the microcomputer but its rigid rules of syntax also make it harder to learn. For this reason Pascal has never gained its anticipated popularity in the area of education or in general personal programming. Its growth to date has been mainly in business applications. Although Pascal itself is not generally considered to be a major CAI language, some Pascal-related languages, notably PILOT, are at the forefront of instructional application.

FORTH

Another of the optional languages available for many microcomputers is called FORTH. In structure it is very much like Pascal and it is sometimes viewed as an easier version of assembly language. FORTH uses single symbols to represent whole words or even whole concepts. It is a very fast and efficient language to program and to run. Unfortunately, it is difficult for the occasional programmer to learn and to keep accurately in mind and for this reason it is considered to be more in the class of professional programmer's languages. As instructional software develops, FORTH may find use in longer CAIs because its programs require considerably less storage space than those written in BASIC. An especially helpful feature of FORTH in certain situations is that it has the capacity to interface easily with other types of peripheral hardware devices and can thus serve to control video display, lab equipment, or other experimental equipment. It is also well suited to making charts and graphics.

Ada

Another of the comparatively new object-oriented languages, along with LOGO, is Ada. Its prime feature is that it puts together object-related concepts and can deal with generalities rather than with the more tedious handling of precisely specific detail found in some earlier languages. Since many details can be omitted, the assembly of programs is speeded up considerably. At present Ada has not yet seen much service as an instructional language, but as games of strategy become more popular in CAIs, this language should have greater educational involvement.

Ada was named after Ada Lovelace, who is credited with being the world's first computer programmer. She used a primitive "computing machine" that was developed in England in the 1800s. The language itself was developed by the United States Department of Defense in 1978 as a language that was to replace the awkward array of other computer languages used by various offices and thus standardize the whole system of computer programming. It was tested extensively over a period of 5 years in order to eliminate major sources of user error. Although it is not quite as easy to learn as is BASIC it is designed around a relatively small vocabulary so as to reduce the need for the new user to memorize a large number of commands to become operational in the system (Saxon & Fritz, 1983). The small programming vocabulary also makes Ada programs efficient to store.

C

C is a relatively powerful language, perhaps on a par with Pascal in terms of learning difficulty. Like Forth, it is considered to be an efficient language in that it employs a very minimal use of words to make up its verbal commands (Plum, 1983), and would, therefore, serve as a good instructional language for microcomputers where RAM storage space is at a premium. In some respects C might be viewed as a tighter and more advanced language in the category of LOGO, because of its use of many single-word commands.

User-friendly computer instruction

In software packages, the term "user-friendly" refers primarily to an abundance of instructions and built-in contingency routines that will prevent the user from making mistakes (Goldes, 1983). Aspects of user-friendly software can be readily identified by the presence of easily understood choices shown on the screen, by a "help" option that can explain different commands, and by the insertion of periodic reminders to run the program properly. The use of specific, plain-language, error statements is also a feature of user-friendly material.

Overall, computerized instructional material is still very much in its infancy. Although it has reached an essentially practical level for the potential user, it still requires a large measure of study and perseverance for its operation. Developmentally, the application of the microcomputer scene and is now hastily striving to catch up both in computer literacy and in knew how to charge the condenser, advance the spark, set the choke, and adjust the throttle. Much is said about user-friendly microcomputers and user-friendly instructional software programs, but a frank and realistic view of the present situation is that not all of the instructional material advertised as user friendly really is user friendly. This condition is particularly true in the field of speech–language pathology and audiology that has arrived only recently in the microcomputer scene and is now hastily striving to catch up both in computer literacy and in critically needed software. Most aspects of microcomputer instruction still require much outside help in setting up the loading commands and in grasping the instructional procedures correctly for the first time. Some materials require frequent and detailed reference to the codebook or user's manual before the essentials are eventually memorized and can be put into operation easily. In addition, most users of instructional programs or would-be instructional programmers cannot shift confidently from one brand of microcomputer to another. Each microcomputer has its own special operating features that must be mastered by the user before its programs will run properly. Aside from a general acceptance of CP/M BASIC language, the obvious advantages of better standardization have been deliberately waved aside by manufacturers. For example, the BASIC commands to clear the screen on an Apple, a Commodore, an Acorn, and an NEC are all different. The commands to run the printer are also different from one system to the next. Hardly any large program can be composed in BASIC without adjusting for small differences in each unit's use of the language. Each has, in essence, its own "dialect" of BASIC that makes the interchange difficult and annoying.

This situation, fortunately, is improving as more and more computer advertisements describe their products as "IBM compatible," as equipment that "accepts Apple software," or that it has "optional CP/M BASIC." Perhaps as computer instruction develops beyond the current stage consumer demand will create a market for the most highly standardized types of products, and the nonadaptive ones will fall by the wayside. In today's computer magazines, the private software companies are already beginning to advertise their wares as being made for about four makes of computers. Already, the narrowing of the field into a few giant industries will establish a functional standard, thereby reducing frustration among consumers and producers of educational software.

Trends in instructional use and development

The multifaceted advances in the use and applications of the CAI cannot readily be foreseen, except to make the obvious observation that the technique is developing at an awesome rate. The best predictions, however, are that the trend in self-instruction by means of the computer will move toward the use of individual, personally owned computers, rather than the facilitation of a large, central computer reached through the channels of locally situated monitor stations. Time-sharing modes of computer instruction based upon large, centralized data banks and information systems have received little use so far, except from commercial office utilization, because the long distance telephone fees are beyond the cost easily afforded by most people on a private basis. Some increased use, however, might be found among those who could access the system late at night or on weekends when the rates are cheaper. For practical purposes, however, time-sharing eductional programs have found better acceptance in the larger populated communities where many people can reach the system through local, rather than the expensive long distance telephone lines. Perhaps as satellite communications replace conventional telephone lines, the concept of long distance calling may actually become obsolete and computer access in that event could be greatly simplified.

Program composer packages

Unfortunately, the programming expertise of the average instructor requires backup from skilled resource personnel and programmers before training software of professional quality can be developed. However, some materials have been introduced to ease the task of the nonprogrammer who is struggling to produce software in his/her own discipline. This assistance is in the form of software known as program composer packages. These are presently very complicated and expensive, and are designed to guide the novice programmer through the composition of CAIs or other types of software on a step-by-step basis. The composer languages—aside from being expensive—are typically "machine-dependent" programs. This means that the program will run only on one type of computer—usually a large mainframe computer, such as those centrally housed in large universities. For example, some of the languages and their computer makes are ASET—UNIVAC, Tutor—Control Data, and Coursewriter—IBM. An additional program, called CAN, has been created for use with a variety of different makes of large computers. On a simpler and fairly inexpensive basis, the various versions of PILOT may serve the immediate needs of the would-be CAI instructor-programmer (Kleinman & Humphrey, 1982). Representing a step beyond PILOT are a host of newer tutorial systems packages, known variously as SCHOLAR, WHY, WEST, SOPHIE, and GUIDION. These are highly interactive with the student, and are therefore sometimes designated as ICAI programs, meaning "intelligent computer-assisted instruction" (Roberts & Park, 1983). A particularly intriguing mode of ICAI is sometimes termed the "apprentice-master" relationship, in which the student is guided through a deductive exercise by the computer. This is exemplified by the MYCIN program for learning the techniques of medical diagnosis (O'Shea & Self, 1983).

A few training and rehabilitation centers have experimented with instructional programs for patients, such as vocabulary programs for aphasics, language programs for children, or sign language programs for the hearing impaired and students in education for the deaf. By far the most technologically advanced program is at the National Institute for the Deaf, which has a microcomputer program interfaced with color television taped samples and displays a visual presentation of sign language or speech reading inserted into the standard computer screen text.

This program, called DAVID, was designed by Sims (1982) for the deaf but its technology holds great promise for all other areas of computer-aided instruction. The user is first shown a video action picture (on disk) of the signed word used in a sentence. The next segment displays another signed scene and the student is asked to choose the correct written sentence from the text appearing on the screen. The result is an excellent blend of written and pictorial presentation for the learning situation; however, the technological hookup is very complicated and considerably beyond the resources of most training institutions at the present time. Although still in its experimental stages, the future of this technique is assured. As its procedures become more easily produced, and its patchwork of equipment becomes more compact and less expensive, its influence in aspects of clinical and academic coursework is a logical consequence (Troutner, 1983).

Interactive video instruction

At an even more advanced level—almost in the realm of science fiction—is the fully interactive video instructor concept. At least in theory, the video screen would converse with students to the extent that students would be unsure that they were actually talking with a computer (Hon, 1983). The hardware is essentially in place now; the software compilation, although entirely possible, represents an extremely ambitious task, not only as high-tech programming, but also as a major piece of artistry (Levin, 1983; Onosko, 1982; Hon, 1983; Kirchner, 1982). The technology of the program involves asking the student a question, then scanning the student's typed answer and finding an appropriate verbal reply within a matter of 3 seconds, and displaying the instructor's image and vocal response. This feat is made possible by storing a very large (54,000) repertoire of spoken segments on video disk, which spins at the rate of 1,800 RPM (Sebestyen, 1982) under the laser optical scanner (Levin, 1983). Unlike video tape, the spinning disk literally has no beginning, middle, or end, so the scanner can pick up any desired segment during any given rotation. Referred to as "level three videodisc systems" (Levin, 1983), these components are available for most common computers that have a video disk card made to be inserted into the microcomputer circuitry. Except for a few experimental samples these packages are not yet available to the regular consumer but the process is underway and the results may appear soon as interactive games and later in the form of very sophisticated tutoring programs.

CAIs, however, may still experience only limited application in some sectors because many instructors are understandably reluctant to expend extra time and resources on methods that could perhaps amount only to a passing fad. One might reason that the popularity of this "new gimmick" might fade as rapidly as it has appeared, much like the CB car radio. On the other hand, many professionals view it not as a new departure from the present way of doing things but simply as a logical step in current development (Holmes, 1982). With its traditional orientation toward equipment, audiology may advance more rapidly into computer instructional uses than will some of the more clinician-centered areas of the field. Active resistance to computer instruction may also be anticipated from those who simply do not function well with mechanical devices in general.

Judging from recent surveys, aphasia and language development will probably be among the first areas to utilize commercially available client-instruction software on a large scale. In most of the instructional settings, students and faculty will probably simply learn to use the software commercially available and may never learn the elements of simple programming at all—much as the secretaries who are highly proficient with word processing may have no concept of how the program itself is made.

Some other fields of learning that are closely allied with communicative disorders, such as statistics and related mathematics, may quite possibly benefit speech-language pathology indirectly in welcoming a new generation of children who reach college without having developed the customary fear of math. The math packages with user-friendly offerings seem to produce learning situations that are more patient with timid students, more tolerant of their fumbling efforts, and more creative and stimulating in the presentation of new material. This experience of more consistently successful achievement from the elementary through high school math courses would seem to instill a better feeling of confidence in approaching new and difficult material in later learning experiences. It is hoped that this attitude will soon be displayed in less avoidance of such recommended courses as trigonometry, calculus, and statistics.

As an additional offshoot of computer utilization, some long-overdue learning of a more subtle nature may appear in the form of better report writing. Some informal reports have indicated that clinicians who learn to write their evaluations and other reports within the constraints of a computer outline have learned to become more concise, to the point, and less vague and rambling in their writing style.

Much of the current computer-oriented instruction is still at a rather fundamental level, being referred to disdainfully as the "electronic flash cards" mode of instruction. Although this application should not be discouraged—it is a good place to start—it does not come close to tapping the real potential of the computer. The microcomputer's internal structure makes it highly adaptable to learning procedures based upon games of strategy (Jay, 1983). So far, these attempts have been fairly elementary and have not been designed in a particularly stimulating format. This is, however, a field where new developments can be anticipated within weeks or months, rather than in years or decades; anything that is not here at the moment is probably just one step over the horizon.

In the field of audiology some hearing aid selection programs are currently available. Designed mainly for hearing aid dispensing, they also serve well as a clinical model for comparison of the selection made by the student clinician. The computer selects the "best aid," which may be compared with the student's choice of hearing aid to be recommended. Further analysis can follow, as to why certain choices were made. In speech pathology a few training programs based upon diagnostic procedures have been made. The program presents a hypothetical clinical case, such as a child's language problem, and asks the student to select the diagnostic instruments that lead to the results of the evaluation and the therapy outline or referral. The program then compares the student's diagnostic procedure with an "ideal procedure" put into the program previously by the instructor. Although in the stage of infancy now, this type of strategy-learning program is considered to be the future of computer instructional techniques.

Recommendations

Instructional software should be developed by at least two instructors in the instructional topic, plus one skilled programmer to add the fine points of the presentation such as special pauses, animation, and other movement and graphic effects. CAIs developed by a single instructor have been found to be least effective in the long run.

Software that has been developed under a short deadline is seldom of lasting value. Some observations of "homemade" software note that only around 5% of such materials are good enough to be passed on to others for general use (Roblyer, 1983). Effective instructional software must first be tried by a group of students and then modified and improved according to their suggestions or complaints. If students enjoy it and run the program even when they do not have to, it will be most effective. By the same token, even the most expensive hardware will tend to collect dust in the training center if the software programs are dull and unchallenging (Roblyer, 1981). The software library should, therefore, be updated at least on an annual basis and the dead wood should be thrown out or otherwise set aside so as not to detract from the more effective and stimulating items in the collection (Golas, 1983).

The breathtaking advances in both hardware and software create a new problem for the instructor. Most materials available are comparatively new and untried. It is nearly impossible to order instructional software that has a documented track record of success. In fact, both hardware and software companies have been justifiably accused of advertising products that are not actually available when the ad first appears. The field is moving so fast that a producer has no way of checking the potential buyer's market except by advertising a product to see how many people would order if it were available.

With such a fast-moving commodity, there is really no proven method to decide which products are valid and reliable. Most authorities recommend cautious planning and evaluation with what appears to be a reasonably good set of materials at any given moment. To hesitate or to wait until the field becomes more stabilized is to wait perhaps in vain and to fall behind completely. To recommend a specific version of today's hardware, for example, is to recommend equipment that may be obsolete within 6 months. Today's instructional software, now written for 8-bit programming, will appear slow and poorly structured next to tomorrow's 16- or 32-bit packages.

SUMMARY

The microcomputer can serve a helpful role as an instructor's aid or tutor, but it cannot replace the live teacher in gaining insight into individual factors that might hamper the learning progress. There are many levels of computer-assisted instruction programs, but most conform to a common format. This involves presenting material, asking test questions of the student, checking the student's answers, and summarizing the student's progress. Communication disorders is just entering the microcomputer era of technology and, aside from several new and relatively experimental programs, the opportunities for computer-assisted instruction are wide open.

In setting up computer-assisted instruction in any training institution, school, or clinic, it is best to designate a coordinator of CAI development. The adoption of computer instruction methodology represents a new and unfamiliar approach to learning and many adjustments must be anticipated before full implementation can be expected.

As the techniques of CAI continue to grow, much more stimulating and thought-provoking learning strategies will be utilized. Futuristic microcomputer languages involving "artificial intelligence" will make learning programs much more interactive for the student and will be able to "discuss" and guide the student through the learning situation. At the present time BASIC is the standard language of the microcomputer, but others, such as LOGO, PILOT, Ada, and Pascal are emerging as needs and applications expand. As the technology of both microcomputer hardware and software develops so will the level of computer literacy within the professional field. As the quality of workshops and other inservice training efforts for computers improve, the benefits from this type of instructional application can be increasingly experienced and evaluated. Computer-assisted instruction offers benefits throughout the field, resulting in better student preparation and more self learning among clients and more efficient training in record keeping among clinicians.

REFERENCES

Dence, M. (1980). Toward defining the role of CAI: A review. *Educational Technology, 11,* 42–46.
Gagne, R., Wagner, W., & Rojas, A. (1981). Planning and authoring computer-assisted instruction lessons. *Educational Technology, 9,* 32–42.
Golas, K. (1983). The formative evaluation of computer-assisted instruction. *Educational Technology, 11,* 24–29.
Goldes, H. (1983). Designing the human–computer interface. *Educational Technology, 10,* 23.
Grossnichle, D. (1983). Profile of change in education: Microcomputer adoption status report. *Educational Technology, 9,* 17–20.
Hazen, M. (1982). Computer-assisted instruction with PILOT on the Apple computer. *Educational Technology, 11,* 36–39.
Herschler, M. (1983). Use of a computer simulation in teaching a college business course. *Educational Technology, 11,* 45–47.
Holmes, G. (1982). Computer-assisted instructions: A discussion of some of the issues for would-be implementers. *Educational Technology, 9,* 26–28.
Hon, D. (1983). Active interaction. *Video Systems, 9,* 19–33.
Jay, T. (1983). The cognitive approach to computer courseware design and evaluation. *Educational Technology, 10,* 18–23.
Kirchner, G. (1982). Design and production of an interactive video disc for elementary school children. *Videodisc/Teletex, 2,* 275–287.
Kleinman, G., & Humphrey, M. (1982). Authoring tools make it easy. *Electronic Learning, 15,* 72–76.
Kurshan, B. (1981). Computer technology and instruction: Implications for instructional designers. *Educational Technology, 8,* 17–22.
Levin, W. (1983). Interactive video: The state of the art teaching machine. *Computing Teacher, 8,* 11–17.
McDougall, A., Adams, T., & Adams, P. (1982). *Learning LOGO on the Apple.* Englewood Cliffs, NJ: Prentice-Hall.
Onosko, T. (1982). Vision of the future. *Creative Computing, 86,* 91–94.
Orwig, G. (1983). *Creating computer programs for learning.* Reston, VA: Reston Publishing Co.
O'Shea, T., & Self, J. (1983). *Learning and teaching with computers.* New York: Prentice-Hall.
Papert, S. (1980). *Mindstorms.* New York: Basic Books.
Plum, T. (1983). *Learning to program with C.* New York: Prentice-Hall.
Price, D. (1983). *Pascal, a considerate approach.* New York: Prentice-Hall.
Roberts, F., & Park, O. (1983). Intelligent computer assisted instruction. *Educational Technology, 12,* 7–12.
Roblyer, M. (1981). When is it "good courseware"? Problems in developing standards for microcomputer courseware. *Educational Technology, 10,* 36–39.
Roblyer, M. (1983). The case against teacher-developed microcomputer courseware. *Educational Technology, 10,* 18–22.
Rushakoff, G. (1984). *Microcomputer-assisted study partner in anatomy and physiology.* San Diego, CA: College-Hill Press.
Ryder, A., Cox, L., & Tilley, B. (1983). Technical specifications for adapting Apple microcomputers for use by students with severe physical disabilities. *Educational Technology, 23,* 20–22.

Saxon, J., & Fritz, R. (1983). *Beginning programming with Ada.* New York: Prentice-Hall.
Sebestyen, I. (1982). The videodisc revolution. *Electronic Publishing Review, 2(1),* 41-89.
Scanland, W., & Slattery, D. (1983). The impact of computer-based instruction upon teachers. *Educational Technology, 11,* 7-13.
Sims, D. (1982). An interactive video system for communication. Scientific Exhibit at the Annual Convention of the American Speech Language Hearing Association, Toronto, Canada.
Steffin, S. (1983). A suggested model for establishing the validity of computer-assisted instructional materials. *Educational Technology, 11,* 32-39.
Steinberg, E. (1983). Reviewing the instructional effectiveness of computer courseware. *Educational Technology, 11,* 25-28.
Trachtman, P. (1984). Putting computers into the hands of children without language. *Smithsonian, 21,* 42-50.
Troutner, J. (1983). How to produce an interactive video program. *Electronic Learning, 11,* 71-75.

Chapter 10

Administrative Applications For Microcomputers

Stephen B. Hood
Leland R. Miller

This chapter deals with administrative applications of microcomputers in communication disorders. The purpose is to describe in detail some of the features that enable microcomputer programs to simplify the administrative demands placed on chairpersons, directors, coordinators, and supervisors, as well as suggest ways in which persons so inclined can develop their own programs. In so doing, attempts are made to avoid any type of "product endorsement." Therefore, subsequent sections dealing with topics such as word processing, spread sheets, and file handling/data base management systems will discuss the specific concepts that are involved, rather than attempt to show what any one specific software program can do (See chap. 5, "Evaluating Software Programs"). Moreover, attempts will be made to differentiate clearly among the various functions served by currently available software programs and those that can be created in the form of custom software.

The first sections of this chapter present a brief overview of administrative functions, followed by an explanation of the development of a mainframe program from computer-assisted management protocols, all of which can be implemented on a microcomputer. The focus then shifts to microcomputer applications based on currently available software packages.

ADMINISTRATIVE FUNCTIONS: AN OVERVIEW

Administration within the professions of speech-language pathology and audiology differs somewhat depending upon the employment setting. Different demands are placed on those who work in the public schools, hospitals, universities, community speech and hearing centers, private practice, governmental agencies, nursing homes, and programs sponsored by agencies such as Easter Seals. Nevertheless, there are several underyling requirements common to all administrators: (1) the need to *gather* different types of information, (2) the need to *manipulate* this information, and (3) the need to ultimately *report* the information in a systematic way. Examples of the types of information to be gathered, manipulated, and reported include such things as client, clinician, student, staff, and supervisor schedules, attendance records, billing,

---

©College-Hill Press, Inc. All rights, including that of translation, reserved. No part of this publication may be reproduced without the written permission of the publisher.

budget management, inventory control, and the writing of clinical, academic, research, and accreditation reports. Frequently, the same or similar information is needed at different times from different sources. Later, this information must be reported to others in a different manner. This means that the information must be produced in a different format. Moreover, few people are able to "do it right" the first time. As a result, schedules, budgets, and written documents must be retyped many times when all that was needed was a minor updating rather than a major overhaul. Consequently, much administrative time is spent in the three areas noted above. Past developments in microcomputer technology have greatly simplified the administrative process. Further developments in microcomputer hardware and software promise to do even more.

Computer functions

Computers may be thought of in terms of three groups that differ with respect to their power: mainframe computers, minicomputers, and microcomputers. Recent research and development have made it possible for the microcomputer to assume many of the more complex functions previously possible only via the minicomputer or mainframe. In addition to the considerations of the size, power, memory, and language (e.g., FORTRAN, COBOL, BASIC, Pascal) one of the most significant differences among computers is their ability to handle multiple functions. For example, if a microcomputer has only one disk, then the operator must waste a considerable amount of time rotating disks. Fortunately, many microcomputers can now handle several external disk drives, a development which greatly simplifies the process and makes it possible for the computer to access more data. In addition, most microcomputers can be expanded and made more powerful. Memory can be increased, floppy disks can be supplemented by peripheral hard disks, and MODEM attachments make it possible for microcomputers to communicate with each other, as well as with mainframes.

In spite of the similarities and differences that exist among mainframes, minicomputers, and microcomputers, and in spite of differences that exist within any one level of computer (i.e., differences in disk operating system [DOS] and memory [48K, 64K, 128K, 256K]), there remains one highly important variable that must be considered: whether the actual application program is *"packaged"* or *"custom."*

Packaged application programs

"Packaged" application programs are those that are commercially available. These programs do everything from balancing the family checkbook and listing dinner recipes to writing individualized education program (IEP) reports and providing cost analyses relative to accounts payable and accounts receivable. Software packages are available to assist with such things as client scheduling, managing a desk top, computing payrolls, graphing data, scheduling appointments, and generating mailing lists. These programs are designed to be "user friendly" and most are, thus allowing a nonprogrammer to use the microcomputer. A blinking cursor indicates what data are to be entered next, and shows precisely where they will be entered. Unfortunately, these packaged programs, while fairly broad in scope, cannot be easily modified to meet specific needs that may be encountered. Moreover, each packaged program is designed to perform essentially one task. Consequently, in cases where entered data are designed for multiple purposes, time is wasted because a single entry cannot be stored in multiple files. The end result is a trade-off between the lowered cost of purchasing an existing software package, and the reduced efficiency of possibly ending up with a program that only partially meets the desired needs.

Custom application programs

"Custom" application programs have the advantage of being generated for specific purposes, but at increased cost. A programmer must be hired to spend the hundreds or thousands of hours necessary to generate the "perfect program." Originally, such programs written for mainframe computers allowed a single entry to serve multiple input functions. For example, a single entry to show that a client received one unit of a specific type of service would simultaneously go to several different subprogram data files that would: (1) credit the clinician with providing the service, (2) indicate the name and certification status of the supervisor, (3) input the clinic location where services were provided, (4) indicate the type of diagnostic or therapeutic service provided, (5) add the cost of the service to the client's bill, and (6) add the service unit to the clinic census report. The increased power of microcomputers has made it possible to create mainframe "look alike" programs; these are the packaged programs referred to above. It is anticipated that in the future these "look alikes" will also be able to "act alike."

The issues are not simply the similarities and differences among mainframe, micro-, and minicomputers; they are also the similarities and differences among packaged and custom application programs.

MAINFRAME DEVELOPMENT OF THE PROGRAM

Recent developments in microcomputer technology have made it possible to convert many mainframe programs to microcomputer software. The program to be described in the initial segment of this chapter was originally developed for use on a mainframe (Digital DEC-SYSTEM 2050) computer available within the Computer Services Division of the university. Programs developed for the DEC, when used for administrative purposes, are available to faculty, students, departments, and programs at no cost; hence, there was a real advantage to selecting this method of data collection, storage, manipulation, analysis, and printing. Moreover, when the program was first conceptualized during the late 1970's, the technology and sophistication of microcomputers were inadequate to handle the scope and complexity of the programs. Some of the factors that influenced the development of the program are listed below, and later in the chapter, in the hope they will help those readers who might wish to develop their own custom packages—either for a microcomputer, or for a mainframe.

The actual program was designed by the first author, based upon standards of the American Speech-Language-Hearing Association, to ensure compliance with the requirements for graduate education as set forth by the Clinical Certification Board (CCB) and Educational Standards Board (ESB). Considerations included external constraints imposed by the need to develop billing modules that would be compatible with the University Business Office, as well as the need to develop forms that would be appropriate for use with third party payment sources such as insurance, Medicaid, Bureau of Vocational Rehabilitation, and Aid to Dependent Children. The actual writing of the master program and subroutines was done in DEC-BASIC by two advanced graduate students in computer science under the direction of the second author. Indeed, the graduate assistantship duties of these two students were partially assigned to the Speech and Hearing Clinic for this project. This agreement was mutually beneficial to the computer science students and the administrators in communication disorders. Rather than develop a textbook project, the students had the opportunity to build a new program from the foundation upward. The final program has saved countless hours of work. By using university students, many thousands of dollars were saved. Those who would consider developing such a custom program, either for mainframe or microcomputer use, should attempt to receive assistance from as many sources as possible, and work to insure an end product that is compatible with already existing institutional policies and procedures, be they in a university, hospital, clinic, nursing home, or some other location. This chapter will show how some of these mainframe functions can now be accomplished with microcomputers.

It is possible to create a package of programs for the microcomputer that is similar in scope and function to the one designed for use on a mainframe. This chapter reviews some of the microcomputer applications already written, and lays the groundwork for creating new ones. The major portions of mainframe programs dealing with client, clinician, billing, and clinical census components serve as reference points. Alternative microcomputer "look alikes" such as financial programs with spreadsheets, file system/data management, and word processing are also presented.

CUSTOM SOFTWARE APPLICATIONS

Student processing

At some point in time all students must be entered into the program. For undergraduate students this is done upon enrollment in the first clinical practicum. For undergraduate students who remain and enter the graduate program, the only modification in already existing data is to change their status from undergraduate (U) to graduate (G). For graduate students who are new to the program, entry is made during orientation week prior to the beginning of classes. The entry procedure accomplishes two essential purposes: (1) demographic information is entered, as is, (2) a summary of previous experience received elsewhere is entered.

Table 10-1 presents examples of the types of information that can be maintained for student clinicians. Demographic information includes such things as name, local address and home address, Social Security and telephone numbers, whether the student is an undergraduate or graduate, and whether the major is speech–language pathology or audiology. These last two entries are especially important. Depending upon whether a "G" (graduate) or "U" (undergraduate) is entered, the clinical clock hours accumulated will be assigned to whichever is the appropriate current level of education. It is essential that a differentiation between the speech–language pathology and audiology majors be entered because of the different ASHA clock hour requirements. The other important entry is whether the person has a car, and if so, how many people it holds. This helps ensure that a driver is available for transportation to off-campus clinic facilities. Finally, note that there are three lines where comments can be entered: for example, "Nancy desires clinical placement in a hospital setting..." or, "Chris needs diagnostic experience with preschoolers..." or, "Beth hopes eventually to work with geriatric clients." All demographic information is modifiable to accommodate changes.

Table 10-1 also summarizes clinical experience obtained to date. The format conforms to ASHA certification requirements and differentiates between hours obtained as an undergraduate and hours obtained as a graduate student. Further distinctions are made pertaining to whether clinical experiences were obtained with a preschooler (A), a school-aged child (B), or an adult (C). Within the disorder categories of articulation, language, voice, and fluency, hours are separated in terms of diagnosis (Dx) and therapy (Tx). Audiology hours are categorized in terms of hearing screening, formal audiometric evaluation, hearing aid evaluation, and aural rehabilitation. The number of hours obtained in the various categories are added, subtracted from ASHA requirements, and the number of hours remaining to be completed is shown at the bottom of the page. The student shown in Table 10-1 has completed all clinical requirements.

Before any data are entered, verification as to the validity of the experience (as per ASHA/CCC/ESB guidelines) is obtained. In addition to tracking the hours of clinical experience obtained, there is a record of the names, certification and licensure status of the clinical

Table 10-1. Student Demographic and Clinical Data

NAME : York, Terry
GRADUATE OR UNDERGRADUATE: G
LOCAL ADDRESS : 616 Knollwood Drive, Bowling Green, Ohio 43402
UNDERGRADUATE SCHOOL : Atlantic University
RACE : Caucasian
SEX : M
PHONE NUMBER : (419) 372-2515
DATE OF BIRTH (MMDDYY) : 10/30/59
MAJOR (S = SPEECH-LANGUAGE   A = AUDIOLOGY) : S
PERMANENT ADDRESS : 21 Fairway Drive, Winchester, Mass. 01890
SOCIAL SECURITY NUMBER : 209-30-8231

DOES STUDENT HAVE A CAR (Y/N)?   Y   HOW MANY DOES IT HOLD?   5

COMMENTS : Terry had no undergraduate experience in voice or fluency. Future interest in neurogenic disorders in adults. Probable thesis candidate. (9-3-84).

CLINICAL EXPERIENCE SUMMARY (Major: SPcL)

		ARTIC DX/TX	LANG DX/TX	VOICE DX/TX	FLUENCY DX/TX	TOTAL DX	HRNG ID	FORMAL AUD DX	HEARING AID	AURAL REHAB	TOTAL
UNDERGRAD	A:	7 /29.5	7.5/14	0 /0	0 /0	14.5	0	0	0	0	58
	B:	0 /0	0 /0	0 /0	0 /0	0	0	0	0	0	0
	C:	0 /8	1 /8	0 /0	0 /0	1	0	0	0	0	17
GRADUATE	A:	5 /31.5	5 /36.5	0 /0	0 /3	10	5	0	0	0	86
	B:	10 /28	24 /50.5	4 /0	5.5 /8	43.5	6.5	0	0	22.5	158.5
	C:	6 /43	2 /64	7 /34	0 /15		4	0	0	0	175.5
RECEIVED		28 /140	39.5/173	11 /34	5.5/ 26	84	15.5	0	0	22.5	495.

ALL UNITS ARE IN TERMS OF FULL HOURS

| ASHA REG: | 25 | 25 | 25 | 25 | 50 | 15 | 0 | 15 | 22.5 | 300 |
| STILL NEEDED: | 0 | 0 | 0 | 0 | 0 | 0 | 0 | 0 | 0 | 0 |

supervisor, and location where the experiences were obtained. This information may be viewed directly from the computer terminal, or can be printed as hard copy as is shown in Tables 10-2 and 10-3.

As may be seen from Tables 10-1, 10-2, and 10-3, extensive information is available. It is possible to determine whether the clinical experiences were obtained with preschool, school-aged, or adult clients, and it is possible to determine whether the diagnostic hours were obtained in speech–language pathology or audiology. Clinical experiences obtained in the disorder areas of articulation, language, voice, fluency, and aural rehabilitation can also be ascertained. Current information is always available regarding how much additional experience is needed to meet the minimum requirements for ASHA certification and state licensure. Upon completion of the program, students are given hard copies of their clinical experience records to submit to any future university they may attend, or use them for sources such as ASHA, state licensure boards, state departments of education, prospective employers, or others. Another hard copy is maintained as part of the student's permanent record.

Client processing

When a client is seen for the first time, basic demographic data are entered. As may be seen from Table 10-4, many routine items are inputted; consequently, they will not be discussed in any detail. Of particular importance, however, are the entries that pertain to billing information. For example, the identification number (typically the Social Security or Medicaid number) is coded as to the type of number it represents. Later, it is this code that determines the format for billing: self pay or third party. Further, in cases of third party payment, it is possible to add data relative to ICDA codes, ADC names and numbers, and insurance names and numbers. This information, whether shown on the computer terminal or printed as hard copy, reveals the client's billing history, the amount of money billed and collected, as well as accounts payable. It is also possible to review the dates of the 60 most recent clinical sessions attended, clinical services rendered, and all charges billed to the client.

The billing program is used to print a single bill, print all bills for all clients, and differentiate among the billing forms used for self-pay clients (which are handled by the business office) and third party payments which are billed directly from the Speech and Hearing Clinic. This program is also used to credit accounts paid. Depending upon local, regional, and/or state requirements, third party payment forms may differ; therefore, an example will not be given. The particular billing form used by the University Business Office is shown in Table 10-5.

Clinic census information

Many university, clinical, hospital, and private practice programs are complex in scope and function. In addition to the on-campus clinic, students frequently engage in practicum experiences at one or several off-campus externship facilities. The Clinic Census Program allows tabulation of the total number of hours of clinical services provided, divided among disorder categories for up to 25 therapy sites (see Table 10-6).

As may be seen from Table 10-6, a summary is provided that shows the total number of hours of clinical service provided in the diagnostic areas (speech–language, hearing and hearing aid), and therapy (articulation, language, voice, and fluency). This information is especially useful for knowing the types of clinical experiences that are predicted for the various clinical settings available for student practicum.

Procedure codes

Those who would develop computer-assisted management programs need to give considerable thought to the procedure codes used. It is imperative that codes used for computer processing be in agreement with those used by local third party payment sources. The procedure

Table 10-2. Clinical Experience Summary: Speech–Language Pathology

8/29/1983	Clinical Experience Summary:	York, Terry		

1) **ARTICULATION**

TOTAL PRESCHOOL HOURS (A):	-U- DX: 7 TX: 29.5	-G- DX: 5 TX: 31.5	
SUPERVISOR'S NAME	PLACE OBTAINED	CCC-SP	LIC-SP
M. PERLMUTTER	BGSU—ON CAMPUS	Y	Y
M. RASTATTER	NAPOLEON CLINIC	Y	Y
J. KLEIN	BGSU—ON CAMPUS	Y	Y
TOTAL SCHOOL-AGE HOURS (B):	-U- DX: 0 TX: 0	-G- DX: 10 TX: 28	
SUPERVISOR'S NAME	PLACE OBTAINED	CCC-SP	LIC-SP
M. WENTLAND	FINDLAY HEARING	Y	Y
M. RASTATTER	BGSU—ON CAMPUS	Y	Y
M. WENTLAND	BGSU—ON CAMPUS	Y	Y
TOTAL ADULT HOURS (C):	-U- DX: 0 TX: 8	-G- DX: 6 TX: 43	
SUPERVISOR'S NAME	PLACE OBTAINED	CCC-SP	LIC-SP
R. JACQUES	NURSING HOME	Y	Y
M. WENTLAND	BGSU—ON CAMPUS	Y	Y
R. OLSCAMP	BGSU—ON CAMPUS	Y	Y
K. MARTIN	TOLEDO HOSPITAL	Y	Y

2) **LANGUAGE**

TOTAL PRESCHOOL HOURS (A):	-U- DX: 7.5 TX: 14	-G- DX: 5 TX: 36.5	
SUPERVISOR'S NAME	PLACE OBTAINED	CCC-SP	LIC-SP
S. DEMARCO	NAPOLEON CLINIC	Y	Y
M. RASTATTER	WOODLANE SCHOOL	Y	Y
R. OLSCAMP	BGSU—ON CAMPUS	Y	Y
TOTAL SCHOOL-AGE HOURS (B):	-U- DX: 0 TX: 0	-G- DX: 24 TX: 50.5	
SUPERVISOR'S NAME	PLACE OBTAINED	CCC-SP	LIC-SP
J. KLEIN	BGSU—ON CAMPUS	Y	Y
M. WENTLAND	FINDLAY HEARING	Y	Y
J. GIDDAN	CHILD RES CENT	Y	Y
TOTAL ADULT HOURS (C):	-U- DX: 1 TX: 8	-G- DX: 2 TX: 64	
SUPERVISOR'S NAME	PLACE OBTAINED	CCC-SP	LIC-SP
R. JACQUES	NURSING HOME	Y	Y
B. SHULMAN	NAPOLEON CLINIC	Y	Y
M. COSMO	PORTAGE HOME	Y	Y

3) **VOICE**

TOTAL PRESCHOOL HOURS (A):	-U- DX: 0 TX: 0	-G- DX: 0 TX: 0	
SUPERVISOR'S NAME	PLACE OBTAINED	CCC-SP	LIC-SP
TOTAL SCHOOL-AGE HOURS (B):	-U- DX: 0 TX: 0	-G- DX: 4 TX: 0	
SUPERVISOR'S NAME	PLACE OBTAINED	CCC-SP	LIC-SP
M. HYMAN	BGSU—ON CAMPUS	Y	Y
TOTAL ADULT HOURS (C):	-U- DX: 0 TX: 0	-G- DX: 7 TX: 34	
SUPERVISOR'S NAME	PLACE OBTAINED	CCC-SP	LIC-SP
R. JACQUES	NURSING HOME	Y	Y
M. HYMAN	BGSU—ON CAMPUS	Y	Y

4) **FLUENCY**

TOTAL PRESCHOOL HOURS (A):	-U- DX: 0 TX: 0	-G- DX: 0 TX: 0	
SUPERVISOR'S NAME	PLACE OBTAINED	CCC-SP	LIC-SP
TOTAL SCHOOL-AGE HOURS (B):	-U- DX: 0 TX: 0	-G- DX: 5.5 TX: 8	
SUPERVISOR'S NAME	PLACE OBTAINED	CCC-SP	LIC-SP
S. HOOD	BGSU—ON CAMPUS	Y	Y
C. DELL	BGSU—ON CAMPUS	Y	Y
TOTAL ADULT HOURS (C):	-U- DX: 0 TX: 0	-G- DX: 0 TX: 15	
SUPERVISOR'S NAME	PLACE OBTAINED	CCC-SP	LIC-SP
S. HOOD	BGSU—ON CAMPUS	Y	Y
R. COLCORD	BGSU—ON CAMPUS	Y	Y

Table 10-3. Clinical Experience Summary: Audiology

8/29/83	CLINICAL EXPERIENCE SUMMARY:	YORK, TERRY				
1)	SCREENING AND IDENTIFICATION					
	TOTAL HOURS OF CONTACT FOR PRESCHOOL		(A):	-U- 0	-G- 5	
	SUPERVISOR'S NAME	PLACE OBTAINED	CCC-A	CCC-SP	LIC-A	LIC-SP
	D. TOWNSEND	CHILD RES CENT	Y	N	Y	N
	S. HOOD	BGSU—ON CAMPUS	N	Y	N	Y
	TOTAL HOURS OF CONTACT FOR SCHOOL-AGE		(B):	-U- 0	-G- 6.5	
	SUPERVISOR'S NAME	PLACE OBTAINED	CCC-A	CCC-SP	LIC-A	LIC-SP
	H. GUTNICK	BGSU—ON CAMPUS	Y	N	Y	N
	D. TOWNSEND	FINDLAY HEARING	Y	N	Y	N
	TOTAL HOURS OF CONTACT FOR ADULT		(C):	-U- 0	-G- 4	
	SUPERVISOR'S NAME	PLACE OBTAINED	CCC-A	CCC-SP	LIC-A	LIC-SP
	H. GREENBERG	BGSU—ON CAMPUS	Y	N	Y	N
2)	FORMAL AUDIOLOGIC ASSESSMENT					
	TOTAL HOURS OF CONTACT FOR PRESCHOOL		(A):	-U- 0	-G- 0	
	SUPERVISOR'S NAME	PLACE OBTAINED	CCC-A	CCC-SP	LIC-A	LIC-SP
	TOTAL HOURS OF CONTACT FOR SCHOOL-AGE		(B):	-U- 0	-G- 0	
	SUPERVISOR'S NAME	PLACE OBTAINED	CCC-A	CCC-SP	LIC-A	LIC-SP
	TOTAL HOURS OF CONTACT FOR ADULT		(C):	-U- 0	-G- 0	
	SUPERVISOR'S NAME	PLACE OBTAINED	CCC-A	CCC-SP	LIC-A	LIC-SP
3)	HEARING AID EVALUATION					
	TOTAL HOURS OF CONTACT FOR PRESCHOOL		(A):	-U- 0	-G- 0	
	SUPERVISOR'S NAME	PLACE OBTAINED	CCC-A	CCC-SP	LIC-A	LIC-SP
	TOTAL HOURS OF CONTACT FOR SCHOOL-AGE		(B):	-U- 0	-G- 0	
	SUPERVISOR'S NAME	PLACE OBTAINED	CCC-A	CCC-SP	LIC-A	LIC-SP
	TOTAL HOURS OF CONTACT FOR ADULT		(C):	-U- 0	-G- 0	
	SUPERVISOR'S NAME	PLACE OBTAINED	CCC-A	CCC-SP	LIC-A	LIC-SP
4)	AURAL REHABILITATION					
	TOTAL HOURS OF CONTACT FOR PRESCHOOL		(A):	-U- 0	-G- 0	
	SUPERVISOR'S NAME	PLACE OBTAINED	CCC-A	CCC-SP	LIC-A	LIC-SP
	TOTAL HOURS OF CONTACT FOR SCHOOL-AGE		(B):	-U- 0	-G- 22.5	
	SUPERVISOR'S NAME	PLACE OBTAINED	CCC-A	CCC-SP	LIC-A	LIC-SP
	M. WENTLAND	FINDLAY HEARING	N	Y	N	Y
	D. TOWNSEND	FINDLAY HEARING	Y	N	Y	N
	TOTAL HOURS OF CONTACT FOR ADULT		(C):	-U- 0	-G- 0	
	SUPERVISOR'S NAME	PLACE OBTAINED	CCC-A	CCC-SP	LIC-A	LIC-SP

codes discussed in this chapter, and shown in Table 10-7, are indigenous to Ohio. If they were to change, then only minor program modifiations would be necessary.

Information on clinical sessions between a client and clinician are entered in such a manner that *a single entry serves multiple functions*. The inputted data are routed to subprograms and subroutines for compilation under a number of different headings: client records, clinician records, and billing and clinical census. The mainframe allows subprograms and subroutines to be properly executed by means of only one entry. It is this "single entry function" that separates mainframe application from currently available microcomputer capability. As will be shown

Table 10-4. Client Demographic Data

10/22/83 Page 47

BOWLING GREEN STATE UNIVERSITY
SPEECH AND HEARING CLINIC

CLIENT NAME:	COX, GREGORY	ADDRESS:		BILLED TO:	COX, M/M DOUGLAS
ID NUMBER	211-48-6164A	STREET	14 HULL ROAD	STREET	14 HULL ROAD
TYPE OF ID	SSN	CITY, STATE	GRAND HILLS, OHIO	CITY, STATE	GRAND HILLS, OHIO
DATE OF BIRTH	082074	ZIP	43412	ZIP	43412
AGE	9	PHONE	823-4991		
SEX	MALE				
PROBLEM:	ARTIC	BILLING INFO:	$7.50/HR, FAMILY RATE	NUMBER OF SESSIONS:	14
DISPOSITION:		SUPERVISOR:	PERLMUTTER	NUMBER OF HOURS:	13.5
DATE OF					
EVALUATION	080383	CASE NUMBER		AMOUNT BILLED	$101.25
SCHEDULE	YES	ADC NUMBER		AMOUNT PAID	$101.25
SCHEDULE MORE					
EVALUATION	NO	ADC 1ST NAME		AMOUNT DUE	$ 0.00
THERAPY INDICATED	YES	ICDA CODE			
OTHER NO DX—ONLY TX					

Table 10-4. Continued

NO.	PROCEDURE CODE	DATE	CHARGE	NO.	PROCEDURE CODE	DATE	CHARGE	NO.	PROCEDURE CODE	DATE	CHARGE
1	92586	081483	$ 3.75	21			$ 0.00	41			$ 0.00
2	92590	081983	$ 7.50	22			$ 0.00	42			$ 0.00
3	92590	082183	$ 7.50	23			$ 0.00	43			$ 0.00
4	92590	082683	$ 7.50	24			$ 0.00	44			$ 0.00
5	92590	082883	$ 7.50	25			$ 0.00	45			$ 0.00
6	92590	090283	$ 7.50	26			$ 0.00	46			$ 0.00
7	92590	090483	$ 7.50	27			$ 0.00	47			$ 0.00
8	92590	091183	$ 7.50	28			$ 0.00	48			$ 0.00
9	92590	091683	$ 7.50	29			$ 0.00	49			$ 0.00
10	92590	091883	$ 7.50	30			$ 0.00	50			$ 0.00
11	92590	092383	$ 7.50	31			$ 0.00	51			$ 0.00
12	92590	092583	$ 7.50	32			$ 0.00	52			$ 0.00
13	92590	100983	$ 7.50	33			$ 0.00	53			$ 0.00
14	92590	101183	$ 7.50	34			$ 0.00	54			$ 0.00
15			$ 0.00	35			$ 0.00	55			$ 0.00
16			$ 0.00	36			$ 0.00	56			$ 0.00
17			$ 0.00	37			$ 0.00	57			$ 0.00
18			$ 0.00	38			$ 0.00	58			$ 0.00
19			$ 0.00	39			$ 0.00	59			$ 0.00
20			$ 0.00	40			$ 0.00	60			$ 0.00

Table 10-5. Billing Invoice

INVOICE

BOWLING GREEN STATE UNIVERSITY

DATE: 10/21/83

DEPARTMENT: SPEECH AND HEARING CLINIC   INCOME: 039027   COST: 04927   OBJECT: 061   INVOICE #: SPH00042
ACCOUNT NUMBER: 402-50-7436   FEI #: 34-6402018

PLEASE INCLUDE ACCOUNT NUMBER WITH PAYMENT.   ** NOTE **   CONTACT THE SPEECH AND HEARING
MAKE CHECKS PAYABLE TO BOWLING GREEN STATE   CLINIC IF THERE IS ANY QUESTION ON
UNIVERSITY AND RETURN WITH DUPLICATE INVOICE   CHARGE.
TO BURSAR'S OFFICE.

TO: SMITH, MRS. PAM
     BOX 263 MAPLE STREET
     BOWLING GREEN, OHIO   43402

QUANTITY		DESCRIPTION	UNIT PRICE	EXTENSION
1	92557	HEARING EVALUATION FOR SMITH, DANIELLE SERVICE PERFORMED ON: 10/11/83	25.00	
1	92567	TYMPANOMETRY FOR SMITH, DANIELLE SERVICE PERFORMED ON: 10/11/83	5.00	
1	92568	ACOUSTIC REFLEX FOR SMITH, DANIELLE SERVICE PERFORMED ON: 10/11/83	5.00	
		TOTAL		$35.00
		AMOUNT DUE FROM PREVIOUS BILLING		$00.00
		TOTAL AMOUNT DUE		$35.00

Table 10-6. Clinic Census Data

Bowling Green State University
Speech and Hearing Clinic
Survey of Clinic Services for the Period: 09/01/82 to 12/10/82

Location	Sp/lang Diag	Hrng Diag	Hae	Total Diag	Artic	Lang	Voice	Fluency	Aural Rehab	Total Therapy	Grand Total
1	210.0	138.5	78.0	426.5	179.5	242.5	202.0	226.5	48.5	899.0	1325.5
2	51.5	0.0	0.0	51.5	61.0	85.5	17.0	0.0	0.0	163.5	215.0
3	29.0	10.0	0.0	39.0	109.0	65.5	0.0	10.5	17.5	202.5	241.5
4	46.0	15.0	0.0	61.0	0.0	0.0	0.0	0.0	0.0	0.0	61.0
5	42.0	27.0	0.0	69.0	48.0	70.5	30.0	44.0	27.0	219.5	288.5
6	0.0	0.0	0.0	0.0	0.0	0.0	0.0	0.0	0.0	0.0	0.0
7	22.0	0.0	0.0	22.0	59.0	75.0	49.5	5.0	39.0	227.5	249.5
8	0.0	0.0	0.0	0.0	0.0	0.0	0.0	0.0	0.0	0.0	0.0
9	15.0	0.0	0.0	15.0	36.0	51.0	32.0	32.5	41.0	192.5	207.5
10	20.0	12.0	0.0	32.0	0.0	0.0	0.0	0.0	462.5	462.5	494.5
11	0.0	0.0	0.0	0.0	0.0	0.0	0.0	0.0	0.0	0.0	0.0
12	0.0	0.0	0.0	0.0	0.0	39.0	0.0	0.0	0.0	39.0	39.0
13	0.0	0.0	0.0	0.0	0.0	52.5	0.0	0.0	0.0	52.5	52.5
14	0.0	0.0	0.0	0.0	0.0	0.0	0.0	0.0	0.0	0.0	0.0
15	0.0	47.0	0.0	47.0	0.0	0.0	0.0	0.0	0.0	0.0	47.0
16	0.0	0.0	0.0	0.0	0.0	0.0	0.0	0.0	0.0	0.0	0.0
17	0.0	0.0	0.0	0.0	0.0	0.0	0.0	0.0	0.0	0.0	0.0
18	0.0	121.0	52.5	173.5	0.0	0.0	0.0	0.0	0.0	0.0	173.5
19	47.0	17.5	0.0	64.5	31.0	79.0	0.0	0.0	28.5	138.5	203.0
20	18.5	10.0	0.0	28.5	0.0	47.0	23.0	0.0	39.5	109.5	138.0
21	0.0	0.0	0.0	0.0	22.5	46.5	33.0	54.5	29.0	185.5	185.5
22	0.0	0.0	0.0	0.0	0.0	0.0	0.0	0.0	0.0	0.0	0.0
23	7.0	0.0	0.0	7.0	13.5	61.0	10.5	0.0	0.0	85.0	92.0
24	0.0	48.0	0.0	48.0	0.0	0.0	0.0	0.0	0.0	0.0	48.0
25	0.0	0.0	0.0	0.0	0.0	0.0	0.0	0.0	0.0	0.0	0.0
Totals	508.0	446.0	130.5	1084.5	559.5	915.0	397.0	373.0	732.5	2977.0	4061.6

Table 10-7. Selected Examples of Procedure Codes and File Maintenance

Clinic facilities		Undergraduate programs	
01	BGSU—On campus	50	Kent State
02	Nursing home	51	Michigan State
03	Head start	52	Toledo Hospital
04	Children's resource center	53	Wisconsin
ICDA codes		**Medicaid procedure codes**	
306.9	Speech—General	92590	1 Hr Therapy, Individual
315.4	Dyspraxia	92593	Spch-Lang Diag. Eval.
389.9	Hearing—General	92557	Hearing Evaluation
784.3	Aphasia	92558	Hearing Aid Evaluation

later in this chapter, many of the applications discussed thus far can be handled on a microcomputer using spreadsheets and data base management programs. Unfortunately, however, these require time-consuming multiple inputs, and at the present time it does not appear possible to merge these diverse programs into a single package. It would appear possible to create a custom software program for a microcomputer if four external drives were available such that one could be used for each of the four subprograms discussed above: client records, clinician records, and billing and clinical census. To date, however, such programs have not been written.

Two-digit codes (01–99) are used to identify the location where services have been provided. As may be seen from Table 10-7, the codes 01–25 are used to identify services provided at our on-campus clinic and at up to 24 additional off-campus externship facilities. These 25 locations ultimately become reported with the clinic census data that are printed (see Table 10-6). However, since many graduate students join programs after having completed their undergraduate education elsewhere, it is necessary that there be some means of entering the clinical experiences that students may already have received. The numbers 26–99 are used to indicate the undergraduate institutions attended by current graduate students. These data are not included within the clinic census data; rather, they serve to give proper credit to students who achieved legitimate clinical experience during their undergraduate course of study.

Two other types of procedure codes are maintained, and these are based on Medicaid and insurance codes used in Ohio. Examples are shown in Table 10-7. *PLEASE NOTE:* only several selected codes are shown. Others are available and used. As may be seen, these include various ICDA diagnostic codes and various procedure codes for direct services provided.

Entering session data

The enter session data program is the mainstay of the computer-assisted program being discussed. A single input is subrouted to the programs that tabulate the student's clinical clock hours, update the client's service history, augment the clinic census report, and provide the date, procedure, and fee for services that will later be needed for billing purposes.

As may be seen from Table 10-8, entries are made for the name of the student, name of the client, date of service, and the procedure codes and fees for up to five different services that might have been provided. Entries also credit the student clinician with the appropriate number of clock hours for services provided under the appropriate supervision of an ASHA certified and state licensed supervisor. Subdivisions differentiate hours obtained in speech-language pathology, as opposed to audiology, and clock hours are subdivided into specific disorder categories.

Table 10-8. Entering Session Data

ENTER SESSION DATA

STUDENT NAME (LAST, FIRST MI.)   HORTON, SALLY J.
CLIENT NAME OR IDENTIFICATION NUMBER: AMES, RICHARD NAME OR ID: N (N/I)
DATE OF SERVICE (MMDDYY)   081383
PROCEDURE CODE   01   92557   02   92590   03____   04____   05____
PROCEDURE AMT   01   1000   02   1000   03____   04____   05____
**NOTE: WHEN NO MORE PROCEDURES ARE TO BE ENTERED, JUST HIT RETURN

Enter Speech or Audiology Date (S/A)?___

SPEECH DATA

1. ARTICULATION
2. LANGUAGE
3. VOICE
4. FLUENCY

DIAGNOSTIC OR THERAPEUTIC (D/T)   T
TOTAL TIME (IN HALF HOUR UNITS)   2
SUPERVISOR'S NAME   S. HOOD
WHERE WAS SERVICE PERFORMED   01
VALID CCC-SP (Y/N)   Y
VALID LICENSE-SP (Y/N)   Y
MODIFY DATA, ENTER NEW SERVICE, OR RETURN (M,E,R) ___

AUDIOLOGY DATA

1. SCREENING AND ID
2. FORMAL AUDIOLOGIC ASSESSMENT
3. HEARING AID EVALUATION
4. AURAL REHABILITATION

TOTAL TIME (IN HALF HOUR UNITS)   2
SUPERVISOR'S NAME   D. TOWNSEND
WHERE WAS SERVICE PERFORMED   01
VALID CCC-A (Y/N)   Y
VALID LICENSE-A (Y/N)   Y
VALID CCC-SP (Y/N)   N
VALID LICENSE-SP (Y/N)   N
MODIFY DATA, ENTER NEW SERVICE, OR RETURN (M,E,R) ___

With respect to audiology data, the entry shows whether the service was in audiometric screening, formal audiometric assessment, hearing aid evaluation, or aural rehabilitation. The length of the session is entered in units (where one unit equals 30 min) and the name of the clinical supervisor is noted. An additional entry signifies the location where the clinical service was delivered, and as may also be seen from Table 10-8, entries are made to show whether the supervisor held the ASHA Certificate of Clinical Competence in audiology and/or speech-language pathology, and was licensed in one or both areas. This differentiation is important because the supervision of formal audiometric testing and hearing aid evaluations *must* be conducted by a person certified in audiology. Supervision of audiometric screenings and aural rehabilitation can be done by a person holding certification in *either* area.

With respect to entering data for speech-language pathology, the specific disorder area is specified (articulation, language, voice, fluency) and whether the service was "diagnostic" or "therapeutic." Then, as with the audiology data, entries are made for the number of units of service provided, the location of service, and the name and certification status of the supervisor.

PACKAGED SOFTWARE APPLICATIONS

Electronic spreadsheets

Several of the applications presented above that use custom application software can also be accomplished using available software packages. Since packages are written to handle a wide range of applications, the user will find that they are more difficult to use and that they also may not perform all of the functions desired. However, software packages are readily available and in the long run are considerably less expensive than having a programmer write the custom software.

One of the more readily available software packages for microcomputers is the electronic spreadsheet. While this software varies from vendor to vendor, it is a package that is available for all microcomputers on the market today.

Definition of electronic spreadsheets

An electronic spreadsheet is a program that manipulates data that can be formatted in a rectangular array (matrix). The user has the capability of entering the data into the matrix and requesting the computer to perform a series of arithmetic operations on the rows and columns in the matrix. The user may elect to have the data displayed on the screen or printed on a printer. Table 10-9 illustrates a simple matrix that can be entered into the computer. After the data are entered, the computer will perform the arithmetic operations and then display the entire matrix on the screen. As is illustrated in this example, the user can label the columns and the rows of the matrix, making it easier to understand the meaning of the data in the matrix. In this example, three income budgets (operating budget, clinic income, and a charitable foundation account) are used to pay five operating budgets (faculty salaries, clinic salaries, clinic supplies, academic supplies, and research equipment).

Spreadsheets are fairly new to the software industry. The first spreadsheet was developed as recently as 1980. Since that time there has been a barrage of spreadsheets that have become available for microcomputers. In general, the price paid for the package represents the quality of the package fairly well.

Spreadsheet applications

Spreadsheets have a wide range of applications, varying from home use to business applications. Any application which makes use of numbers that can be arranged into a rectangular array can be entered into the microcomputer, using a spreadsheet package to be used for projecting budgets, planning expenditures, accounting, processing inventory, and classifying information. The data shown in Table 10-1 could be set up in a spreadsheet which would aid in keeping records of clinical hours according to various categories. Likewise, Table 10-6 contains a matrix of numbers that could also be established and stored using a spreadsheet.

Table 10-9. Spreadsheet Example of Five Expense Categories Funded from Three Income Sources

EXPENSES	OPERATING	CLINIC	FOUNDATION	TOTAL
FACULTY SALARIES	278,000	0	0	278,000
CLINIC SALARIES	48,000	13,000	0	61,000
CLINIC SUPPLIES	1,250	7,390	2,210	10,850
ACADEMIC SUPPLIES	7,394	600	300	8,294
RESEARCH EQUIPMENT	12,506	453	320	13,279
TOTAL	347,150	21,443	2,830	371,413

The calculations to obtain the totals would be performed automatically by the microcomputer. As new and revised data are entered into the matrix, the microcomputer updates the calculations to reflect the most recent data.

How to use

Spreadsheets are very simple to implement. Most manuals that accompany the software are easy to read and in several hours a user would have the basic knowledge to set up a simple spreadsheet. The first task in implementing the spreadsheet for a particular application is to establish the template. This involves labeling the rows and columns and giving the arithmetic operations. Each row and column is assigned either a number or a letter as is illustrated in Table 10-10, where the five rows represent student clinicians and the four columns represent clock hours obtained in the therapy categories for articulation, language, voice, and fluency. Any element in the matrix can then be represented by giving its row letter and its column number. For example, C4 refers to the third row and the fourth column. Arithmetic calculations can be given in terms of the element representation. For example, by placing B1 + C5 in element D4, the microcomputer will automatically add the two elements and place the sum in D4. Likewise, D4 can be added to C4 and that sum can be placed in F5. Therefore, F5 contains the value of B1 + C5 + C4. Operations can be performed other than simple addition. Spreadsheets vary from each other as to the different arithmetic functions that can be performed, but most can subtract, multiply, and divide. This implies that the user can have the computer calculate averages and percentages. Some spreadsheets come equipped with trigonometric functions.

After the template is prepared, the spreadsheet can be displayed on the screen so that the user can enter the data. A cursor can be moved to the different slots in the matrix that informs the microcomputer where the data are to be placed. Most spreadsheets allow the user to give the element representation, such as D3, which causes the cursor to move to the corresponding location. After the data are entered, the calculations are performed and again the spreadsheet is displayed on the screen. If the user prefers a hard copy, the spreadsheet can be printed. Several recently developed spreadsheets will then search through a row to find a given entry. The cursor will be left at the location of the row if the search was successful.

Disadvantages of spreadsheets

Spreadsheets are generally not as easy to use as custom-built packages. Since spreadsheets are applicable for wide ranges of applications, the user must enter more commands to carry out the different functions. A custom-built package can immediately request the required information. The spreadsheet user may need to enter commands that are meaningless to the particular application, while custom-built packages can request information without additional commands.

The one main advantage of a spreadsheet is that purchasing it is considerably less expensive than paying a programmer to develop and debug a custom-built system. Also, by purchasing

Table 10-10. Spreadsheet Examples of Four Clock-Hour Categories for Five Student Clinicians

	1 HOURS	2 ARTICULATION	3 LANGUAGE	4 VOICE	5 FLUENCY	6 TOTAL
A						
B	OLSCAMP, R	12	15	7	8	42
C	BLOOD, G	11	13	4	6	34
D	MILLER, R	16	14	4	5	39
E	HAYNES, W	18	14	6	7	45
F	KEMPF, D	19	16	7	9	51
G	TOTAL	76	72	28	35	211

a spreadsheet, it is possible to avoid having to wait a long time while the system is being programmed. Another advantage for purchasing a spreadsheet is that it comes with documentation which would otherwise have to be developed by the user.

Selecting a spreadsheet

Spreadsheets are now available for use on microcomputers. The better known microcomputers have a variety of spreadsheets that may be selected. Microcomputers with a CP/M disk operating system have even more choices. In selecting a spreadsheet, the following items should be taken into consideration:

1. The spreadsheet must handle a matrix that is large enough for the application. Each spreadsheet lists the maximum number of rows and columns that it can store. The number of rows and columns needed will limit the number of the available spreadsheets. There are several spreadsheets that have "virtual memory" and allow the user to have a matrix of essentially any size. The system stores the matrix on a disk whenever the microcomputer's memory is filled. Likewise, the computer brings that portion of memory back into the system whenever the user references it.

2. Some spreadsheets interface with word processors to permit constructing a table in a spreadsheet and using the table in a document that is prepared with a word processor. This may be of particular value to administrators who need to combine these two functions such as might be needed for annual reports, research proposals, accreditation documents, or grant applications.

3. A few spreadsheets produce graphics from the matrix such as pie charts, line graphs, and bar graphs. Again if the user employs spreadsheets to generate data for documents, this could be a very useful feature.

4. The spreadsheet must be accompanied by a readable manual with many examples (see Schwartz, chap. 6).

5. Before purchasing a spreadsheet, it would be beneficial to talk with other people who use spreadsheets and get their opinion of the spreadsheets they use. There are several articles on spreadsheets which address the advantages and disadvantages of spreadsheets that the user may wish to consult (Bishop, 1982; Grushcow, 1983; Spindler, 1980; Stiefel & Simpson, 1983).

Data base management system

A data base management system (also known as File Handler or Information Management System) is a package of programs that can be beneficial to administrators who have large amounts of related data that must be stored and then retrieved at some later time. In selecting a data

base management system it is important to realize that there are three main types of data base management systems:
1) file management systems
2) relational data base management systems
3) network/hierarchical data base management systems.

The order in which the three systems are presented above represents the level of difficulty in using the system. The file management system is the easiest to use (i.e., the most "user friendly") in situations where a specific program is needed for routine use. On the other hand, a beginning user would have a fairly difficult time implementing the network/hierarchical system. The next section of this chapter will present an overview of these three systems.

File management systems

A file management system is the simplest of the three data base management systems to use, and can be used by most nonprogrammers. The disadvantage of this system is that it is restrictive in its use. This system is applicable only if each record in the file has the same format. Also, if two or more files are needed there cannot be any referencing either between or among the files. This implies that the files are independent of each other; therefore, any reports generated can be based only upon information obtained from one file. If the user would like to store information on each client, such as name, address, dates of the client's visits, type of treatment used, and name of clinician, then a file management system would satisfy this need. A file is created by specifying the name and length of each item (field) in the record. During the creation of the file an identification number, letter, or word must be specified which the microcomputer can subsequently use to locate a particular record within the file. In the example of the client file, the client's name would serve as a unique identification for each record. This creation procedure is accomplished by choosing one of the options displayed on the menu when the system is first loaded. Initialization is performed once, and only once, for each file that is created.

After records have been entered, the user has several options. Modification of any of the records that were previously entered is accomplished by giving the identification of the particular record to be modified. The microcomputer searches the records until it finds the correct record and then displays the contents of the record on the screen. The system then allows the user to modify the contents of the record. Although the identification item is the only item that cannot be modified, the user may delete an entire record or add another record to the file. Another option available on the system's menu allows the user to define and print reports. The user specifies the fields to be printed, the headings for each column, and the report's title. These specifications can be stored on a disk so that if the same report is to be printed at a later time, the specifications can be retrieved.

Several components of the mainframe program, discussed earlier, are appropriate for file handling systems. For example, the student demographic data shown at the top of Table 10-1, or the client demographic data shown at the top of Table 10-4, could be maintained on a file management system. Retrieval of client information could be based upon any one of a large number of identifying characteristics: name, age, disorder classification, name of clinical supervisor, source of payment, or zip code. The retrieval of student information could be accomplished for any one of a number of variables: name, undergraduate school attended, whether the student had transportation to off-campus clinics, or status as a graduate or undergraduate. Two other uses of file management deserve brief discussion to show additional ways in which such programs can be used. Table 10-11 illustrates an example of inventory maintenance. This table shows one inventory *file* which contains eight *records* (Visipitch, Microcomputer, Spectrograph, etc.), each of which contains three *fields* (Item Identification, Date of Last Calibration or Repair, and Date of Next Scheduled Calibration). In this example, the delimiter could be keyed to a particular identification item, the date when calibration or

Table 10-11. Equipment Inventory—Maintenance Checks

Item Identification	Last repaired or calibrated	Next repair or calibration
Visipitch	September, 1983	March, 1984
Spectrograph	November, 1983	May, 1984
Viscorder	January, 1984	July, 1984
Beltone #1	January, 1984	May, 1984
Maico #3	February, 1984	June, 1984
Grason Stadler	March, 1984	July, 1984
DAF #2	March, 1984	August, 1984
Microcomputer	April, 1984	July, 1984

repair last occurred, or the date when the next calibration is scheduled. The program could then respond by printing a report to show all items needing calibration in "July, 1984" (i.e., Visicoder, Grason Stadler, and Microcomputer).

Table 10-12 presents a file management system to track employee information. A form of this type could be designed for the particular data required based upon institutional policy. This example shows information such as name, address, academic degrees earned, date hired, rank, and tenure status. Depending upon the information required, a listing could be requested of all personnel hired in 1976, who hold the rank of associate professor and who are tenured. In all of these cases, the file of Michael Curran would be retrieved. On the other hand, Michael Curran would not be retrieved if the request were for full professors, those who were untenured, those who held the Certificate of Clinical Competence in Audiology, or those hired in 1984.

Relational data base management systems

A major disadvantage of the file management system is that once the record has been initialized, additional fields cannot be added. This is the advantage that a relational data base system has over the file management system. In other words, the user need not anticipate all the field and all of the requirements of the system in advance, since they can be added later. Relational data base systems have a language of their own which allows the user to refer to items in a record and these items can represent identification names in other records.

Some relational data base systems are easy to use because the initialization of the files is menu or query driven. This means that the user does not have to be a highly sophisticated computer programmer to initialize the files, but simply answer the questions that are given on the screen by the initialization program.

Network/hierarchical management system

The third data base management system is the network/hierarchical system. This is the most difficult for a user to implement since the initialization of this system is neither menu nor query driven. Instead, the user must learn a data description language which describes the structure of the data. To add to this problem, the user will also have to use a host language such as BASIC or COBOL to implement the system once the data base has been defined.

Most program applications that can be implemented on a relational system can also be implemented on a network/hierarchical system, and vice versa. What the network/hierarchical does permit is fast execution time. This is a major benefit if the user has a very large data base and does not want to wait a long time while the computer searches through several files to find a particular item. This happens when a relational system has an exceptionally large data base. In a network/hierarchical system the user enters the relationships of the items which form a network within the data. This network contains "pointers" that the computer uses for

Table 10-12. Employee Personnel Form

NAME:		Curran, Michael F.	
ADDRESS:		2418 Falcon Place	
CITY/STATE/ZIP:		Weston, Ohio 43412	
PHONE:		(419) 668-2937	
SOCIAL SECURITY:		243-09-0221	
DEGREES —	BA/BS	Michigan	RESEARCH INTERESTS:
	MA/MS	Kent State	Aphasia, Voice
	PhD	Wisconsin	
DATE HIRED:	Asst. Prof.	1976	ASHA CCC: SP
	Assoc. Prof.:	1976–1982	LICENSE: #1922
	Professor:	1982–	ASHA MEMB:#00091728 09
TENURE STATUS:		Tenured	
GRADUATE FACULTY STATUS:		Active. Renew in 1986	

searching and printing routines. The network/hierarchical system allows for fields of data to be modified, as in the relational system, but the network during the initialization cannot be changed. The billing information shown in Table 10-5 could be implemented using either a relational or network/hierarchical management system.

Those considering use of a data base management system should first determine whether their purposes are more in line with the functions served by a file management system, or the more sophisticated form of a relational or network/hierarchical management system. In addition to considering the skills of the user, it is important to consider how many storage fields are needed per record, and the maximum field size in characters. File handlers allow the user to update only one file at a time; however, some data base systems allow the updating of more than one file simultaneously. Other considerations might be whether the user wants the ability to perform various mathematical calculations, perform logical or relational comparisons, and finally whether one data base can be used to update another.

Data base software is rapidly changing, so that many problems encountered today should not exist in the future. Furthermore, some of the data base packages that can be purchased may not fit precisely into one of the three types described above. They will basically be one of the three types but may contain aspects of the other types. There are several recent articles and books on data base systems that the reader may wish to consult (Hartmann, 1983; Kruglinski, 1983; Martin, 1983; Page & Roberts, 1982).

Adaptations of software programs: An example of financial management

Those who have used commercially available software programs have possibly learned that some programs can serve purposes other than those for which they were originally designed. As was shown earlier, spreadsheets can arrange data in a rectangular array (matrix) where rows and columns are used to differentiate among numerous categories of data. Other software programs, designed for other purposes, can be adapted to accomplish similar functions.

An informative example is personal financial management, which was originally designed to help the user manage family financial records for deposits and expenses throughout a 1-year period (Gold, 1980). The user simply enters the current date to set a "flag" to input the data into the proper month. Entries can be made for funds received, and funds expended according

Table 10-13. Year-End Budget Review: Total Expenses

	Total budgets	Budgets $ spent	Budget %
Jan	2,875.00	2,604.09	91%
Feb	3,290.00	3,630.69	110%
Mar	7,430.00	7,416.10	100%
Apr	4,000.00	4,174.10	104%
May	13,300.00	14,762.75	111%
Jun	11,715.90	12,130.69	104%
Jul	4,145.00	4,893.78	118%
Aug	2,750.00	3,705.16	135%
Sep	2,185.00	5,067.17	232%
Oct	2,185.00	3,374.41	154%
Nov	2,195.00	3,466.68	158%
Dec	2,700.90	6,432.17	238%
Total	58,771.80	71,658.67	122%

to specific budget subcategories. Data can be recalled to show receipts and expenses both on a per monthly basis, as well as in terms of "current year to date."

The first step is to initialize the program by setting up the various budget categories needed for receipts and expenses. For purposes of explanation, only *expenses* will be discussed.

Expenses

Faculty Salaries
Staff Salaries
Telephone
Utilities
Rent
Office Supplies
Clinical Supplies
Academic Supplies
Research Equipment

Access to the data entry mode allows the user to enter the appropriate receipt or expense category by date and function. Within function would be a notation of the source of the specific receipt or expense. As needed, records are immediately available to show the current status of any or all budget accounts, and these may either be viewed on the screen or printed.

With respect to total budget expenses, it is possible to determine how much money has been expended on a month-by-month basis or, as is shown in Table 10-13, as a total year-end budget review. For each month the total amount of money budgeted, the total spent, as well as the actual percentage of budget expended is given.

It is also possible to examine each specific budget category for one specific month. As may be seen from Table 10-14, each budget category is listed vertically in the first column (arbitrarily labeled A through L in this example). The second column shows the actual amount budgeted and the middle column shows how much money was actually spent during the month. Column four shows the percentage of the budget that was spent, and the last column shows what percentage of the *total budget* was spent per budget category.

It is often helpful to know, within a specific budget category, how much has been expended on a monthly basis, and how this amount compares with the actual amount budgeted. Table

Table 10-14. Budget Category Summary for June

Budget Ident.	Budget	$ Spent	Budget %	Total %
A	1,000.00	982.00	98%	2%
B	450.00	450.20	100%	1%
C	1,800.00	1,752.76	97%	4%
D	480.00	505.34	105%	1%
E	685.00	546.75	80%	1%
F	600.00	616.36	103%	1%
G	675.00	654.95	97%	1%
H	100.00	95.01	95%	0%
I	1,020.90	1,074.41	105%	2%
J	1,250.00	585.94	47%	1%
K	775.00	760.00	98%	2%
L	etc.	etc.	etc.	etc.

10-15 shows a monthly summary of expenses for part-time student employment during each of the twelve months of the year. The months are shown in column 1 and the total of all budget expenses is shown in column 2. Column 3 shows the actual amount budgeted per month (in this case, $80.00) and column 4 shows the amount actually spent. Column 5 shows what percentage of the budget was actually expended, and the last column shows what percentage of all expenses was used for this particular budget category (i.e., part-time student employment).

Finally, it is sometimes necessary to determine the expenditures on a cumulative basis, throughout the year. Table 10-16, again using part-time student employment as the example, shows these cumulative amounts. Thus, whereas Table 10-15 represents just 1 month, Table 10-16 is for the entire year. The column labels are identical.

Personal finance manager programs also allow the user to search, sort, and edit data that have been previously entered. Consequently, errors can be easily corrected. The information can be viewed directly from the screen or a permanent record can be printed. In either event, the information is saved on the diskette.

In cases where the management system is used for specific accounting and bookkeeping purposes, it is possible to reconcile the expense account, as well as show a listing of the current balance. Finally, budget categories can be added (up to the ceiling imposed by the particular software program used), deleted, or modified during the year.

Word processing

Definition of word processing

Anything that can be typed on a typewriter can be typed into a word processor. Moreover, information stored via word processing is available to reuse, or reuse after modification. The features of word processing result in significant time saving. Since word processing capabilities vary as a function of the make, model, and memory of the microcomputer, the particular software program being used, and type of printer available, it is difficult to give a universal definition of "word processing." Therefore, what follows should be considered a general description rather than a specific definition.

A word processing system may be conceptualized as a program or collection of subprograms that permits the user to *enter*, *edit*, *delete*, and *print* textual material. Such material may be temporarily stored within the memory of the computer, or permanently on some external medium

Table 10-15. Specific Budget Category Summary for Part-Time Student Employment

	Total Spent ($)	Monthly results Budget	$ Spent	Budget %	Total %
Jan	2,604.09	80.00	72.86	91%	3%
Feb	3,630.69	80.00	83.54	104%	2%
Mar	7,416.98	80.00	69.00	86%	1%
Apr	4,174.10	80.00	73.49	92%	2%
May	14,762.75	80.00	102.95	129%	1%
Jun	12,130.69	80.00	103.50	129%	1%
Jul	4,893.78	80.00	63.23	7%	1%
Aug	3,705.16	80.00	71.77	90%	2%
Sep	5,067.17	80.00	121.88	152%	2%
Oct	3,374.41	80.00	62.14	78%	2%
Nov	3,466.68	80.00	54.64	68%	2%
Dec	6,432.17	80.00	140.37	175%	2%

such as a hard disk or floppy diskette. The ultimate purpose is to produce a formal written document. Word processing software makes it possible to quickly correct errors, move words, lines, and paragraphs, and effect formatting tasks without retyping each revision by hand. Examples include setting or changing left and right margins, setting or changing paragraph indentations, determining single or multiple spacing, setting top and bottom page margins, programming page headers and footers, determining the number of lines to be printed per page, and automatic pagination.

Word processing software allows the user to store and modify written information. The initial step is to enter (type) the information as on a conventional typewriter. Periodically, it is important to "save" the information held in the computer's memory on the data diskette to guard against losing the information held in the computer's RAM (random access memory) should there be a power failure or some other malfunction. Once saved, the user has the information available for future use. It is wise to make periodic backups of the diskette. Thus far, the operation of typing information into the word processor is identical to typing the information on a typewriter. This is where the similarity ends. Every typist knows the frustration of proofreading a document only to discover errors in spelling, punctuation, wording, syntax, and grammar, and places where sentences or paragraphs might better fit elsewhere. With conventional typing, this means that the page must be fixed (often a messy procedure) or completely retyped. In the case of a long document, fixing errors that occur early in the text sometimes results in the necessity of retyping many subsequent pages simply because earlier error corrections resulted in pages being out of alignment.

Word processing allows the user to "scroll" from one section of text to another so that what has been entered can be readily accessed and viewed. It is possible to make the job of editing easier by using a "split screen" function so that portions of text that occur at different locations can be viewed simultaneously. It is not necessary to obtain a hardcopy of text unless a hardcopy is needed. In addition, it is possible to "jump" from one text segment to another or to "search" for items to modify. Many word processing programs have a "glossary" function that allows the user to automatically insert a specific word, string of words, or sentence(s) from the computer's memory buffer simply by typing a predetermined designator character. Within

Table 10-16. Specific Budget Category Summary for Part-Time Student Employment

		Year-to-date results			
	Total Spent ($)	Budget	$ Spent	Budget %	Total %
Jan	2,604.90	80.00	72.86	91%	3%
Feb	6,234.78	160.00	156.40	98%	3%
Mar	13,651.76	240.00	225.40	94%	2%
Apr	17,825.86	320.00	298.89	93%	2%
May	32,588.61	400.00	401.84	100%	1%
Jun	44,719.30	480.00	505.34	105%	1%
Jul	49,613.08	560.00	568.57	102%	1%
Aug	53,318.24	640.00	640.34	100%	1%
Sep	58,385.41	720.00	762.22	106%	1%
Oct	61,759.82	800.00	824.36	103%	1%
Nov	65,226.50	880.00	879.00	100%	1%
Dec	71,658.67	960.00	1,019.37	106%	1%

the actual text it is possible to format the desired output with respect to such things as margins, paragraphs, and the number of lines to be printed per page. The text may be left justified, right justified, center justified, or full justified (see Table 10-17). It is possible to automatically print page headings and page numbers, either at the top and/or at the bottom of the page, without manually retyping it on each and every page.

Finally, it is possible to use a "form feed" function so that at predetermined locations the printing will automatically begin at the top of a new page. A special form feed function will begin printing a new page if, *and only if*, there are fewer than "X" lines left on the page currently being typed. Therefore, if FF10 were entered, the command to begin typing a new page would be executed *only* if there were fewer than 10 lines remaining on the current page. This feature is particularly helpful when sufficient space must be saved to insert a table or figure.

Proofreading is also made easier with word processing. In addition to the user's viewing the final copy for visual aesthetics, other software programs are available to "proof-read" the text for errors in spelling. In cases where the professional terms are not listed among the thousands of words stored in the "spelling checker's" memory, it is possible to enter additional terms. Some programs will access mailing lists, produce multiple copies, and perform still other functions such as the typing of form letters.

The many functions of word processing can be subdivided into four essential components. First, there must be the ability to *insert* new data into what is already in memory. This may involve adding leltters, words, sentences, and paragraphs. Second, there must be the ability to *delete* characters, words, lines, sentences, and paragraphs. These "editing features" save countless hours of retyping major sections of documents, as is so frequently the case with conventional typing, when it has been necessary to make changes in an earlier draft. The third major function of word processing is the ability to *search* and find specific locations within the text. Finally, there must be the ability to *print* the document. Depending upon the microcomputer used, the particular word processing software program available, and which printer is employed, it is possible to do such things as: underline, switch from regular to bold-face, use subscripts and superscripts, change the print font, insert footnotes, ensure that there is at least a given amount of space at the bottom of a page, maintain continuous pagination, print headers and/or footers on each page, and insert tables and figures at the appropriate location. Other optional add-on features include spelling checkers, the ability to perform mathematical calculations within the text, and the ability to merge the text with form letters and mailing lists.

Table 10-17. Examples of Printed Output

LEFT JUSTIFY

This is an example of left justification. See how it works.
All left margins are to the left side of the paper.
Even with a short line.
Or, with a longer line, it will be printed like this one is printed.

RIGHT JUSTIFY

This is an example of right justification. See how it works.
All right margins are to the right side of the paper.
Even short lines.
Or, with a longer line, it will be printed like this one is printed.

CENTER JUSTIFY

This is an example of center justification. See how it works.
All margins are justified to the center of the paper.
Even short lines.
Or, with a longer line, it will be printed like this one is printed.

FULL JUSTIFY

This is an example of full justification. See how it works. All margins are justified to both margins, left as well as right. Whether short or long, the line will attempt to fill itself in with extra spaces in order to give the effect of a fully justified series of margins. This, as well as the examples noted above, can be programmed within the text with an embedded print command. See how much fun it is!! And, see how much your secretary will enjoy these extra features.

Administrative applications

Depending upon work setting, different administrative reports will be needed. Whether they are for use in hospitals, schools, clinics, private practice, universities, government, or some other setting, the simple fact of the matter is that the preparation of administrative reports and documents is a necessary part of the job! The possible administrative uses documented in the following paragraphs are not meant to be exhaustive, but rather, to give a general orientation to ways in which word processing may be useful to administrators, department chairpersons, clinical directors and coordinators, clinical supervisors, and staff and students.

It should be emphasized that several underlying factors make word processing especially useful. First, it is frequently the case that numerical data and written documentation are used for multiple purposes. That is, the information that may be needed for a report to the ASHA Educational Standards Board this week may be needed as part of a grant application next month. Word processing allows this information to be stored, recalled, used, reused, moved, modified, merged, or appended with other documentation in order to best meet the specific and current needs of today, as well as the anticipated needs of tomorrow. Second, there are instances where interim reports are needed and where the actual format of the report will not change. All that must be changed are a few modifiers, adjectives, and numbers. Rather than totally retype the entire report, word processing allows the simple deletion of sections that are to be expunged and the addition of new information that is requested. Word processing allows greatly improved efficiency with respect to writing and editing, revising and merging information, and allows a "clean copy" without extensive retyping.

A word processing program can be beneficial to an administrator or staff member who needs to produce many copies of a document, but where each copy of the document will be slightly different. The basic "core document" can reside on a floppy or hard disk, be loaded into the microcomputer's memory to be modified as needed, and then be printed. This saves typing the document each time a copy is needed. An example illustrating this is the process of writing letters of recommendation for a student that must be sent to several different graduate schools or prospective employers. The "core document" can be typed and saved on a diskette. Then, all that needs to be changed is the address and salutation of the person to whom the letter is sent.

Listed below are examples of word processing functions with administrative significance.
1. Documentation for accreditation of reaccreditation.
2. Preparation of grant applications.
3. In-House documents and reports for central administration.
4. Form letters and mailing lists.
5. Modification and updating of staff resumes, curriculum vitae, performance evaluations, job descriptions, and position vacancy announcements.
6. Modification of academic and clinic schedules, course syllabi, and classroom examinations.
7. Reports for certification or recertification by third-party payment agencies.
8. Research reports, manuscripts for publication, articles, and book chapters.
9. General correspondence.

Clinical applications

Many custom software packages have become available for clinical use (see Rushakoff, chap. 7). This is true both for use in the clinic, with respect to the assessment and treatment of communication disorders, and for administrative purposes. The American Speech-Language-Hearing Association established a Committee on Educational Technology. More recently, and partially as an outgrowth of this committee, a Computer Users in Speech and Hearing group (CUSH) has been formed. Since it is impossible to obtain a *current* listing of available state-of-the-art software programs, readers are referred to CUSH for a current list of available packages (Fitch, 1984). Programs are now available to assist clinicians with a variety of uses such as generating diagnostic and therapy reports, summarizing IEPs, and correspondence packages for use with clients, families, and administrators.

Since this chapter has been concerned with "Administrative Applications," the reader is referred to other chapters in this *handbook* for clinical (see Rushakoff, chap. 7), research (see Mahaffey, chap. 8), and instructional (see Shearer, chap. 9) applications. Word processing will clearly be a significant benefit to those who write reports for these purposes. Additional information regarding word processing is available from other sources (Adams, 1983; *Consumer Reports*, 1982; Glatzer, 1981; Lutus, 1981, 1982; Miller, 1982; Rodwell, 1983; Rosen, 1983; Schmeltz, 1983; Stanton, Wells & Rochowansky, 1983).

SUMMARY

In this chapter, attempts have been made to explain the transitions that have occured in the evolution from mainframe to microcomputers. Applications that were available only on mainframes a few years ago are now becoming available for microcomputers. It is certain that new developments in software in the next few years will expand the capabilities of the microcomputers still further.

In this chapter, the reader has been exposed to the use of computer-assisted programs for the management of words (word processing), numbers (spreadsheets), and data bases. Examples have been provided for both "packaged" and "custom" programs that can assist in the collection, manipulation, and repeating of data in some systematic way.

REFERENCES

Adams, S. (1983, November). Commodore word processors. *Popular Computing,* 181–188.
Bishop, J. (1982). Beyond the peaks of Visicalc. *Byte, 7,* 29–39.
Computer as a super-typewriter. (1983). *Consumer Reports, 48*(10), 540–551.
Glatzer, H. (1981). *Introduction to word processing.* Berkeley, CA: Sybex Publications.
Gold, J. (1980). *Personal finance manager.* Cupertino, CA: Apple Computer Company.
Grushcow, J. (1983). *The Visicalc applications book.* Reston, VA: Reston Publishers.
Hartmann, J. (1983, December). Aura 5: A new integrated database system. *Popular Computing,* 114–115.
Kruglinski, D. (1983, October). Database management systems. *Personal Computing,* 117–134.
Lutus, P. (1982). *Applewriter IIe operating manual.* Cupertino, CA: Apple Computer Company.
Lutus, P. (1981). *Applewriter III operating manual.* Cupertino, CA: Apple Computer Company.
Martin, J. (1983). *Managing the data-base environment.* Englewood Cliffs, NJ: Prentice-Hall.
Miller, J. (1982). Word processing for movies and popes. *Softalk, 3,* 72–78.
Page, J., & Roberts, D. (program authors) and Bedke, J., & Doerr, C. (manual authors) (1982). *Personal file system.* Mountain View, CA: Software Publishing Company.
Rodwell, P. (1983). *The personal computer handbook.* Woodbury, NY: Barron's Educational Publishing.
Rosen, A. (1983). *Getting the most out of your word processor.* Englewood Cliffs, NJ: Prentice-Hall.
Schmeltz, L. (1982). *Word processing with your personal computers.* Blue Ridge, PA: Tab Publishers.
Spindler, L. (1982). Electronic worksheet. *Radio Electronics, 53*(9), 80–108.
Stanton, J., Wells, R., & Rochowansky, S. (Eds.) (1983). *Apple Computer Software.* Los Angeles: The Book Company.
Stiefel, M., & Simpson, D. (1983, September). Minicomputer spreadsheets take advantage of hardware capabilities. *Mini-Microsystems,* 172–178.

REFERENCE NOTES

Fitch, J. Computer Users in Speech and Hearing (CUSH). University of South Alabama. Mobile, AL 36688.
Mahaffey, R. (1983, November). *Computer technology: The revolution has started without us.* Paper presented to the annual convention of the American Speech-Language-Hearing Association, Cincinnati, OH.
Punch, J. (1983, November). *Computer technology: The revolution has started without us.* Paper presented to the annual convention of the American Speech-Language-Hearing Association, Cincinnati, OH.

SECTION IV
A BROADER PERSPECTIVE

Chapter 11

Issues and Controversies in the Use of Microcomputers

Kent J. Wilson

The microcomputer is becoming an important informational, educational, clinical, and recreational tool. While some claim that the microcomputer is comparable to the teaching machine or instructional television, widespread applications of microcomputers are more of a societal than an educational phenomenon (Hoffmeister, 1982).

Actually, microcomputer applications to communication disorders are just beginning to develop, and the speech/language pathologist and audiologist must be wary as well as knowledgable about its capabilities and limitations. This chapter discusses a number of issues and controversies that are confronting us at the present time with the use of the microcomputer. It is hoped that by understanding some of these arguments, we may avoid an uncritical embrace of the technology that may turn to rejection when it fails to meet unrealistic expectations.

COMPUTER LITERACY

One of the most important issues facing us today is the growing concern that our knowledge and acceptance of computers are lagging far behind the use of computers in so many facets of our daily lives. Computers are used when cashing a check, paying a bill, buying a new car, using a telephone, or traveling on a bus, train, or plane. They have been adopted in virtually every aspect of business, cultural, social, and even religious organizations as a means to improve the effectiveness and efficiency of operations. Computer manufacturers and authors who write for computer magazines have been telling us we need to be "computer literate" if we are to survive in this technological age.

Computer literacy, however, means different things to different people. Some argue that it is the ability to program, while others believe it is the ability to use specific applications such as word processing, or just knowledge about microcomputers in general—ROMs and RAMs, bits and bytes. There are still others who would insist that it includes all three areas. While there may be general agreement that computer literacy is the ability to understand and work with computers, there is no consensus on the precise knowledge, skills, or attitudes that an individual needs to function adequately in this technological society.

Computer literacy is not only ill defined, but much debated. It is believed that with all levels of education, starting perhaps as early as kindergarden and continuing through the school

©College-Hill Press, Inc. All rights, including that of translation, reserved. No part of this publication may be reproduced without the written permission of the publisher.

system, university, and adult education, individuals in our society need to understand the various ways the microcomputer can be used. It is also argued that they need to understand the positive and negative consequences of those applications.

Few full-scale computer literacy courses exist. Many colleges and universities offer computer literacy workshops and inservice training opportunities, but what often passes for computer literacy is vague history or learning to program in a simplified way. Specialized courses are needed for each group addressed. Technologically and media-based arguments for a single type of computer use are entirely misleading. Microcomputers in speech/language pathology and audiology can be used in a variety of ways, as discussed in previous chapters of this book, and should be adapted to the individual situation being considered.

Speech/language pathologists and audiologists need to understand and appreciate the roles, functions, benefits, and limitations of the microcomputer. As we become more comfortable with the technology, new ideas, approaches, and additional applications for microcomputers will hopefully be initiated.

CYBERPHOBIA

"Cyberphobia" is a term that is growing in usage and incidence (Anderson, 1983). Fear is a common emotion of people as they first begin to use a microcomputer. They may be afraid of making a mistake, erasing a program, or making the microcomputer "self-destruct." They may suffer from an ingrained fear of the technology as well as a fear that, by attempting to use the microcomputer, they are treading into technological territory that will be overwhelming. One pictures oneself with the machine set up and ready to go and suddenly getting the feeling, "Suppose I press the wrong key—what will happen?" Or "Will I lose all my information or muck the whole system up dangerously?"

Cyberphobia is an issue that affects many of us when we first consider using microcomputers. Most people want to know more about microcomputers and anticipate feeling comfortable using them. But if we become intimidated and fearful of microcomputers, effective learning can be blocked. Speech/language pathologists and audiologists need to overcome any inhibitions concerning microcomputers before being able to direct their utilization more effectively.

Working with a personal computer too often has been difficult and tedious for users. Rothfeder (1983) suggests that much of the blame for this difficulty is attributable to the aura surrounding microcomputers, as well as to the fact that microcomputers were invented by technologists who had built and worked with mainframe computers. The first generation of personal computers, with their keyboards, operating procedures, and manuals, were complicated by an electronic shorthand that was better suited and more understandable to mainframe computer users than to individuals who wanted to plug the microcomputer into an AC socket and make it perform. This has certainly contributed to the frustrations of many who have purchased a microcomputer as well as dissuaded many would-be users from buying a microcomputer at all.

Many people become more fearful when trying to learn how microcomputers work. Relatively little about the machine's technology needs to be understood to be able to use it quite effectively. Certainly, one can use a telephone without understanding much about how it works. In fact, few persons posses a thorough understanding of the telephone's mechanical operations. This is also true of microcomputers. Users can decide how much or little to learn about its internal workings.

Figure 11-1.

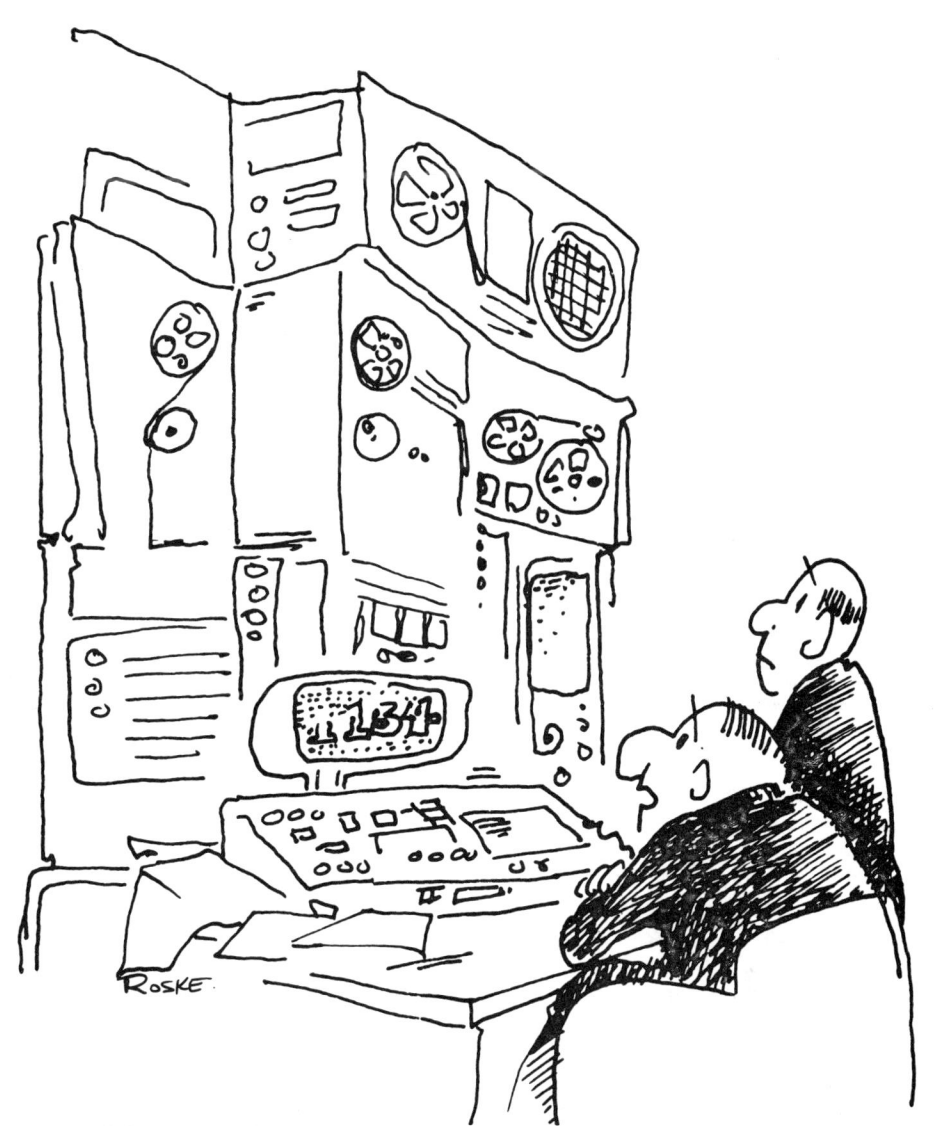

Now, that's what I call magic!

One possible reason people feel intimidated by microcomputers may be the terminology used, sometimes referred to as "computerese." Unfortunately, a new user who is not familiar with the terminology can become confused and may misunderstand a great deal of information. People often object to computerese, in particular, because it makes them feel left out. New users cannot digest much of the information contained in magazine articles, advertisements, and other sources without an understanding of the terms used.

However, every field has particular words and concepts that communicate specific information about the equipment, operation, and basic concepts of that field. Unquestionably, microcomputer literature is characterized by a highly specialized vocabulary that can be initially confusing and threatening to many people.

Cyberphobia can be overcome in a number of ways. Many individuals read books and magazines that describe the workings of microcomputers, or study tutorial programs of microcomputers that teach a new user how it operates. These methods often succeed in making users less intimidated by a microcomputer, but they involve a significant amount of time and effort.

Hoffman (1983) argues that an open mind is vital in overcoming the fear of microcomputers. He explains that microcomputers are neither like most other technology in people's experience nor like what people expect them to be. It usually takes a certain amount of time for people to feel comfortable working with microcomputers. To accomplish this, Hoffman teaches students new ways of thinking and new ways of learning. It is his belief that what computer science instructors can teach students can be used in other areas also.

The effort to make computers intuitively easy to use and less threatening has been summed up in a little two-word piece of microcomputer jargon: user friendly (Shea, 1983). As speech/language pathologists and audiologists become more comfortable with its technology, they will expand the range of applications for the equipment and will discover options not even imagined currently.

ISSUES IN SELECTING SOFTWARE

Given the amount of available software, one's particular objectives for use, the lack of standards, and the high costs, selecting software and its documentation can be a major obstacle and a problem faced by many professionals today. There are no distinctive criteria for selecting software, just as there is no set formula for selecting other instructional materials. Selecting software requires time, thought, and certainly some degree of expertise. This is particularly true in the areas of content needs for individual learners and practical applicability for classroom settings (Hannaford & Sloane, 1983).

Documentation that accompanies software has often been characterized by reviewers as incomplete, poorly organized, and miserably written. This intimidates and frustrates new and experienced microcomputer users alike. Skills for creating a program are not the same as skills for telling someone how to use that product. People who develop software for microcomputers are product experts, not user experts. All too frequently the product-oriented engineers may have significant say over documentation.

Why have manuals been so disorganized, ill-conceived, poorly rendered, and unclear? Collopy (1983) believes that when personal computers were first unveiled, the job of writing documentation was often given to the least knowledgeable member of the programming staff. The vendor did not wish to use more experienced programmers for this task. Thus, documentation took a back seat to every other meaningful job.

Documentation should answer questions regarding software needs and expectations. Some documentation may explain basic features clearly, but contain an advanced section that is virtually impossible to decipher, even after learning the basics. The current trend is to employ professional writers in the development of software documentation. Many of these writers usually have a strong computer background but will, by design, know little abut the specific program being developed. Therefore, the nonprogrammer can analyze the program more objectively and develop the documentation without making inappropriate assumptions.

Figure 11-2.

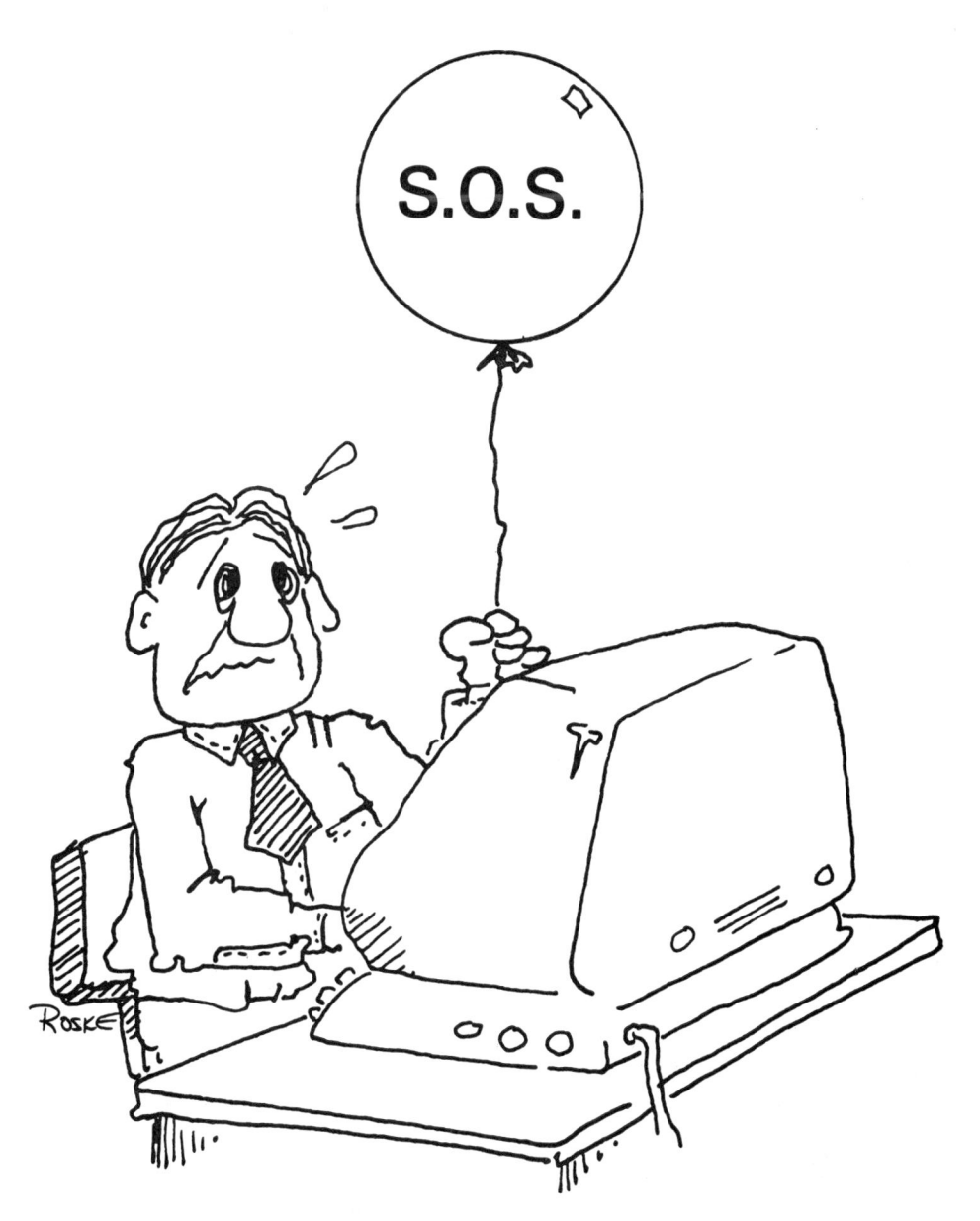

Stephens (1983) argued that if consumers of software want good, high-quality documentation they must accept some responsibility for it. He offers the following **nine-point plan** for pressuring software publishers to invest the necessary resources to assure better documentation.
1. Keep documentation in mind when shopping for hardware and software. Evaluate documentation by reading reviews, asking to look at the user's guide from the local vendor, and talking with friends about their experiences with the program.

2. If contracting for customized software, make the completion of satisfactory documentation one of the terms of acceptance.
3. When working with newly purchased software, make notes about specific discrepancies or weaknesses in the user's guide. Then write to the software publisher to report these specific faults.
4. Provide editorial input to a favorite magazine or journal.
5. Clip and send reviews in which documentation is mentioned to software publishers.
6. Bring up the subject of documentation at a users' group meeting.
7. Write software reviews that also discuss documentation for the user's group newsletter.
8. Assume responsibility for "word-of-mouth" advertising. When discussing software with others, tell them about the documentation as well.
9. When making a software purchase in which the quality of the documentation is a factor, be sure the right people become aware of it. Write directly to the developer.

There is a need for independent reviews and evaluations of the software now being marketed in our field. At the present time, however, there is no comprehensive, systematic, or effective way to accomplish this task. Also needed are the critical judgments of professionals in our field who are familiar with programming procedures on the quality and utility of programs offered commercially. With the thousands of programs being produced, substantial resources will be necessary.

CONTROVERSIES IN SOFTWARE DEVELOPMENT

Many, if not most, persons developing software are not familiar with the established goals and objectives in our profession, a shortcoming that is likely to be reflected in their products. Some of the programs may be useful and effective, but most will not meet the quality standards we should expect. The production of effective software is a difficult task, requiring a high level of training and experience. Software development involves careful specification of objectives, selection of programming strategies, detailed analysis of content structure and sequence, and development of pretests and posttests, preliminary drafts, revisions, trials, validation, and documentation (Gleason, 1981).

Hannaford and Taber (1982) have outlined a number of prerequisites that should be considered in the development of software for handicapped individuals in order for them to gain maximum benefit from the microcomputer. They suggest that software material be built around a user's specifically identified goals and objectives. Not only should the knowledge and skills of the user be specified, but provision should also be made for the user to enter a program at his level of microcomputer proficiency with subsequent branching available to appropriate, more advanced levels of content.

Special attention should also be given to how material is presented, for example, the size of letters, their clarity, spacing, and whether they are upper or lower case. In addition, the way the user obtains, maintains, and controls the system can be an important consideration. One should also determine if the stimuli are presented in such a way that selected sensory modalities may be used. The use of various features of the computer such as color, animation, and sound may also facilitate the gaining and holding of some patients' attention, another important factor in learning. With proper programs, a learner can be stimulated to recall previously learned information or processes, thereby enhancing the retention and transfer of learning.

The processes used in presenting stimuli should also be scrutinized carefully. Such factors as the pacing and length of a program, the clarity of its directions, and the language used should be considered. Is the program humanistic? For example, does it use the patient's name, appropriate feedback, and reinforcement?

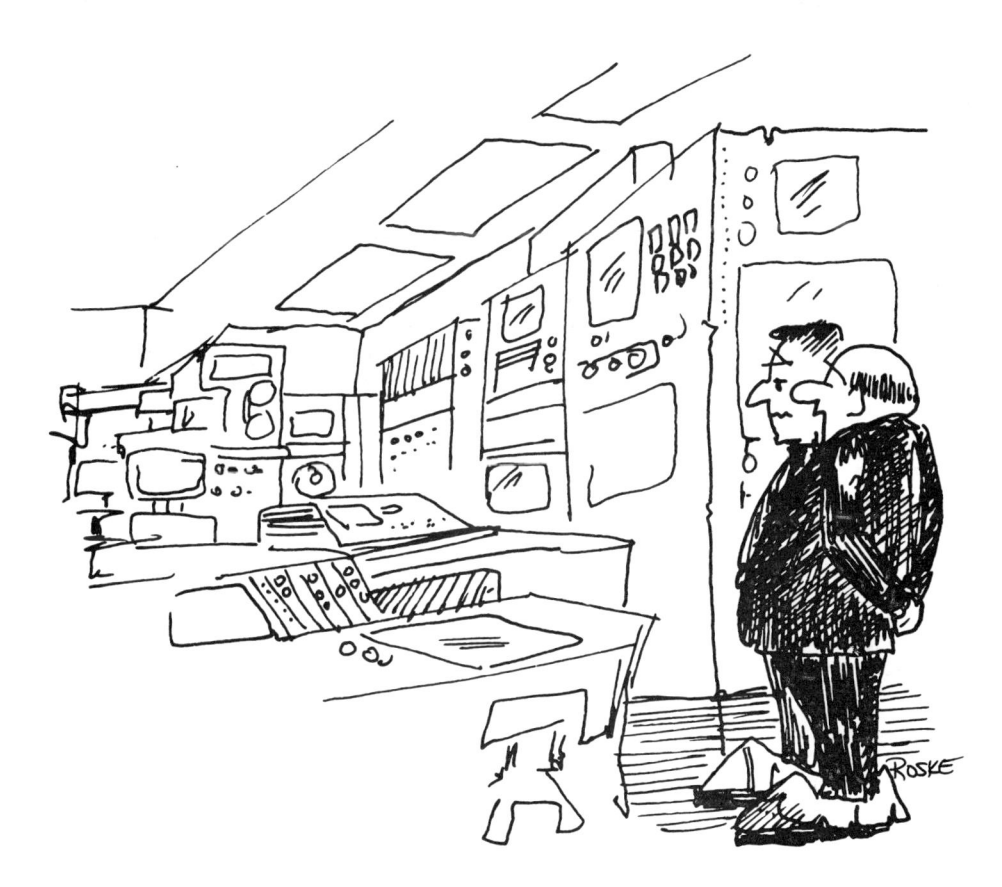

Figure 11-3. **Now we just need a Computer Programmer. . .**

Another possible benefit is that the computer can be programmed to interact in a number of ways, ranging from strict stimulus/response, found in most drill and practice programs, to more elaborate interactions such as those found in simulation programs. Depending on the program, the computer is able to present a stimulus, accept a response, evaluate the response, present appropriate feedback and reinforcement, and then move to the next appropriate segment. Such interaction can be nonthreatening and especially beneficial to those who have previously faced failure.

Another consideration is response handling. What types of reinforcement and feedback are given? Does the type of reinforcement vary? Is reinforcement personalized? What type of feedback is given an incorrect response? Is it appropriate and does it provide additional information? What occurs with repeated incorrect responses? Is the client provided feedback for correct responses which reiterates why the response was correct, or is feedback simply a single word or phrase? Are provisions made for reporting cumulative results of the client's performance to him, and are these results permanently stored for future reference?

One should ask if the method of user response is appropriate for a given patient's abilities. Does the user respond by using the keyboard, a paddle, a joystick, touching the screen, or using a light pen? Does he have to type a word, a phrase, a sentence, or only a letter or number?

Evaluating the technical adequacy of software also involves determining the extent to which it can be controlled by the clinician or client. A clinician should be able to individualize software for a client by modifications in the program or setting certain parameters. However, due to problems with unauthorized duplication of commercial software, this flexibility is prevented by developers or publisher who "lock" access to their software. Ideally the client should be able to begin a program, choose the desired selection from a menu or index, enter this selection, obtain help or clues from the program if problems arise, and exit the program whenever desired.

Another issue of technical adequacy is whether the software is "error trapped." Software that is vulnerable to random input and unskilled handling will quickly become unusable. The software should be immune to damage likely to be incurred through normal use by clients and experienced users.

Clinicians will have to work with computer programmers to ensure the availability of clinically appropriate and usable technology (Budoff & Hutten, 1982). One perplexing problem involves the "compatibility" of software. Almost every make of microcomputer uses a particular language, dialect of a language, or operating system. Software developed for one make of microcomputer may not operate on another. Many unwary and uninformed people have learned of this only after much unnecessary frustration and expense. A second major problem is that more emphasis is generally placed on the technical aspects of software than on their educational aspects. In other words, some programs are written that make extensive use of the various capabilities of the microcomputer, e.g., animated graphics, but which neglect the educational considerations necessary to facilitate learning. Nor is it unusual to find programs with poorly sequenced instructions, inaccuracies, misspellings, or incomplete sentences in the instructions given on the monitor or in the documentation. This problem may reflect the fact that much software is currently produced by individuals who have expertise in computer programming, but little, if any, in education.

PIRACY

Software piracy is becoming an increasing controversy in the personal computer field. Software publishers are scrambling to find new ways to protect their products. The casual copying of programs by microcomputer hobbyists, although not epidemic, is commonplace. Many people apparently fail to see that the practice is not just unethical—it is also illegal.

Software piracy is an ambiguous term that means different things to different people. Software executives see it as a violation of their rights, while others argue that it is the only way to deal out justice to greedy program peddlers.

A 1980 amendment to the Copyright Act allows owners to copy programs that are considered an essential step in the use of a microcomputer program. This exemption only applies to copies of programs that are sold, however. On the other hand, if a copyright owner chooses to make the program available only by lease or by license arrangement, copying is permitted only under the terms and conditions specified by the copyright owner. Violation of these conditions constitutes infringement.

But is software piracy ever justifiable? Many individuals making duplicates seem to be doing so as insurance, in case something goes wrong with their original, as it often does. What happens if a direct-mail program "dies"? Without a backup, the only recourse is to return the disk to the manufacturer and hope that it will not take longer than a few weeks to get a replacement.

Manufacturers understand such problems, and many have designed some floppy disk-based programs that allow users to make one backup copy. After one copy is made, software "jamming" information is automatically added to the original floppy disk to prevent, at least theoretically, additional illegal copies. In practice, though, enterprising software pirates can crack the protection mechanisms and make copies at will. Some individuals are giving copies away by the dozen; others are selling them. By one estimate, unauthorized copying has risen to cut annual sales of the ($200 million) microcomputer software publishing industry by $12–36 million. There are also network systems which connect thousands of microcomputers to one another via telephone lines. Through these systems it becomes possible to send a program from New York to Arizona in a matter of minutes (Shaffer, 1982).

Until recently, copying was limited to computer buffs who used their knowledge of electronics and programming to outwit the protection schemes. "Copy-all" programs were born, and now anyone with such a program can make unlimited duplicates of almost any other program. With the advent of such programs, retailers and makers of microcomputers report that corporations, government agencies, and educational institutions are buying several microcomputers at a time, but only one copy of certain important software. But they do not call what they do piracy and, in a sense it is not. Software vendors complain most about illegal copies that are sold to third parties.

The industry is faced with a dilemma: how do the manufacturers serve their customers' legitimate needs to make backup copies, while protecting an expensive software investment? There are at least two possibilities: put the would-be software pirate at a disadvantage if he makes an illegal copy, or better still, make it virtually impossible for pirates to make a copy (Morgan, 1981).

Legal protection methods

The most common legal mechanism for software protection is the copyright law. Copyrights have been clearly established, both by statute in 1980 and by case law, as a method for protecting computer software programs (Carrick, 1983).

A copyright is essentially the right of an author to control the copying of his or her work by others. Copyrighting offers protection as a legal remedy and a deterrent to piracy. A copyright covers the expression or program listing of software but not the idea, procedure, or concept underlying the software. A competitor could, for example, use the copyright owner's basic procedure or method of solution without infringing upon copyright if a different but equivalent program were developed. Also, the copyright owner is provided no protection against competitors who independently develop the same program; a copyright offers protection only against actual copying (Becker, 1981).

If an individual pirating a program can be identified, copyright law permits monetary recovery of the profits pirates made from the program or of any losses suffered as a result of their copying it. Copyright law also allows statutory damages even if the author cannot prove the amount of damages by the pirates and the court can, at its discretion, award from $100 to $50,000. A developer can also request an injunction that would prohibit pirates from continuing their copying, as well as cover court costs and perhaps attorney's fees (Remer, 1982).

The term of a copyright encompasses the lifetime of the author plus 50 years. In the case of a work made for hire, the term is the earlier of two periods: 75 years from the year that the program was published, or 100 years from the year that the program was written.

There are basically two requirements for establishing a copyright. First, the developer should include a notice of copyright on the program which should appear on the monitor when the program is loaded or a listing is printed. The copyright notice should include the internationally recognized copyright symbol, (C), the year of publication (the year it becomes available to the public or to distributors), the copyright owner's or the program developer's name, followed by All Rights Reserved. Second, the copyright owner must obtain, complete, and return Form TX to the US Copyright Office, Library of Congress, Washington, DC 20559, along with a copy of the source code and a check for $10.00.

There are a number of speech/language pathologists and audiologists developing and marketing software who need to be aware of how to protect their software. There is nothing more frustrating than to discover, after having invested time and effort, that someone has pirated ideas or the software itself without compensating the author for his work or the money it cost to develop it. First, the author must decide what it is to be protected, and then determine what method is the best way to assure that protection.

Daniel Remer recently published an excellent guide to legal considerations designed especially for program developers and software publishers (Remer, 1982). It clearly and simply sets forth the law relating to the development, protection, and marketing of computer software.

Trade secrets and copyright protection are two of the basic forms of legal protection that are applicable to software development. A trade secret is commonly defined as a formula, process, mechanism, compound, or compilation of data known only to certain individuals using it in business to obtain a commercial advantage (Becker, 1981). For a trade secret to be upheld by the courts, a secret must exist. In addition, there must be an obligation on the part of all persons who learn the secret not to disclose it. Confidential relationships are generally established between employers and employees, or between businesses cooperating in technical development by a type of contract known as a disclosure agreement.

One advantage of trade secret, in contrast to copyright, is that a trade secret exists as long as the secret is maintained; it does not expire after a predetermined period of time. There are no formal procedures, applications to fill out, or government fees to pay to establish a trade secret. Furthermore, there are no delays, because a trade secret becomes enforceable as soon as it exists.

Anyone who has access, or potential access, to a program while it is in the developmental stages should sign a nondisclosure statement before given access to the trade secret. This offers several advantages. First, it stresses that the trade secret is being taken seriously and insists that anyone with access do the same. Second, it legally binds the signer from disclosing the secret. Third, if the signer should disclose the secret to someone else, that person cannot legally make use of it without facing the possibility of monetary damages, court injunctions, and so forth. The law does not recognize a trade secret if there are individuals who have seen the secret without obligating themselves not to divulge it. Unlike copyright law, trade secret is not a federal law. Each state has its own version (Remer, 1982).

Copy protection

Another possible solution to the piracy problem is to make it so difficult and costly for pirates to make copies that the problem disappears. The concept of the so-called ID ROM is a recent development now being used in England. Built into the control is a special ROM containing an identification number that is duplicated on the program's floppy disk. The program periodically checks for the presence of ID ROM. If it's not found, the program crashes (Morgan, 1981). This technique puts one more stumbling block in the way of the pirate, and it does not add appreciably to the total cost of software (the ID ROM costs about $20.00).

Two of the more promising solutions to the software protection problem come from inventor Marc Kaufman. He has filed a patent for an "execute only ROM," a new type of read-only memory which produces a sequence of executable code in the normal manner but which prohibits the user from randomly accessing memory addresses. As Kaufman explains, the user begins execution of the program at a known address. A "secret" executive routine, built into the ROM, contains a table of the next legal steps for every given step in the program. Only those steps listed in the table can be accessed by the user. For example, if the program contains a branch to one of two places, only those two places can be examined by the programmer at that time. If a program contains enough branches, it would take an inordinate amount of time for the user to run through every permutation of the program to get a complete listing of the code, even if a computer did the searching. An unreadable EPROM is also in the works, enabling the do-it-yourselfer to create secure programs (Morgan, 1981).

Kaufman's second idea is to add a "black box" to a personal computer. Every piece of software would come with a magnetic key (or other type of hard-to-duplicate key) that plugs into the black box and contains a coded ID number that matches the ID number on the floppy disk. The program resides on the disk in encrypted form. To decode the program, the key must be plugged into the box. With this scheme, the user can make as many backup copies as desired, but only one of them can be used at a time. The drawback to such a system is the need for the black box. But if the idea catches on, the price would probably be competitive (Morgan, 1981).

CONCLUSION

The microcomputer has found its way into many offices, schools, and homes. It is also beginning to be used in a number of rehabilitation settings throughout the country. This "information revolution," which was predicted by many, has arrived, bringing with it the promise of dramatic changes in the way people live, work, and perhaps even think. But a number of issues and controversies need to be considered.

It has been predicted that by 1990, 75% of the nation's work force will be dependent on microcomputers. With such increases in their use will come an inevitable increase in the number of cyberphobic cases (Chin, 1983).

There is a need to improve our understanding and acceptance of the roles and potential of microcomputers in society as a whole and in the speech/language profession specifically. The development of computer literacy courses and workshops for the general public and, in particular, for speech/language pathologists and audiologists, will require a major effort during the next several years. Of major concern is the need to incorporate computer literacy courses into curriculum requirements. These courses will hopefully reduce resistance, fear, and anxiety created by the use of microcomputers.

The task of developing appropriate and acceptable software must be faced by our profession and by all levels of the educational establishment. Literally thousands of programs are being written, but few of them are acceptable because they lack certain prerequisites. There is also a desperate need for impartial review and evaluation of these programs to determine their value and effectiveness. At the present time, there is no comprehensive, systematic, or effective organization to accomplish this task.

Another major problem in the development and distribution of software relates to the federal copyright law. The latest revision of the law has been interpreted in several different ways and has been violated by many individuals. The need to incorporate appropriate copyright and copy protection methods into the development of software by our professionals will hopefully curtail such violation.

REFERENCES

Anderson, J. J. (1983, August). The heartbreak of cyberphobia. *Creative Computering*, 114–128.
Becker, S. A. (1981, May). Legal protection for computer hardware and software. *Byte*, 140–146.
Budoff, M., & Hutten, L. (1982). Microcomputers in special education: Promises and pitfalls. *Exceptional Children*, 40(2), 123–128.
Carrick, R. (1983). Guarding against software piracy: The legal problem. *Infoworld*, 5(33), 41–44.

Chin, K. (1983). Cyberphobia, fight or flight reactions to computers. *Infoworld, 5*(29), 22-24.
Collopy, D. (1983). Software documentation: Reading a package by its cover. *Personal Computing*, 124-144.
Gleason, G. (1981, March). Microcomputers in education: The state of the art. *Educational Technology*, 7-18.
Hannaford, A., & Sloane, E. (1981, November). Microcomputers: Powerful learning tools with proper programming. *Teaching Exceptional Children*, 54-57.
Hannaford, A., & Taber, F. (1982). Microcomputer software for the handicapped: Development and evaluation. *Exceptional Children, 49*(2), 137-142.
Hoffmeister, A.M. (1982, October). Microcomputers in Perspective. *Exceptional Children, 49*(2), 115-121.
Hoffman, R. (1983). Teaching computer concepts to the terrified masses. *Infoworld, 5*(38), 15-16.
Morgan, C. (1983, May). How can we stop software piracy? *Byte*, 6-10.
Remer, D. (1982). *Legal care for your software: A step-by-step guide for computer software writers*. Berkeley, CA: A Nolo Press Book.
Rothfeder, J. (1983, February). Striking back at technological terror. *Personal Computing*, 62-66.
Shaffer, R. (1982). Software makers losing sales to program pirates. In Broadwell, B., & Edwards, P. (Eds.), *Data processing: Computers in action*. Belmont, CA: Computer News.
Shea, T. (1983). Jolts and joys are the fallouts of computer jargon. *Infoworld, 5*(28), 22-23.
Stephens, J. G. (1983). Documentation users, unite! *Infoworld, 5*(20), 55.

Chapter 12

Microcomputer Applications: A Perspective in the Development of the Profession

James M. Mullendore

REFLECTIONS ON THE STATE OF THE ART

In the preceding 11 chapters, the authors have provided a detailed description of the functions of the microcomputer in the clinical, research, instructional, and administrative areas of the field of communication sciences and disorders, and have also identified numerous useful funding and informational resources for professional users.

Considering the scope of this coverage, it is legitimate to question why a final chapter dealing with "perspectives" is necessary. If the microcomputer were merely an extension or improvement in one of the forms of technology previously used, there would be no need to examine it in perspective. If the microcomputer represented merely a contemporary advancement without profound long-range ramifications, a critical examination of its implications would not need to be undertaken. If the microcomputer were an instrument with capabilities limited narrowly to some clinical, research, or administrative function, it might deserve a more superficial treatment than it has been given. On the contrary, the microcomputer is a unique technological achievement which, even in its early stages of development, has demonstrable applications in an incredible variety of human activities with the capability of extension beyond the present scope of human imagination.

However, it does possess limitations and requires intelligent and carefully planned utilization to achieve optimum results. It is capable of being misused, and users could become disillusioned with it if they failed to comprehend both its capabilities and limitations. Still, it is just one more instrument in a long list of the technological advances in recorded history and, as such, must be treated in many respects as similar to the developments which preceded it. Thus, the most appropriate view of the application of the microcomputer to the profession dealing with communication sciences and disorders should be one taken with a perspective which will enable users to comprehend the new technology from an objective viewpoint concerning its role in their professional lives.

As an identifiable profession with a formal national organization representing it in the United States, the field of communication sciences and disorders spans only six decades, a fleeting moment in the existence of the human race. It is significant, however, that this brief period

---

©College-Hill Press, Inc. All rights, including that of translation, reserved. No part of this publication may be reproduced without the written permission of the publisher.

of time has been the most productive technologically in the history of mankind. The opportunities to improve communication have been amplified by modern scientific developments. During this century radio, and more recently television, with its ability to transmit both words and pictures electronically, have expanded the scope and influence of human communication dramatically. The recording of the human voice has progressed from low-fidelity impressions on rubber cylinders to magnetic and electronic impressions of the highest fidelity.

Present professional view of microcomputers

The advent of the technology leading to the development of the computer provided the means for an even more rapid acceleration in the rate of technological progress. The addition of a memory component to the transmission of information provided the basis for a quantum leap in the management, manipulation, processing, and utilization of human knowledge.

The microcomputer was a predictable product of this aspect of technological progress. It was inevitable that individuals working in communication sciences and disorders would discover the potential usefulness and application of the microcomputer to their field. However, the users have barely scratched the surface of this instrument's capabilities. In fact, many of the present microcomputer clinical applications reside only at the "Dick and Jane" level of sophistication. To some scientists and information specialists with considerable previous experience with the microcomputer, this may suggest that the members of this field are incredibly unsophisticated. There may even be questions as to why communication specialists were not in the forefront of developments in information processing. On serious reflection, however, there appears to be no reason for an indictment of the profession. On the contrary, it has moved systematically to the utilization of the microcomputer, and has found its potential importance and impact on the field to be sufficiently significant to justify major efforts to educate the membership from the most basic level onward into increasing levels of sophistication.

It is interesting to speculate how the present level of knowledge will be viewed by those who will be living in the twenty-first century. With the incredible rapidity of developments in the computer field, it can be assumed that, even ten years from now, elementary written instruction on the applications of the microcomputer will be an historical curiosity. For these future historians, then, it should be noted that virtually all of the people presently active in the field of communication sciences and disorders were educated in colleges and universities where the only computers available were mainframes used primarily for administrative and advanced scientific purposes. Only a minority within the profession now have access to a microcomputer. Those who utilize such instrumentation acquired that knowledge and proficiency outside of and beyond the formal educational process. Informal instruction and, often, self-instruction provided the background knowledge for those in the profession whose fingers have recently come in contact with a microcomputer keyboard.

The conditions just described are in the process of a dramatic change. Presently there is a major trend toward the acquisition and use of microcomputers in the elementary and secondary schools of this country that will make present and future generations of children as familiar and comfortable with microcomputers as present and past generations have been with typewriters. Thus, elementary information about microcomputers will be largely unnecessary in the future. Subsequent editions of this book, or similar ones, will deal with specific applications of the microcomputer at levels of sophistication which have not yet been developed.

As applications of microcomputers are considered, it is apparent that the information is timely but not timeless. It is timely because it captures the profession in a moment of transition. By its very nature, the profession deals with people who have problems. Remediation does not involve the prescription of a pill, but involves the establishment of rapport, the identification of the problem through face-to-face verbalization, and application of therapy procedures requiring careful personal counseling. However, instrumentation has always been used to assist and expedite clinical efforts. Clinics are replete with audiometers, tape recorders, and a variety of other devices which have been considered necessary in evaluative and remedial work.

Except perhaps in the case of the audiometer, books have not been available in the early stages of the development of the instrumentation to provide instruction in the utilization of the instruments. In the case of the microcomputer, however, elementary instruction for the profession has become available almost at the instant in time when the device itself began to appear in the clinics. In the evolution of the field, none of the previous instrumentation, however, displayed the complexity yet universal applicability of the microcomputer. Hence, it has become particularly important to possess the broadest possible range of information about it from the moment of its appearance.

Professional clinical programs using the microcomputer are still primitive. Consequently, there are relatively few examples of innovative clinical applications presently available for purposes of illustration. This promises to be one of the more rapidly developing aspects of the field. Handbooks are needed which will introduce individuals to the microcomputer; they will stimulate development, and that in itself will be a significant contribution.

Within the past 2 years, the shelves of libraries and bookstores have rapidly filled with books on the uses and applications of microcomputers in business and education. The references range from rudimentary instructional manuals to complex treatises on programming and mathematical applications. Over 50 popular microcomputer magazines and journals have appeared within the past few years. Thus, a reader of almost any skill level should be able to find information to enable progress to a higher level of sophistication. However, individuals who work with communication disorders need sources of information that deal with the relatively diverse ramifications of a profession involving clinical, administrative, educational, and research components, all of which are richly endowed with tasks inviting the utilization of microcomputers.

By their very nature, microcomputers are fascinating instruments. No instrument previously invented has possessed the versatility to enable one to play games, plan the family budget, solve mathematical problems, display learning programs, make statistical projections, and accomplish many other tasks, all with the same hardware. Only a short time ago microcomputers were identified primarily as instruments of business and research. Today they are projected as necessary adjuncts to education and valuable "appliances" for the home. It is little wonder, then, that the communication sciences and disorders profession has embraced the microcomputer and demonstrated the determination to make it a vital tool by providing specialized instruction books that describe its application.

There is another observation to be made upon reflection about the present state of the art in the microcomputer field, namely the inevitable realization that there is so much yet unknown and so much still to learn about microcomputer utilization. With the microcomputer one is dealing with a subject that one must start from "scratch" with in terms of future professional applications.

The information on applications of the microcomputer clearly suggests the necessity for users both to understand the general theoretical concepts and, at the same time, be able to operate the instrumentation. However, there is still no unanimity of opinion as to the optimum extent of preparation and knowledge which should be recommended for individuals in a profession such as this. For instance, there is active debate concerning the necessity for learning to program microcomputers or which computer language should be used. Perhaps the most useful premise for the present may be to suggest that due to its intricacies, computer science must be considered as a separate and distinct profession, and that the assistance of skilled professionals from that field should be used whenever it becomes necessary to move beyond relatively elementary levels of application. However, this dividing line will vary from individual to individual, and criteria for determining it have not yet been firmly established.

One final observation concerning the state of the art is required to establish a proper perspective. Presently available material deals only with this (1984) generation of microcomputers. The rate of progress appears to be accelerating, and the present instruments that seem so fascinating are probably comparable to Alexander Graham Bell's early version of the telephone. The big difference in using this analogy, however, is that the standard telephone, a century after its invention, still has a transmitter, receiver, and a system of wires connecting it to other telephones. Wireless versions and the numerous refinements of the system required many decades of development, but some of the basic concepts still remain. By contrast, progress in both the technology and the applications in the microcomputer field appears to be capable of acceleration at a pace infinitely more rapid than that of the telephone. In fact, there will probably not even be such an item as a microcomputer a century from now. Instead, the future clinical scientist will be dealing with complex instrumentation of which the microcomputer components will comprise only a small part. The sophistication of the instrumentation will be extensively multiplied by the interaction of the various components. Indeed, the principal location of the 1984 microcomputer will be in a museum.

Does this suggest that it should be considered a waste of time to learn how to apply the microcomputer to professional needs? Not in the slightest. The basic concepts must be learned to provide a frame of reference for the more complex applications which will follow. The mastery of the presently available microcomputers opens the door to the remarkable advances in the management of information, which are certain to evolve by the end of this century.

MICROCOMPUTERS IN PERSPECTIVE

Historical point of view

Looking at the profession from the vantage point of history is another way to place the emergence of the microcomputer in perspective. It is particularly important to note that the motivating force in this profession has always been the desire to understand, diagnose, and treat the disorders of human communication. The focus has been on the close contact between the clinician and patient. Activities have involved direct personal or interpersonal relationships designed to improve the quality of life of those who seek help. The key element in this relationship is the clinician, whose understanding of the process of communication and whose skill in evaluating and managing deficiencies and disorders makes the eventual difference. Thus, when the microcomputer arrived on the scene, a key question was, "What can the microcomputer do for the clinician?"

This approach is typical of the professional attitude taken throughout the history of the field of communication sciences and disorders. Characteristically, methods, procedures, and instruments have been employed as they became available. In some cases, achievements that preceded the formal development of the profession by many decades, including the works of pioneers such as Garcia, Scripture, and Helmholtz, were rediscovered.

Perhaps the best example of the application of advancing technology to professional needs has been in the field of electronic amplification, transmission, and recording. The invention of the vacuum tube enabled a quantum leap in communication media so that, by the time the profession became established, devices for recording and scientific examination of the processes of human communication had become available in growing numbers. Making voice recordings on hard rubber discs is a task that still lives in the memories of the senior members of the profession. Later on, recorders used thin, rapidly moving strands of wire (which had the ugly habit of occasionally skipping the spool and winding up in a metallic bird's nest). Early tape recorders used easily torn and low-fidelity paper tape, which, fortunately, was quickly replaced by more durable and efficient plastic tape. These machines were, however, relatively large and heavy and typically had only a moderate lifespan. However, clinicians embraced them and made use of their ability to record and replay the sounds of speech. Members of the profession were grateful for the fact that they were relatively cheap to operate by virtue of the capability of erasing and reusing the tapes; hence, clinicians used them as a means of achieving important clinical and research objectives.

Developments in the World War II era produced a miniaturization of the vacuum tube, enabling such advances as smaller recording and playback apparatus, more sophisticated laboratory instrumentation, such as the instrumentation used for speech analysis and synthesis, and major improvements in hearing aids. During this period, the profession also welcomed the development of the cathode ray tube and capitalized upon its application in the oscilloscope, which enabled the conversion of the sounds of speech into a visible medium. Then came the epic discovery of the transistor and the fantastic miniaturization of electronic instrumentation through the use of printed circuits. By that time, the profession had significantly increased its research personnel, and clinicians were routinely trained in the utilization of instrumentation. The professional adaptation to the transistor age, which brought new solutions to professional problems, was virtually instantaneous.

As a half century of progress is viewed from the vantage point of time, an inescapable observation is that there has been a phenomenal acceleration in the rate of development and availability of applicable technology. It is equally important to note that clinicians have always utilized this technology as a means to achieve clinical objectives rather than as an end in itself or as a substitute for personal involvement. While it is probably an exaggeration, it appears that the rate of technological progress is almost exponential. Although few individuals realized it at the time, these trends and achievements were the forerunners of the present microcomputer, which must be viewed with the same perspective as the technology preceding it.

Despite such rapid progress, all clinicians and researchers have, at one time or another, become impatient with the lag of time between the laboratory development and the practical utilization of instruments and materials. The microcomputer appears to have bridged this gap more quickly than some of the earlier technology as evidenced by the clinical applications that have already appeared and the new software that is being produced at an accelerating rate.

In any event, it is evident that the development of the microcomputer is an excellent example of incredible technological growth, for its forefather was a bulky, room-sized, heat-generating monster of limited capability, whose functions have been effectively miniaturized into a fingernail-sized chip. Here is a use for that age-old aphorism in the observation that the microcomputer is indeed "a chip off the old block." The phenomenal rate of advancement toward universal acceptance of the microcomputer may have analogies, but no exact parallels, in the history of human technological progress.

Reflection of trends in society

As the microcomputer is viewed from a historical perspective, the conclusion is inescapable that its phenomenal increase in numbers and acceptance may well be a reflection of larger trends in society itself. John Naisbitt presented a convincing case for what he described as "megatrends" in his recent work of the same name (Naisbitt, 1982). In his conclusion (p. 215), he observed that, "We are living in the *time of the parenthesis,* the time between eras." One of the trends he described in the first chapter of the book is the transformation from an industrial society to an information society, a change which has been accelerated by computer technology.

One such trend has magnified the importance of the role played by the field of management of human communication disorders. Oral communication is far and away the most frequently utilized mode of transmitting information, and individuals with speech disorders or deficiencies are seriously disadvantaged in a world where oral communication is increasingly important. The microcomputer is becoming vital to virtually all aspects of human activity, including the field of communication sciences and disorders. This trend and the profession's relationship to it appears obvious and inevitable.

Cost effectiveness as a professional issue

One of the concerns which cannot be ignored is that professional survival depends upon being (or becoming) cost effective. This is a relatively recent trend in clinical speech, language, and hearing services. In earlier times, the provision of services for human communication disorders existed mainly in the public schools, university clinics, or through community agencies such as the Easter Seal Society. Fees were nominal or nonexistent, and there were only a few isolated private practitioners or free-standing clinics where the fee schedule truly reflected the cost of the services provided.

This state of affairs has changed dramatically, particularly within the last 10 years. The public school systems are receiving less tax support, and consequently have found it necessary to reexamine their traditional services and activities from the point of view of whether their costs are justified by their value. As a consequence of legislation mandating that educational services be provided to all children, specifically including those with various disabilities, the public educational system has felt the impact of markedly accelerating costs. This change has occurred in an era characterized by an unusually high rate of inflation in the economy as a whole. Special education, including services to the communicatively handicapped, is an area of high educational cost, and has been the target of increasingly critical examination. Thus, even the public school speech clinician, long sheltered within a system where no special requirements for economic efficiency existed, has become a target for examination. Even the definition of what constitutes a clinically significant defect requiring specialized services has become one of the focal points of this examination. The utilization of the microcomputer must therefore be considered as a means of improving the efficiency and extending the services of the clinician. As an adjunct to the clinician, it has the potential to take over some of the time-consuming processes involved in speech and language instruction, facilitate record keeping, and improve the diagnostic and evaluative procedures required in public education.

Other facilities for service delivery in the field have also been challenged to demonstrate that they are able to generate income commensurate with their cost. An increasing proportion of the membership has entered private practice or taken positions as employees within medical or clinical practices, depending upon fees for services for continued existence. University clinics, which have traditionally provided the supervised practicum facilities for students, have been challenged in many instances to generate higher income to offset some of their operating cost. Microcomputers are particularly well adapted to these settings. In addition to the functions previously mentioned, they provide a highly efficient means of maintaining student and clinic records, facilitating scheduling, doing word processing, manipulating data, performing complex statistical calculations, developing projections, and conducting research. In perspective, it may be suggested that the greatest immediate impact of the microcomputer will be upon the academic area of the field, for it is here that its versatility will be most fully utilized.

This profession has been (and still is) labor intensive. The income required to provide competitive salaries has increased sharply as a result of the unusual increases in the cost of living experienced during the last decade. The profession has resisted, perhaps with good justification, measures which might control costs, such as the increased use of supportive personnel. Traditional professional practice has consisted primarily of an individualized approach with a consequently heavy time commitment of the clinician. Before the advent of the microcomputer, there were relatively few kinds of programmed instruction or individualized independent practice devices which would enable a clinician to delegate work to unskilled personnel or to automation. Indeed, clinicians have taken justifiable pride in the fact that they have always demonstrated a special concern for those they served, as evidenced by the time devoted personally to each individual.

However, as the world changes so must the profession change. As positions develop in locations where the work is more exposed to the challenges of cost effectiveness and appropriateness of outcome, it will be increasingly necessary to design and use more efficient and effective procedures. The microcomputer appears to have arrived in time to provide the possible answer to such a problem. It has the capability and capacity to help develop programs that will make the profession more cost effective. The employment of these programs will enable clients to learn by using the microcomputer, thus freeing the professional clinician's time for other clinical activities.

The significance of this development may be that it offers the potential for increased productivity under professional control in the clinical setting. Although existing microcomputer programs do not, for the most part, enable the implementation of this potential, it may be confidently predicted that newer and more effective ones will emerge.

Need for increased program adaptability

As the gap between existing professional software and the capabilities of the microcomputer is viewed in perspective, there are several areas in which it appears that progress must and will be achieved. The most obvious of these is the need for programs with more complex feedback to the users. Rather than a simple acknowledgment of "correct" or "incorrect," learners should have additional information in the form of explanations as to exactly what the error was and why it was made, in order that subsequent efforts will be more than random trials. It is also obvious that modalities of present microcomputer programs function within too narrow a range, and thus are limited to use only by certain groups of clients. For example, it is impossible for nonreaders, or those with limited reading ability, to respond to written explanations. Those with hearing impairments likewise would be severely penalized by programs in which the response is only in an oral mode. Clients who are colorblind possess a limitation which would impair their success in managing programs where color is a critical feature.

While it may be difficult to find any single common denominator of stimulus and response, it is entirely possible for flexible programs to be developed with the modifications needed to adapt their use to a broader range of individuals.

There is also a need for an extensive and carefully validated development of programs appropriate to developmental, age, or skill levels. Innovative formats must also be developed to accommodate different kinds of personal interests and the variables resulting from individual differences in socioeconomic as well as racial and ethnic backgrounds.

Specific applications to various types of communication disorders must also be investigated closely to determine what would be needed and useful for therapeutic application. The software should undergo the careful design and validation which has been given to some of the paper-and-pencil tests presently in general use by the profession. As yet, there is no national or international clearing-house for evaluating and judging the software as it becomes available and, in fact, there are no existing standards against which it may be judged. As the present status of software utilization is examined in perspective, this looms as a major area of deficiency.

Increased administrative efficiency through the use of the microcomputer has already been demonstrated, as discussed in detail by Hood and Miller (chap. 10). The increase in cost effectiveness and efficiency in this area has almost limitless potential. In research, too, capabilities exist which are beyond the limits of present visualization.

As the present status of the use of the microcomputer in the field of communication disorders is further examined and attempts are made to predict trends, there are reasons to suggest that the greatest future impact during the final years of this century will be on its clinical applications. This is not to suggest that administrative, academic, and research functions will be significantly less important, but merely to observe that computers in one form or another have had a longer history of utilization in these areas, and that microcomputers will accelerate and broaden those functions that have already been instituted. Clinical applications, however, are still only in an early and rudimentary state of development, and thus offer the greatest potential for innovation and progress.

The microcomputer as evidence of a technological achievement

There is another important trend in society which has ramifications affecting the use of the microcomputer in the field of communication sciences and disorders, namely the growth in the quantity of available data and information. Each advance in modern technology increases the ability to produce and disseminate information, and the consequent expansion of the data base results in a disproportionate increase in published reports. The very technology designed to increase efficiency actually has had the effect of multiplying the problems resulting from the accumulation of data.

One example of such a trend is in the accumulated clinical files. For many years, the only defense against the tidal wave of paper was the purchase of additional filing cabinets. Various data management systems were tried from time to time as they became available, but they were crude and largely unsuccessful. As records accumulated, it became obvious that data retrieval was even more of a problem than its storage. Unless motivated by a need for carefully planned longitudinal research studies, the data in the case files almost defied systematic retrieval.

It is evident that the immense capacity for storage, retrieval, and analysis through microcomputer utilization has arrived none too soon for application to this problem. More specifically, microcomputers offer the possibility of sophisticated data management to individuals and smaller programs which would not otherwise have access to computer capabilities. Additionally, it should be noted that the microcomputer also enables simplicity of entry of data and versatility in its management through the utilization of a wide variety of programs.

As the microcomputer is further viewed in perspective, one must be particularly impressed by the technological achievement which it represents.

Minifie (1981) emphasized its impact on the profession in an address to the directors of the academic training programs with the following observation:

> We are in an era where digital logic circuits are reshaping the potentials for clinical diagnosis and clinical management processes in very dramatic ways. Juxtapose that idea with the fact that most clinical fields change slowly. If the technology continues to advance at breakneck speed, then deliverers of clinical services either must develop sufficient knowledge about these devices so they can be utilized toward goals which are clinically sound, or the practitioners will become slaves to someone else's technology and lose control over the direction of the clinical process.

As Minifie's observations suggest, there is a notable contrast with earlier technological advances. In the earlier technology, the objective was to produce better things for mankind to use. In heavy industry the production of goods was thought to be necessary to *assist* mankind. By contrast, computer technology appears to be designed to *augment* and perhaps even *replace* human personnel in increasingly complex occupations. Computer technology has become so sophisticated that it is not just self-perpetuating but actually self-accelerating. Computers are used to design better computers which, in turn, will be used to design still better ones. The obvious conclusion, then, is that present generation of microcomputers will be quickly replaced by future generations of instruments of radically improved design and with infinitely greater capabilities.

The potential for acceleration seen in computer technology and its application to the microcomputer has no parallel in history. Whereas the industrial and agricultural revolutions (or evolutions) were measured in centuries, the microcomputer evolution is measured in decades or less. What, then, does this mean for our profession?

IMPACT OF THE MICROCOMPUTER ON THE PROFESSION

Captivation by the hardware and immersion in the software of a microcomputer may tend to reduce an individual's objectivity concerning its role in professional work. It is equally likely that the user's impression of its applicability is dependent upon his or her individual needs and personal skills. Therefore, it may be useful to examine systematically the present status of microcomputer utilization in the profession and attempt to make some projections into areas of future use.

Present status of utilization

First, the area of research, and clinical research in particular, must be examined. The clinical problem of bulging filing cabinets packed with data concerning thousands of cases has been previously described. Collectively, professional clinicians have treated literally millions of communication disorders with varying degrees of success. It is acknowledged that members of the profession still do not understand many facets of etiology and remediation, and concede that some of the important answers reside in the voluminous data previously amassed, if only the information could be retrieved and analyzed systematically. Unfortunately, most of these data are beyond retrieval. It is disconcerting to observe how many published research studies are conducted with 5, 10, or 25 subjects instead of the thousands which might be more meaningful.

The microcomputer provides a means by which this deficiency can be remedied. It is reasonable to expect that, in the future, readers will see an increased number of published studies involving significantly larger numbers of cases, and it is hoped that there will be an increased proportion of clinical research emanating from practicing clinicians who are not primarily researchers. If this does not happen, the profession will have no one but itself to blame.

As recently as 5 years ago, investigators doing research in communication disorders were limited in their computer utilization to the time and facilities of centralized units to which they had access through local terminals. The advantage of such an arrangement was the availability of the potential power and storage capacity of the centralized facilities. However, there was also the sometimes frequent difficulty of getting access to the computer from the remote terminals. This and some of the other disadvantages of the mainframe can be eliminated by the acquisition of microcomputers, and consequently their number has rapidly increased in research facilities. With the anticipated increase in the power and versatility of microcomputers in the future, their utilization may be expected to become the method of choice in scholarly work. This will be particularly true when the microcomputer is integrated as a part of a complex research process or system and functions as a component rather than as a freestanding unit.

The use of the microcomputer for administrative purposes has become so widespread that observers tend to underestimate its importance and significance. It should also be noted that its use in the profession is not significantly different from administrative use in the business field in general.

As the administrative use of the microcomputer is reviewed, it appears not only to provide the means to achieve a more advanced state in the instrumentation and automation of basic and routine functions, but, more importantly, it also sets the state for development of an entirely new kind of office where electronic memory replaces paper, and virtually instantaneous data management is substituted for laborious and time-consuming clerical functions. This should provide the means, therefore, for an improvement in the cost effectiveness of clerical functions, thus satisfying an increasing demand upon the profession. However, it should be observed that the use of the microcomputer will not automatically bring order out of chaos. The user is obligated to develop systematic procedures, the use of which will be enhanced and accelerated by the microcomputer. Finally, it should also be noted that a potentially significant cost will be incurred in the process of conversion to the new system, including the staff retraining required.

The most obvious expansion of the use of the microcomputer is in clinical activities. The growth of interest in clinical use has been dramatic. One need only compare the American Speech-Language-Hearing Association convention programs of 1980 and 1983 to observe this recent trend. From only a few isolated papers in 1980, the program grew to more than 20 short courses, miniseminars, technical sessions, poster sessions, and videotapes on the microcomputer in 1983. There was also an impressive increase in the number of software exhibits at the 1983 meeting; these were almost totally lacking in previous years. There have, of course, been a variety of computer applications to specialized areas of the field in the past, such as those utilized in brainstem-evoked response testing and speech synthesis, but it is obvious that the microcomputer has opened a wide range of new applications with the capability of adaptation to clinical work.

Recently developed microcomputer programs, such as those identified in the preceding chapters of this book, suggest the possibility of new dimensions in clinical applications. A growing wave of new programs encompassing both diagnostic and therapeutic applications is emerging. Programs involving instructional and tutorial processes as well as simulation are in evidence. However, the overriding weakness of these programs is the elementary level of their sophistication. Predominant among those presently on the market are programs which are, in effect, only electronic flashcards. While there may be some time saved and even the possibility of improved therapeutic efficiency, the utilization of a microcomputer at such an elementary level is analogous to using a sledgehammer to put a thumb tack in the wall.

Assuming the continued rapid improvement of the microcomputer, it is reasonable to doubt that the field can fully tap the potential of the instrument in the near future. With the limited number of programs available, it is also possible that the use of the microcomputer may be sporadic and occasional rather than an integral part of a continuing and systematic clinical process. In making such observations, there is no intent to minimize the efforts or disparage the good intentions of those who develop software or the clinicians who use it. It is a simple factual observation, on the other hand, that in the present state of the art, the limitations lie more in the capability of the users than in the microcomputer itself.

Professional reaction to technological advances

Historical trends provide a point of view for the further evaluation of the microcomputer. Though young, the field of communication sciences and disorders has witnessed spectacular technological advances both in its own field and the world at large. For example, in the little more than half century of its organized existence in this country, the life spans of its practitioners have encompassed international events ranging from the first solo flight across the Atlantic ocean by Charles Lindbergh to man's landing on the moon, as well as the almost routine flights of the Challenger into outer space. In the same span of time, the horse-drawn plow gave way to mechanized agriculture and the crystal set grew into global radio and television.

Remarkable skill has been shown by members of the profession in the development and use of the products of technology. The advances in audiological instrumentation during the past 20 years exemplify this characteristic. Communication scientists have employed in the laboratory, and then later in the clinic, a remarkable variety of technology including recording media ranging from discs to videotape, x-rays, stroboscopes, high-speed photography, oscilloscopes, speech synthesis equipment, and a long list of other instrumentation.

Realistically, the microcomputer is one more such product. Like many other products, it has been rapidly embraced, but its application thus far has been elementary and minimal. The professional reaction of wide-eyed wonder at its potentialities is likewise comparable to responses to earlier inventions. (Some can still remember the excitement evoked by early commercial television as viewers watched the snowy black and white picture on the 12-inch screen in the living room.) Recalling the contrast between that picture and the large, slick color transmission of today, it becomes obvious that people are living in a truly dynamic world where nothing is ever really constant except change, and where accelerating technological progress is essentially routine.

Examine for a moment the microcomputer hardware presently in use with its space-consuming components. Now think back to the audiological testing booth of 20 years ago with its separate pure tone, speech and Bekesy audiometers, the GSR unit, and a variety of special testing devices, then visualize that same booth today with the specialized components neatly packaged into an efficient solid state instrument, perhaps with a computer interface. One may speculate about the future generations of the microcomputer by the same measure. Just as the evolution of microcomputer hardware may be visualized, so too it must be realized that the true significance of contemporary professional involvement is that it lays the groundwork for future developments of infinitely greater sophistication.

A number of writers have analyzed contemporary trends in microcomputer hardware and software and have attempted to predict the nature of future developments. One of the more concise statements applicable to the field of communication sciences and disorders was made by Gleason (1981) in his discussion of the state of the art in the microcomputer field as it applied to education:

> Realistically speaking, most knowledgeable people agree that hardware development is considerably ahead of software development and implementation. However, the current micros are really only first-generation devices, which will become outmoded in a few years. Already available improvements, such as touch-sensitive screens, light pens, "bubble" memory systems, videodisc interfaces, random access audio devices, etc., will enhance greatly the performance capabilities of micros, but quite likely with attendant cost increases.

Utilization of the microcomputer

With improved hardware and increased software assured in the future, it is appropriate to examine the professional utilization of the microcomputer. Such questions must be asked as: Is the use actually an improvement? Are clinicians sacrificing important individual attention by relying excessively on instrumentation? Does the microcomputer introduce a troublesome artifact in the clinical process? Have some members of the profession become so infatuated by the microcomputer that they risk the possible neglect of the other avenues and approaches to problems?

Each of these questions should be examined briefly. Cohen (see chap. 2) has argued that if a microcomputer cannot perform a task better or faster than the present method of doing it, its use should be questioned. Take just one example which may or may not be appropriate to any particular clinic: Clinical schedules are frequently developed by charting the times, clients, and assigned clinicians on some sort of a large board displaying the entire weekly schedule in a highly visible fashion. This could easily be transformed into a microcomputer program if the advantages of such a program outweighed the disadvantages. However, for some clinics, the maintenance of the large wall display may be the superior method, and this would be particularly true if it required more time to enter and retrieve data from the microcomputer than to revise the manual display which was replaced (Punch, Levitt, Mahaffey, & Wilson, 1983).

The question of the importance of intensive personal clinician-client contact also introduces a judgment area into microcomputer utilization. An appropriate criterion would be to evaluate whether the eventual gains for the client would be greater with the use of the microcomputer as a clinical tool than the possible losses in rapport and stimulation which might be achieved through continued personal contact. Even the most sophisticated software possible for a microcomputer is no match for the flexibility, clinical intuition, and human creativity available from a skilled clinician. Those almost indefinable subjective factors involved in the rapport between individuals in the clinical setting must also be considered. The synthesized voice presently used in microcomputer programs is mechanical, impersonal, and lacks the inflections of warmth and affection of human speech.

To continue answering the questions posed above, the possibility is raised that inappropriately used technology may inhibit rather than facilitate human interaction. Perhaps the most familiar traditional clinical example of such a possibility is in the use of the tape recorder. Virtually everyone has had the experience of achieving some therapeutic objective with a client which merited recording, only to find that, with the recorder turned on, the client experienced a relapse. For optimum use, it is suggested that the microcomputer should be placed and employed in such a way that it becomes a permanent and familiar part of the environment, so that its use will become an integral and normal part of a continuing therapeutic process.

Finally, it is not unreasonable to assume that some people will become so infatuated with the microcomputer that they will lose sight of the fact that it is only one instrument or avenue of approach to the management of clinical problems and processes. It is unlikely that any presently active clinicians will see the day when humans are removed from the system and replaced by robots and totally mechanized processes. It is conceivable, however, that with the anticipated growth in the quantity of available software for clinical use and with the expected simplification of the operation of the microcomputer, clinicians might design therapy plans employing disproportionate amounts of time on microcomputer utilization and thus fall short of achieving optimum clinical results.

The reader must be alert to the possibility that other misapplications of the microcomputer are also possible. For example, adequate research data are lacking concerning the possible emotional and psychological effects of computer-assisted instruction upon individuals. Unless programs are imaginative and challenging, the operation of a microcomputer in clinical applications can quickly become boring and tedious. Studies of these factors and of the relative rates of progress for comparable materials between clinician-administered and computer-administered programs are needed. In the long run, it appears certain that the impact of the microcomputer on the field will be profound and positive, but it still cannot be assumed that it will be 100% positive.

Awareness of limitations

Still other questions must be asked in response to an inquiry as to why a microcomputer needs to be used. These include: Is it a labor-saving device? Does it provide an improved learning method? Will it improve data management in the particular facility for which it is being acquired? All of these questions and many others have been addressed in the previous chapters, and it must be emphasized that a prospective user must be prepared to answer them both when the instrumentation is sought and after it has been acquired.

When using a microcomputer, it is important to maintain a proper professional perspective. Obviously, people can get "hooked" on microcomputers. They seem to possess almost magical qualities, and the rapidity with which they solve problems and manage data generates a feeling of almost superhuman power. Thus, the user must be careful not to ascribe to them capabilities or uses for which they were never intended. Furthermore, it must be recognized that there is a possibility that, in clinical settings, inappropriate use may result in a depersonalization of the clinical process which could be more detrimental than useful. Clinicians must not lose sight of the fact that, with or without microcomputers, this is still a "hands-on" profession. Instrumentation is useful to the extent that it serves as a labor extender; it enables a job to be done better or performs activities that clinicians personally cannot or will not do. For example, as yet there is no electronic substitute for good clinical judgment. However, there is a reasonable expectation that computerized enhancement of clinical skill will become routinely available in the future. In the field of medicine, for example, programs are available, though not yet in widespread use, to assist the physician in diagnosis. While results obtained through diagnostic instrumentation may be fed directly into the system, the interface between the physician and patient constitutes the most important and sensitive link in the evaluative process.

There are still other considerations that professionals must become aware of. The development of a program, whether it be for record keeping or language development, freezes the process at a point in time, just as does the publication of a book or test. Change will not occur until the program is modified or a new one substituted. It is therefore possible, paradoxically, that the very instrumentation which has enabled phenomenal progress might, with inappropriate utilization, tend to arrest or discourage it.

Papert (1981) voiced his concern about the possibility that the early and unsophisticated uses of microcomputers in education might tend to become permanent as a result of the availability of elementary levels of software and particularly because of programming instruction limited to BASIC. As an analogy, he cited what he called the "QWERTY phenomenon." He defined this as ". . . a tendency for the first usable, but still primitive, product of a new technology to dig itself in." He explained:

> The top row of alphabetic keys of the standard typewriter reads QWERTY. For me this symbolizes the way in which technology can all too often serve not as a force for progress but for keeping things stuck. The QWERTY arrangement has no rational explanation, only a historical one. It was introduced in response to a problem in the early days of the typewriter: The keys used to jam. The idea was to minimize the collision problem by separating those keys that followed one another frequently. Just a few years later, general improvements in the technology removed the jamming problem, but QWERTY stuck.

The same word of caution is appropriate with respect to existing commercially available software. It is based on present concepts and theories and, in most instances, unimaginative utilization of peripherals and add-on hardware, and there is no necessary reason why it should survive as the standard or established practice of the profession merely because of its availability. On the contrary, the survival and much of the success of the profession in the future depends upon its ability to translate its theories and practices into useful software for clinical work.

A present condition which may be subject to change in the future is that of the competence (incompetence) of the members of the profession as computer programmers. Presently, the professionals who deal with communication sciences and disorders and individuals who are trained computer scientists are in two separate and distinct professions. Different skills, interests, and aptitudes are evident. Hence, creativity in the development of software for use on the microcomputer is markedly different from the more traditional course of action involving the use of a paper and pencil or typewriter. Software productivity requires a unique combination of professional technical skills and the utilization of teamwork to translate ideas into a new medium. This is one of the considerations that gives rise to the persistent question of what and how much clinicians should know about microcomputers. This question, or variations of it, is being asked in many quarters at the present time. There is, for example, considerable debate concerning the meaning of the term "computer literacy." An article in the *Chronicle of Higher Education* included an effort by George W. Baughman, Director of Special Projects in the Office of Fiscal Affairs at Ohio State University to clarify the various levels of knowledge, which he placed into three classifications:

> Computer literacy, the most basic, includes familiarity with the terminology, some knowledge of how a computer works, and what it is used for.
>
> Computer competence means being able to use a computer as a tool in a particular field—what computer people usually call "applications." A person who is computer-competent can use a computer at least three different ways to solve problems in his field.
>
> The third category encompasses the computer or information scientists, "the guy who says 'My profession is computing.'" (Baughman, 1984)

An effort to put the microcomputer in perspective as it relates to the profession would not be complete without a few final observations concerning the ownership and personal utilization of the instrument. Just as the advent of computer technology has rendered many items of previously used hardware obsolete, so too the acquisition of the microcomputer has made previous budgetary patterns inappropriate. When capital equipment requests were limited to such relatively low ticket items as calculators and typewriters, it was possible to spread these requests over more than a single fiscal year, if funds were limited. Although there is a comparatively large price range, a microcomputer of appropriate quality and its necessary accessories introduce a new dimension into many of the budgets typical of the smaller clinical service facilities. It must also be observed that, in some instances, more than one microcomputer is deemed necessary. This requires a new and different form of fiscal planning, for the maintenance and acquisition of software requires an outlay at a level well beyond the range of the typical supply budget. In academic institutions, such software may exceed in expense the annual library appropriation for the program. Also, at this stage in history, one must exercise particular concern about the fact that the present generation of microcomputers will become rapidly obsolete as successive generations of instruments are produced. Replacement, therefore, will be an important consideration. Fortunately for those contemplating the purchase of a microcomputer at this point in history, it appears that the present generation possesses improvements and refinements based on user experience and advancing technology which models of only a few years ago did not possess. Capabilities have improved to the point where the many uses described in this book, and also many others yet to be devised, may be accomplished with present generation models. This in itself should suffice for the continuation of professional activities in the immediate future. However, it is a safe bet that enthusiastic users will find themselves with their noses pressed flat against the display window at the microcomputer store, drooling over the improvements of the new models and their capabilities within 3 years of their initial purchase.

Thus, the factor of rapid obsolescence, the certainty of development of new methods of microcomputer utilization with the software accompanying it, and the fact that the profession is already playing "catch-up" makes it a certainty that it will be necessary to run at double speed just to catch up with yesterday's advances in microcomputer technology.

CONCLUSION

On a more positive note, this chapter must conclude with the observation that the profession devoted to working with individuals with communication disorders has once again distinguished itself by the rapidity of its recognition of a valuable tool which will serve as a continuing support system for the countless variety of functions required to fulfill future professional obligations.

This chapter has attempted to place the microcomputer and its professional utilization in perspective. The past has been explored in an effort to find comparable technological achievements and examined to determine the manner in which the profession handled them.

The present state of the art has been reviewed both from the standpoint of the development of the instrumentation and the status of available software. The chapter has also presented at least a limited commentary on the professional utilization of presently available microcomputers and programs. By grasping the relationships between events of the past and the present, it has been possible to establish a perspective to serve as a frame of reference for the future. Attempts to delve into the future, however, were undertaken with understandable timidity, particularly where the development of hardware is concerned.

Microcomputers will continue to become more powerful, more efficient, more compact, and simpler to operate in the years to come. Their use by members of the profession will increase with predictable rapidity and immense effectiveness. The microcomputer may provide the most significant advancement in instrumentation which has yet become available for use in the speech-language-hearing profession. The ultimate winners, then, will not be the professional clinicians themselves, but rather those who are served—the individuals with disorders of speech, language, and hearing who need professional help.

REFERENCE NOTES

Minifie, F. D. (1981). Graduate education during a technological revolution. (Unpublished) Proceedings of the second annual conference on graduate education of the Council of Graduate Programs in Communication Sciences and Disorders. St. Louis, MO.

Punch, J., Levitt, H., Mahaffey, R., & Wilson, M. (1983). Computer technology: The revolution has started without us. Miniseminar presented at the Annual Convention of the American Speech-Language-Hearing Association. Cincinnati, OH.

REFERENCES

Baughman, G. W. (1984, January 11). Ohio State eyes "computer literacy"; Who needs it? Who should teach it? *The Chronicle of Higher Education, 27*, 14.

Gleason, G. T. (1981, March). Microcomputers in education: The state of the art. *Educational Technology, 21*, 7-18.

Naisbitt, J. (1982). *Megatrends*. New York: Warner Books, Inc.

Papert, S. (1981, March). Computers and computer cultures. *Creative Computing, 7*, 82-92.

SECTION V
MICROCOMPUTER TERMINOLOGY

Chapter 13

Glossary of Microcomputer Terms

Michael R. Chial

Accumulator: one or more data registers available to the arithmetic logic unit (ALU) of the central processor of a computer to temporarily store the results of mathematical and logical operations. See also Arithmetic logic unit and Central processing unit.

Acoustic coupler: a device (hardware) that allows a computer or a computer terminal to be connected to the handset of a telephone for purposes of communicating data, programs, or messages. Information is transmitted through the coupler by means of coded tone pulses. Acoustic couplers usually contain MODEMs. See also MODEM.

Address: a particular location in computer memory identified by a number. On a computer with 64K bytes of primary memory, an address is represented by a number between 0 and 65,536.

Address bus: a communication channel (i.e., a set of electrical connections) internal to a computer by which the central processing unit can access particular input devices, output devices, or locations in memory. See also Central processing unit, Control bus, and Data bus.

Addressing mode: any of several different ways of selecting or referring to memory addresses, including direct (by specific numerical address) and indirect (by a symbol which "points to" a place where the numerical address can be found).

Alphanumeric: all printable numbers, letters, punctuation marks, and special characters (for example, "%" and "#").

Alpha testing: a phase in the development of commercial application programs, prior to distribution, in which experts or sympathetic users identify problems and make recommendations for improvement. Also called "formative" evaluation. See also Beta testing.

Algorithm: a step-by-step procedure for solving a particular class or type of problem. Algorithms may be expressed as equations, verbal "recipes," flow charts, or in a particular computer language.

Alternate (ALT) key: a nonstandard key on a keyboard which, when used simultaneously with another key, issues a special command to the computer. Similar in use and effect to the control key. See also Control key.

American National Standards Institute (ANSI): a nongovernmental organization which develops and distributes technical standards for use by all segments of society. ANSI committees are staffed by representatives of trade and professional associations, government agencies, and individuals who arrive at consensural standards for measurement, instrumentation, procedures, and practices in a wide range of technical areas. ANSI Committee S1 deals with acoustics, Committee S3 with bioacoustics, Committee S12 with noise, and Committee

©College-Hill Press, Inc. All rights, including that of translation, reserved. No part of this publication may be reproduced without the written permission of the publisher.

X3 with information systems. Previously known as the American Standards Association (ASA) and the United States Standards Institute (USASI).

Analog: an event which varies from small to large in a continuous manner, or in infinitely small increments. Examples of analog signals include sound, heat, light, and length. Examples of analog machines include wrist watches with hands, phonographs, slide rules, dimmer switches for electric lamps, and tuning dials of radios. See also Digital.

Analog-to-digital converter (ADC): a device (hardware) that translates continuous, time-varying analog signals into discrete digital signals, usually for subsequent processing by a computer. See also Digital-to-analog converter.

Application software: a class of computer programs designed to solve problems of specific interest to computer users. The same (or similar) application programs often are available for different hardware configurations. Examples include accounting programs, word processing programs, data base management programs, and program generators (i.e., programs that write programs). See also System software and Utility software.

Architecture: any ordered design. More specifically, the functional, logical, and physical design of a computer system or component (e.g., a microprocessor).

Arithmetic logic unit (ALU): a functional component of a central processing unit which accomplishes simple mathematical and logical operations on data. More complex operations (e.g., multiplication) are managed as a series of simple operations (e.g., addition). See also Central processing unit.

Artificial intelligence (AI): a category of computer application focusing on the study of sensory and cognitive processes, particularly in the area of decision making. One class of AI is robotics, another is expert systems, and another is natural language processing.

ASCII: ("askee") acronym for "American standard code for information interchange." This 7-bit binary code assigns a unique decimal value from 0 to 127 to each of 128 letters, numbers, punctuation marks, control characters, and special characters. For example, the symbol "@" is represented by ASCII code 64, while ASCII code 7 is "control-G" (originally called the "bell" command because it activated the bell of teletype machines—today, buzzers replace bells). See also Baudot.

Assembler: a system software program which translates code written in assembly language into machine language. See also Assembler language, Disassembler, and Machine language.

Assembly language: a class of low-level computer languages that use mnemonic symbols (operation or "op" codes) instead of numbers to tell a computer to do something. Operation codes are commands which invoke actions by a central processing unit (for example "JMP," which means "jump to a new memory location"). Different central processors employ different (and usually incompatible) assembly languages.

Asynchronous: without a time keeper. Asynchronous communication protocols (such as RS-232) do not require that the two ends of the communication channel share a common clock or pacemaker. Instead, only the sending (source) end of the system requires a clock.

Authoring language: a class of high-level computer languages used primarily to create lessons for computer-assisted instruction. These languages typically employ shortcuts for entering, scoring, and grading test items, and for managing branching to particular program locations as a function of student performance. PILOT is an example of an authoring language.

Background: a second-priority task in a multitask or multiprogram system environment, less important or less active than a foreground task.

Backup: a plan for avoiding problems. Backup copies of data or programs are machine-readable duplicates held in reserve against possible loss or damage of original copies. Backup procedures usually involve storing original copies of programs and data in protected locations.

Bandwidth: the difference between the lowest and highest frequencies that can be transmitted by an analog communication channel, expressed in hertz (Hz) or cycles per second. Bandwidth also refers to the number of digital pulses that can be transmitted by a digital communication channel, expressed in bits per second.

Baseband: a class of digital communications network employed in local areas and using two-conductor (coaxial) cables. Baseband systems typically have transmission bandwidths up to 10 megabits per second. See also Broadband.

BASIC: acronym for "Beginners' All-purpose Symbolic Instruction Code," a high-level computer language invented by Kemeney and Kurtz at Dartmouth College in 1963. Originally designed as a teaching tool, it is the most common programming language available on microcomputers. BASIC exists in several dialects which differ in their ability to index variables, handle fractions, and perform logical operations on string variables. Most versions of BASIC are interpreter oriented.

Batch processing: a style of computer use common in large computer centers in which users submit programs to be run on a first-come, first-served basis. The time required to execute a program (turn-around time) is largely determined by clerical and accounting activities. Batch processing optimizes the use of computer resources and can be very efficient for large or complex problems. It is often wasteful of user time for more modest problems. See also Dedicated processing, Distributed processing, and Time-sharing.

Baud: colloquial term referring to the number of bits per second that can be transmitted in serial mode. For example, "300 baud" is a transmission speed of 300 bits per second. If 10 bits are required for one alphanumeric character, this rate transmits 30 characters per second. Serial transmission rates range from 110 to 9600 baud for MODEM communication (110, 300, and 1200 are most common), and up to 19000 baud for short-distance communication.

Baudot: a character coding system used in early teletype communication. This 5-bit binary code assigns a unique decimal value from 0 to 32 to each letter of the alphabet and each of several punctuation marks. A letters versus numbers "shift" allows a total of 64 distinct alphanumeric characters. Because this coding system was designed for electromechanical devices, it assumes a relatively slow rate of data transmission (six characters per second). It is incompatible with ASCII, the major coding system used for modern electronic telecommunication. However, the Baudot code is the traditional system for telecommunication devices for the deaf (TDDs). See also ASCII, telecommunication, TDD, and TTY.

Benchmark: any specific program used to make direct comparison of computers or computer systems. The results of benchmark tests are usually expressed in terms of execution time (less is better) and, where computations are involved, accuracy (more is better).

Beta testing: a phase in the development of commercial application programs prior to distribution in which samples of the intended (target) audience of users exercise a program to assess effectiveness, efficiency, accuracy, speed, and friendliness. Also called "summative" evaluation. See also Alpha testing.

Binary: two. Referring to the base-2 number system in which a place holder can assume the value 0 or the value 1. Each digit in a binary number represents a power of 2. A binary (or digital) signal is characterized by the presence or absence of something, such as an electrical voltage. Internally, all digital computers use binary numbers.

Binary-coded decimal (BCD): an organization of bits to express a value (number). A single BCD has four digits or place holders and can express base-10 values ranging from 0 (0000) to 16 (1111). A four-digit BCD is sometimes called a nibble. Two nibbles (8 bits) are a byte.

Binary file: a "chunk" of information (usually on a disk) stored in the form of binary-coded decimals. If the information stored in a binary file is a program, it is in machine language form and can be directly executed by the central processor.

Bit: a single digit (place holder) of a binary coded decimal.
Bit-mapped graphics: a method for implementing graphics on a display screen or printer in which each of a large number of dots can be addressed and turned on or off. See also Character graphics, Raster graphics, and Vector graphics.
Black box: any hardware device that accomplishes a customized function or operation, the details of which are considered unimportant.
Bomb: an unexpected and undesirable termination of a program. Bombs are catastrophic in the sense that they destroy data and (sometimes) programs. Also called a "crash."
Boot(strap): a system program (usually in firmware) invoked immediately after a computer is turned on which "tells" the central processor what hardware resources are available to it. When this program is executed, the computer is said to be "booted."
Branch: the ability of a computer to move from one part of a program to another, or to "pass control" from one location in a program to another. Branching may be either unconditional or conditional. For example, each time a program is executed, control may be passed to a part of the program that displays the title of the program (unconditional branch). Similarly, if a user types the letter "O" when the number "0" is expected, control may be passed to a routine that tells the user a mistake has been made (conditional branch). Most high-level languages include control structures to facilitate branching. Examples include the "GO TO" and "IF—THEN GO TO" structures of BASIC.
Broadband: a class of analog communications network employed in local or distinct areas and using two-conductor (coaxial) cables. Broadband systems can carry many varieties of signals, including audio, video, and data. Communicating devices are connected to broadband systems by means of MODEMs. See also Baseband and MODEM.
Bubble memory: a contemporary information storage technology which alters the magnetic charge of "bubbles" of semiconductor material. Bubble memory uses no moving parts and thus is faster and more robust than magnetic disks. Bubble memory is also nonvolatile, that is, information is retained even when electrical power is removed.
Bundling: a marketing strategy in which hardware and software are sold as an inseparable unit. Unbundled systems are those in which hardware and software components are priced and sold individually.
Buffer: a device (hardware) or a software routine that temporarily holds information, or which reserves memory for later occupation by information. For example, a print buffer accepts information from a computer at high speed, then passes that information to a lower speed printer.
Bug: colloquial term for error. Hardware bugs are caused by design errors, by physical or electronic malfunction, or by misuse. Software bugs are caused by logical, syntactical, or typographical errors in programming.
Bulletin board: see Electronic bulletin board.
Bulk memory: see Mass memory.
Bus: a set of electrical connections in a computer which carry information from one place to another. Some of these connections are used for data, while others are used to identify particular hardware devices, and still others are used to control the direction of data flow. See also Address bus, Control bus, and Data bus.
Byte: a fundamental unit of storage in computer memory equivalent to one ASCII character; 8 bits addressed as a single unit. Microcomputers typically contain at least 64 kilobytes (65,536) of memory.
C: a high-level computer language developed by Bell Laboratories in the 1970s. C is a structured (i.e., it requires precise problem analysis and precise solution planning), compiler-oriented language, especially well suited to tasks involving large amounts of input and output operations.

Calculator: an electromechanical or electronic device which performs operations on numbers, as distinct from a computer, which performs operations on any type of symbols (including numbers). See also Computer.

Call: a command which passes program control to subroutine, often with the intent to return to the place where the call occurred.

Canned: off-the-shelf. A canned program is one that is expected to work appropriately in many situations.

Carriage return key: see Return key.

Cartridge disk: a relatively new disk medium employing a rigid protective case and a 3-inch or 3.5-inch magnetic storage surface capable of recording as much information as a 5.25-inch floppy disk. The 3-inch version is a proprietary development of Sony Corporation. Cartridge disks are more robust, but more expensive and less common than floppy disks. See also Disk and Disk drive.

Cathode-ray tube (CRT): a display device in which an electronically aimed stream of electrons strike phosphorous material, thus causing visible images. Also, any device containing such a tube (e.g., television monitors and receivers, oscilloscopes, video terminals).

CBASIC: a version of the high-level computer language BASIC which employs a compiler to translate source code into object code.

Central processing unit (CPU): the "central nervous system" of a computer, typically placed on a single chip. CPUs accomplish primitive logical and mathematical functions, store intermediate results of symbol manipulations, and direct the flow of data and instructions to and from peripheral devices which act as sensors and effectors. See also Arithmetic logic unit, Clock, Master control unit, Program counter unit, and Register.

Centronix bus: a parallel transmission system developed by Centronix, Inc., in support of that firm's printers. The Centronix bus has become a de facto standard for interfacing computers and printers.

Character: any graphical symbol that has meaning. See also Alphanumeric.

Character graphics: a method for implementing graphics on a display screen or printer in which characters are used to build images. In this context, characters are standardized groups of dots. See also Bit-mapped graphics.

Character printer: a type of printer similar to a typewriter that produces characters as entire shapes, typically in different sets (fonts) of shapes. Character printers are slower and more noisy than dot-matrix printers, but produce excellent quality images. Most such printers use changeable symbol mechanisms (e.g., daisy wheels or type balls). Virtually all character printers use inked ribbons and impact mechanisms. See also Daisy-wheel printer and Dot-matrix printer.

Chip: colloquial term for integrated circuit, referring to the form and material (usually silicon) used to make such circuits.

Circuit board: a piece of rigid insulating material upon which conductive copper traces and integrated circuits are placed. Circuit boards are also called "printed circuit (PC) boards" in reference to the manufacturing process used to make them.

Clock: a functional component of the central processor of a computer which acts as a pacemaker to synchronize operations and the flow of information (data and instructions) among other components. The clocks of different microprocessors operate at different frequencies (speeds), ranging from 1 to 10 megahertz. See also Central processing unit and Real-time clock.

CMOS: ("seemoss") acronym for "complementary metal-oxide semiconductor." A category of semiconductor technology used in the design and manufacture of microcomputers. CMOS-integrated circuits are relatively immune to electrical noise and require relatively little electrical power. See also TTL.

COBOL: acronym for "COmmon Business-Oriented Language." COBOL is a high-level computer language developed in the early 1960s. It is more structured than BASIC and FORTRAN, but less structured than Pascal or C. COBOL is a compiler-oriented language.

Code: the written form of a computer program. More generally, any systematic method for representing something in terms of symbols. See also Source code and Object code.

Cold start: the process of starting up a computer by applying electrical power.

Command: a symbolic instruction that tells a computer to do something.

Command-driven software: a type of computer program that requires the user to communicate with the program through the use of a set of explicit commands. Commands are consistent within programs, but usually not between programs. Programs of this type are hard to learn, but relatively flexible. See also Menu-driven software.

Communication: in this context, the transmission of information between one computer and another computer, or among computers and other hardware. Such transmission may employ analog signals or digital signals, but must employ hardware, software, and a communication network of some sort. See also Baseband and Broadband.

Compiler-oriented language: a category of computer languages that accomplish translation of source code (written by a programmer) into object code (required by the computer) at the level of the entire program. In other words, all the individual statements of the program are translated into machine language at one time. The resulting object code can be stored, recalled, and executed very quickly because no time is devoted to translation. FORTRAN, Pascal, and CBASIC are examples of languages of this type. See also Translator.

Composite video: a method of conditioning video signals which combines a synchronizing signal with the video information signal. The "sync" signal causes the CRT electron beam to scan across and down the surface of the tube at a constant rate, thus producing a stable, legible image. In the United States, the standard for composite video assumes an image of 525 horizontal lines and a scanning rate of 30 screen images per second.

Computer: a machine that accepts, stores, and manipulates symbols. Some symbols are instructions; others are data, the subject matter on which instructions operate. Both instructions and data can be modified. The idea of a stored-instruction computer was developed by John Von Neumann in 1945.

Computer-aided design (CAD): the application of computers to the design of products such as automobiles, appliances, and electronic devices. The output of the most sophisticated CAD systems becomes input to computer-aided manufacturing (CAM) systems which numerically control robots and other manufacturing machines.

Computer-assisted instruction (CAI): the application of computers to the interactive delivery of instructional services, including simulation, drill work, "programmed" instruction, Socratic dialog, and didactic testing. Programs designed for CAI are often called "courseware," a word properly reserved for fully integrated applications. See also Computer-managed instruction.

Computer-augmented communication (CAC): a category of computer application which focuses on solving the communication problems of the handicapped. Examples include text-to-speech translators for the blind, teletypes (and related devices) for the deaf, and voice-output communication aids (VOCAs) for the cerebral palsied or laryngectomized.

Computer idiot: (1) an invention of the mass media. (2) A soon-to-be unemployed person, usually over the age of 30, whose laziness, limited mental flexibility, or negative attitudes preclude computer literacy.

Computer language: a group of artificial (i.e., invented) systems for machine manipulation of symbols and relations among symbols. Computer languages differ from natural languages (English, French, German) in that they are *designed* to enhance certain functions (processing numbers, processing letters and words, processing data organized in lists, etc.). Such languages, however, exhibit all of the features of natural language, including a symbol set (a "phonology"), the ability to concatenate symbols, rules of structure (syntax), semantics, and pragmatics. Computer languages differ in speed, syntax, pragmatics, friendliness, and other respects. Examples include ALGOL, APL, BASIC, C, COBOL, Forth, FORTRAN, LISP, LOGO, Pascal, PILOT, and about a hundred others. See also High-level language, Low-level language, and Translator.

Computer literacy: elementary understanding of the functions, applications, operation, and programming of computers.

Computer-managed instruction (CMI): the application of computers to the administration of instructional services, including record keeping, construction and scoring of tests, monitoring of student progress, and the scheduling of instructional personnel and events. See also Computer-aided instruction.

Computer nerd: (1) an invention of the mass media. (2) An often-hired, often-fired person, usually under the age of 30, whose excessive fascination and skill with computers and related technology preclude meaningful interpersonal relations and effective social function.

Computer science: a discipline which focuses on (1) the design, analysis, and application of computer hardware, system software, and programming languages; (2) the definition, utility, application, distribution, and management of information by means of computers; and (3) the analysis, design, and evaluation of systems for managing information and processes.

Computer system: a central processing unit, primary memory, all related peripheral devices for input, output, and secondary storage of information, and the system software required to allow communication among devices and between the system and the user. See also Microcomputer, Minicomputer, and Mainframe computer.

Computer terminal: see Terminal.

Concatenation: stringing things together, such as phonemes in spoken language, letters and words in written language, or characters in fields, records, and files of a data structure.

Console: a computer or computer terminal consisting of a keyboard and some sort of display screen (e.g., video receiver, video monitor, or liquid crystal display monitor).

Control (CTRL) characters: a group of ASCII characters which are usually not displayed, but which cause certain events to occur. For example, on most computers and computer terminals "CTRL-G" causes a buzzer to sound and "CRTL-M" causes a carriage return. Control characters have ASCII code numbers in between 0 and 26.

Control bus: a communication channel (i.e., a set of electrical connections) internal to a computer by which the central processing unit can determine the direction and speed of information flow to and from peripheral devices. See also Address bus, Central processing unit, and Data bus.

Control (CRTL) key: a special key on a keyboard which, when used simultaneously with another key, issues a control character to the computer. See also Control character.

Coprocessor: an ancillary integrated circuit placed in a microcomputer to assist the central processing unit (CPU) in performing specialized tasks (e.g., mathematical operations). Coprocessors are designed to work with particular CPUs. When properly supported by software, coprocessors can significantly increase execution speed. See also Central processing unit.

Core memory: an information storage technology heavily used in mainframe computers and minicomputers built during the 1960s. Tiny doughnut-shaped "cores" of magnetically sensitive materials were woven into matrices with wires which sensed, placed, and erased magnetic charges on individual bits of memory. More generally, any primary memory system in a computer.

Courseware: see Computer-assisted instruction.

CP/M: acronym for "control program for microprocessors," an operating system developed by Digital Research, Inc., for 8-bit computers based upon 8080, 8085, and Z80 microprocessors. CP/M is the most common such operating system now in use. Variations are now available for other microprocessors (e.g., CP/M-86 for the 16-bit 8086 and 8088 processors and CP/M-86K for the 68000 processor). MP/M-II is a multiuser version of CP/M and concurrent CP/M is a version which allows multitasking (up to four programs running simultaneously).

Crash: see Bomb.

Cursor: a special display screen symbol which indicates the location at which the next character will appear. Cursors are usually in the form of a blinking square, bar, or underline character.

Cursor keys: special keys on a computer keyboard which permit the cursor to be moved up and down, or right and left on the display screen. In some computer systems (or programs), cursor keys are destructive (i.e., they erase displayed characters); in other applications, they are nondestructive. See also Cursor.

Cybernetics: a discipline which focuses on the similarities and differences between organic and machine processes, especially in areas involving sensing, cognition, communication, control, learning, decision-making, and abstract reasoning. Cybernetics was founded by Norbert Wiener in 1948. See also Artificial intelligence and Robots.

Daisy-wheel printer: a character printer employing a changeable print element in the form of a daisy. Daisy-wheel printers are commonly used to generate business and professional correspondence indistinguishable from typewriter copy. They are slower and more expensive than dot-matrix printers; some do not allow output of graphics.

Data: reports (plural) of observations of events or phenomena expressed with numbers or other symbols; information of any kind.

Data base: a collection of information that can be organized, reorganized, managed, and maintained by electronic means. By connotation, a data base can be accessed by a number of different users.

Data base management system: a category of application software that allows entry, editing, deletion, organization, sorting, merging, and tabulating of information in a data base.

Data base service: a category of computer application involving telecommunications which allows paid subscribers access to large, mainframe computers and a variety of data bases, including popular and technical literature bases, financial reporting services, census information, news "wire" services (e.g., Associated Press), and others. Examples include Telenet, Tymnet, the Source, and Lockheed Data Services.

Data bus: a communication channel (i.e., a set of electrical connections) internal to a computer by which the central processor can exchange information (data or programs) with peripherals. See also Address bus, Central processing unit, and Control bus.

Data communication equipment (DCE): a device (hardware) which establishes and maintains communication between computers or computer terminals (i.e., data terminal equipment). A MODEM is an example of a DCE. DCE connectors are specified by the RS-232 asynchronous serial standard in terms of signals levels, signal functions, and connector pins. See also Data terminal equipment (DTE).

Data terminal equipment (DTE): a device (hardware) which serves as a source or receiver of data in a communication network, usually either a computer or a computer terminal. DTE connectors are specified by the RS-232 asynchronous serial standard in terms of signal levels, signal functions, and connector pins. See also Data communication equipment (DCE).

Daughterboard: a secondary printed-circuit board of a small computer which plugs into a connector on the primary circuit board (motherboard).

Debug: to find and correct errors (bugs).

Decimal: ten. Referring to the base-10 number system in which a place holder can assume a value from 0 to 9. Each digit in a decimal number represents a power of ten. The decimal number system is the system most often used by people. See also Binary, Octal, and Hexadecimal.

Dedicated processing: the use of a relatively simple computer system used for only one class of application. Examples include computerized audiometers. More generally, dedicated computer systems are those used for limited classes of applications, or by single individuals. See also Batch processing, Distributed processing, and Time sharing.

Delimiter: a character which serves to signal separation of one datum from another. For example, in a list of mean length of utterance scores, the symbol "/" (backslash) might be used to indicate the end of one datum and the beginning of another: "3.2/6/4.7". Computer programs and programming languages employ different delimiters for different purposes. By convention, the most common delimiters are commas, spaces, and the return character.

Default: a set of standard conditions in effect until explicitly changed. For example, the default output device for a computer may be a display screen, even though an alternative output device (e.g., a printer) is available and can be selected.

Digital: an event which varies from small to large in a discrete manner and which can assume only limited values. Examples of digital signals include the presence versus absence of a voltage or a magnetic field. Examples of digital machines include wrist watches with numerical displays, music boxes, an abacus, a simple on–off switch, and push-button tuners on radios. See also Analog.

Digital tablet: see Graphics tablet.

Digital-to-analog converter (DAC): a device (hardware) that translates discrete, digital signals into continuous, time-varying analog signals. See also Analog-to-digital converter.

Digital plotter: a device (hardware) that draws pictures, graphs, characters, and other images under computer control.

DIP: acronym for "dual in-line package," the most common physical housing for integrated circuits. DIPs are available in configurations with 8 to 40 pins for connection with other circuit elements.

Direct memory access (DMA): a method by which primary memory can be read from or written to without involving the central processing unit. DMA is necessary in applications which require very high speed movement of data (e.g., sampling single-unit nerve potentials in neurophysiological research).

Disassembler: the opposite of an assembler. A system software program which converts code expressed in machine language into code expressed in assembly language. See also Assembler, Assembly language, and Machine language.

Disk: a secondary memory system common to microcomputers. Disks can store more information than the primary memory of a computer; thus, they are called "bulk memory" devices. They are also nonvolatile: information remains even when electrical power is removed. There are four major disk technologies: floppy, hard, cartridge, and reflective (video). These differ in recording methods, physical size, memory capacity, access speed, erasability, and cost. See also Cartridge disk, Floppy disk, Hard disk, Video disk, and Disk drive.

Disk drive: the device (hardware) that allows a disk to be accessed. Disk drives are connected to computers or computer terminals by means of a cable and an interface card (hardware) and controlled by means of a disk-operating system (software). Different disk media and technologies (floppy vs. hard, magnetic vs. optical), and disk sizes (3-inch, 5.25-inch, 8-inch) require different disk drives. Drives contain a stepper motor which moves a small "head" to record (write) and retrieve (read) information, and another motor which causes the disk to rotate, thus minimizing the time required for the head to locate any particular point on the surface of the disk. Magnetic disk systems employ a magnetic head similar to (but much smaller than) that used in audio tape recording. Video disk systems use a laser source to read holes burned in the surface of a disk at the time of manufacture. Magnetic disk systems are read–write systems; video disk systems are read-only systems.

Disk-operating system (DOS): generic term for a system software program (usually written in assembler language and stored as machine code) which manages communication between a central processing unit, disk drives, printers, and other peripheral devices. Disk-operating systems simplify such communication by allowing user-specified names for data and program files, and by keeping track of housekeeping details. Most DOSs permit creation and deletion of files of various types (e.g., sequential vs. random data files, binary code vs. ASCII code files) as well as file cataloging and transfers of files from one disk to another. Disk-operating systems are typically command driven, rather than menu driven. This feature allows creation of special "executive" files consisting of commands to the DOS which can do a series of complex tasks under program control, rather than direct user control. DOSs range from simple to complex. More complex systems support several high-level languages and various utility programs. The ideal DOS is "transparent," that is, it works unobtrusively and automatically.

Display screen: a device (hardware) used to output textural or graphical information. Display screens may use any of a variety of display technologies, including the cathode-ray tubes found in video monitors and video receivers, and the liquid crystal systems found in many portable computers and computer terminals.

Distributed processing: a relatively complex system of computers linked together by means of a communication network. Each computer "shares" parts of a large processing job. See also Batch processing, Dedicated processing, and Time sharing.

Documentation: instructions for using hardware or software. Software documentation includes hardcopy (paper) instructions separate from the program, as well as instructions to the user encountered when the program is executed and annotations contained in the source code of the program itself. Good documentation accurately anticipates the sophistication and needs of the user and is a crucial aspect of user friendliness.

DOS: see Disk-operating system.

Dot-matrix printer: a type of printer that produces characters and graphics by means of individually activated dots arranged in an X-Y coordinate pattern. Image resolution and quality depend upon the number of dots in the matrix. The 5-by-7 and 9-by-13 dot-matrices are common. Dot-matrix printers are generally faster and cheaper than character printers (e.g., daisy-wheel printers). Some allow the use of multiple type fonts (including user-designed fonts), but they may produce poorer-quality images than character printers. Dot-matrix printers employ various techniques to place images on paper: inked ribbons and impact mechanisms, ink-jet mechanisms, electrode and thermally sensitive paper systems, or electrode and electrosensitive paper systems. See also Character printer.

Download: the process of directing data files or program files from a large computer to a smaller computer, computer terminal, or other device via a communication network.

Down time: an interval during which a system does not function.

Drive: see Disk drive.

Driver: a computer program or subroutine written in a low-level language which manages the details of communication with an input device or an output device.

Dumb terminal: a computer terminal (hardware) entirely dependent upon a remote computer for data processing. Dumb terminals (e.g., teletypes and some video terminals) exchange data with computers via communication networks, most often those using asynchronous serial protocols (ASCII character codes and RS-232 signals).

Dump: see Memory dump.

Duplex: see Full-duplex and Half-duplex.

EEPROM: acronym for "electronically erasable programmable read-only memory." EEPROMs are similar to EPROMS, except that ultraviolet light is not necessary for erasure of old information. See also EPROM.

Electronic bulletin board: a category of computer application employing communication networks to allow users to enter, store, and receive notices of general interest to the users of the system. Electronic bulletin boards may involve local or distant sites and make use of existing telephone systems. They differ from data base services in that users do not pay subscription or connect-time fees. Electronic bulletin boards may become the CB radio of the 1980s. See also Data base services.

Electronic mail: a category of computer application focusing on the use of computers to enter, edit, transmit, and receive textual information (primarily correspondence) via communication networks. These networks may involve local or distant sites, dedicated lines, or common carriers (i.e., existing telephone systems). Electronic mail differs from electronic bulletin boards in terms of the privacy of communications shared by users of the system.

Electronic Industry Association (EIA): a trade association of companies involved in manufacturing electronic devices and support systems. The EIA promulgates standards for mechanical housings and mountings for electronic instruments.

Emulator: something that acts like something else.

End-of-file (EOF): a special character placed at the end of a file of data which signals termination of the file.

End-of-record (EOR): a special character placed at the end of a record in a file of data to signal termination of the record.

Endless loop: a process, routine, or task which repeats itself indefinitely. Although some endless loops may be intentional, they are often the result of logical errors in programming. Hence, the phrase has a negative connotation.

End-user: a user of computers, as opposed to a programmer, designer, or administrator of computers.

Enter key: see Return key.

Entry point: a location in memory containing the first executable instruction in a machine-language program. Also, the number of a statement in a computer program at which a subroutine begins.

EPROM: acronym for "erasable programmable read-only memory." EPROMs are integrated circuit devices (hardware) which store binary information indefinitely, or until that information is erased by exposure to ultraviolet light. Once erased, new information can be stored. EPROM is nonvolatile: information is retained even with loss of power.

Ergonomics: a discipline which focuses on the physical interaction of people and machines, that is, the person–machine "interface." Ergonomic design tries to make machines fit people, rather than the other way around.

Error recovery: the process of identifying and correcting errors without losing data and without having to reexecute a program. Error recovery is a characteristic of friendly programs and systems.

Error trap: a software routine designed to "intercept" error messages from an interpreter or operating system without forcing the program to cease operation. Error trapping is used extensively in program development and is necessary for error recovery.

Escape (ESC) key: a special key on a keyboard which, when used prior to another key, issues a command to the current program. The ASCII code number for the escape key is 27.

Ethernet: a proprietary baseband communication used for local area networks (LANs). Ethernet was developed by Xerox Corporation and is also used by Digital Equipment Corporation (DEC).

Execute: to cause a program or process to operate.

Execution time: the time necessary to complete a process or program.

Expansion interface: a device (hardware) connected to a computer which allows a user to connect more peripheral devices to the system than would be possible without the expansion interface.

Expert system: a category of computer application that relies upon a very large data base to solve problems much the way human experts solve them. Expert systems employ specialized data bases called "knowledge bases" which include histories of problems, successful solutions, unsuccessful solutions, and inference logic. Expert systems are still largely experimental. See also Artificial intelligence.

Extensible: a property of some computer languages by which it is possible to define entirely new types of variables, logical relations, or processes. These can then be permanently incorporated into the language. Pascal and Forth are extensible; BASIC and FORTRAN are not.

Fatal error: an error which causes a program to terminate execution prior to completion of the task, usually with the loss of data.

FIFO: acronym for "first-in, first out." Information stored in a serial buffer or sequential data file is managed on a FIFO basis.

Field: a category of information found in all the records of a file. The smallest meaningful, manipulable unit in a record. In a file of names and addresses, one field might be reserved for zip code numbers, another for first name. See also File and Record.

Fifth-generation computer: a not-yet-realized development proposed by the Japanese government in 1982. This development will require extremely fast microprocessors, extremely large capacity primary and secondary memory systems, and significant advances in artificial intelligence. The distinguishing feature of fifth-generation systems is to be the integration of functions through a new approach to problem solving. This approach will incorporate (1) a knowledge base (relational algebra, data-intensive "scenarios"), (2) context data (about specific problem situations), and (3) an inference "engine" (which derives abstract methods for problem solving). Other features include talker-independent speech recognition and natural language processing. To materialize, this development must invoke a fifth major technology for computer memory (the first was vacuum tubes; the second, magnetic cores; the third, transistors; and the fourth, MSI and LSI circuits). See also Expert system.

File: an organized set of data treated as a unit. Files are unified by relations shared by the elements of the file. Computer files are analogous to office file cabinets (not individual file folders). In a file of names and addresses, several fields (e.g., name, street number, street name, city, state, zip code) make up each of several records (e.g., all the address information for a given person). A set of related records then constitutes a file (e.g., all the records—persons—belonging to a particular organization).

Financial maintenance: the process of entering, editing, and discarding data stored in files. An especially important aspect of file maintenance is "garbage collection," the active discarding of information that no longer has currency or value.

File management system: see Disk-operating system (DOS).

File protection: any of several methods for ensuring that stored information will not be inadvertently lost or tampered with. Because most magnetic storage media (disks, tape, bubble memory) destroy old information whenever new information is recorded, many file protection schemes are designed to prevent unintended "overwriting." No file protection scheme is foolproof. Thus, backup procedures are necessary. See also Write-enable and Write-protect.

File management: a category of computer application used to guide and effect fiscal operations such as client billing, tax accounting, and payroll production. Previously in the domain of mainframe computers, a large number of financial management and general accounting software packages are now available for microcomputers.

Firmware: software stored in nonvolatile main memory such as PROM, EPROM, or EEPROM.

Flag: (1) an electrical signal or signal channel (hardware) which signals the occurrence of an event. For example, an interface circuit might reserve one channel (wire) to tell another device that data can or cannot be accepted. (2) A variable used in a computer program (software) to indicate a particular state of a process or task. For example, a variable named "TALLY" might be used to count the number of times a process has been repeated. When a predetermined value (a "sentinel value") is reached, the process is terminated.

Floating point: a positive or negative number consisting of an integer (whole number) part and a fractional (decimal number) part. Floating point numbers (also termed "real numbers") are so called because the position of a decimal point can "float" from one location to another in a string of digits. See also Integer.

Floppy disk: the most common type of secondary memory used with microcomputers, so called because the storage medium (a Mylar substrate surfaced with magnetically sensitive particles) is pliable. The disk is placed inside a protective plastic envelope that can be inserted and removed from a disk drive. Data can be recorded (written) and retrieved (read) under machine control and are organized via concentric tracks and radial sectors. Floppy disks come in two sizes (5.25-inch diameter and 8-inch diameter) and in different "densities" (information capacity based upon the amount of magnetic particles per unit area). They also come in several hard (mechanically marked) and soft (marked by software) sector configurations. Some can store data on both sides; others on only one side. Floppy (or flexible) disks can store between 80 and 580 kilobytes, depending upon diameter, density, and the number of functional sides. See also Disk and Disk drive.

Flow chart: a graphical representation of an algorithm, process, or program. Flow charts employ standardized symbols to signify actions (e.g., input from keyboard, output to printer) and are one of several methods used to plan, debug, and document computer programs. They are most useful for problems that are linear or hierarchical in structure and less useful for problems that employ a networked structure.

Footer: a sequence of characters appearing at the bottom of a page. Many word processing systems let the user define a footer, then automatically place it at the end of each page.

Footprint: the physical space occupied by hardware. Large microcomputers, printers, and disk drives have larger "footprints" than small ones.

Foreground: a first-priority task in a multitask or multiprogram system environment, more important or more active than a background task.

Format: a predetermined structure of some sort, independent of the information to be placed in that structure. For example, the format of a business letter includes a date, address, salutation, and signature; a speech includes an introduction, body, and conclusion; a data file includes a set of data records, each consisting of a set of data fields. The fact that certain kinds of information conform (or can be made to conform) to a format is what makes information processing possible.

Form feed: a control character that causes a printer to eject the current page and position the next page.

Forth: a relatively low-level, compiler-oriented computer language developed in the mid 1970s and available on some microcomputers. Forth is very fast and has been successfully used in real-time process control tasks.

FORTRAN: acronym for "FORmula TRANslation." FORTRAN is a high-level computer language originally developed in 1956 for mathematical processing of scientific and engineering data. It is available on virtually every mainframe computer and is still used extensively. FORTRAN exists in several standardized versions (e.g., FORTRAN III, IV, V) which are nominally upward compatible with each other. A compiler-oriented language, FORTRAN has the advantage of very fast execution. It is now available on several microcomputers.

Friendliness: a user's perception of how easy it is to work with something (e.g., documentation, a program, or a computer). A friendly system places minimal demands on a user in terms of learning, memory, and recovery from mistakes arising from any source. Also called "user friendly."

Full-duplex: a serial asynchronous communication protocol which permits simultaneous sending and receiving of information. An example of a full-duplex system is a two-way telephone conversation. In full-duplex data communication, a character is sent from a data source along a communication channel to a data receiver which then echoes the character back to the source. This provides feedback about whether the signal sent was actually received. This "echo-back" feature is useful in noisy communication situations. Full-duplex is optional with most MODEMs and most time-shared computer systems. See also Half-duplex and Simplex.

Function key: a nonstandard key on a keyboard which accomplishes a special task, such as clearing the display screen or outputting the information shown on a display screen to a printer. Because such keys are nonstandard, they vary across devices. Programmable function keys are those whose functions can be changed with software. User-definable function keys can be modified by programs written by the user of the system.

Game paddle: a control device (hardware) consisting of a potentiometer (variable resistor) wired as a voltage divider and connected to an analog-to-digital converter. A knob is used to turn the "pot" and send one-dimensional information to a computer, primarily to control the position of images depicted on a display screen. Game paddles were first used in an early video game ("pong") and are so called because paddles are used in the game ping pong.

Game port: a connector, plug, or socket found on some microcomputers by which various manipulanda (game paddles, joysticks, pushbuttons, trackballs, etc.) can be attached to allow input of information from the user. On some computers, game ports also accommodate simple display devices (lamps and other low-power devices) to allow output of information to the user.

General purpose computer: a computer of any class (micro-, mini-, or mainframe) which is capable of performing unrelated programs for unrelated purposes. General purpose computers typically support several different computer languages and a range of input and output peripherals. See also Special purpose computer.

GIGO: acronym for "garbage-in, garbage-out." Contaminated data or erroneous processes can produce only contaminated or erroneous outcomes.

Graphic display: any of several electronic devices (hardware) used to show graphic images (pictures rather than text). Some graphic displays product hardcopy, others produce softcopy.

Graphics: any nonalphanumeric information. Graphics include charts, graphs, pictures, and animated figures. Several techniques exist for displaying graphics on display screens and printers. These differ in image resolution, speed, flexibility, and other characteristics. See also Bit-mapped graphics, Character graphics, Raster graphics, and Vector graphics.

Graphics preparation: a category of computer application designed to allow entry of numerical information for subsequent rendering in graphical form. Most graphics preparation programs provide for entry and editing of data, designation of labels (quantities and units), and specification of graph format (pie chart, line graph, bar graph, etc.) independent of other operations on data. Some allow fitting of general classes of equations (linear, exponential, or logarithmic least-squared error) to data points. Depending on the program, finished graphics can be saved and retrieved in either numerical or image forms to be displayed on a terminal screen or printer. Also called "presentation graphics."

Graphics tablet: a device (hardware) used to input graphical information for subsequent processing or transmission. Graphic tablets typically employ a stylus (non-drawing pen) to trace over images or shapes. The tablet senses the position of the stylus, converts positional information into X-Y coordinate values, and sends those values to a computer via an interface. Also called "digitizer" and "digital tablet."

Hacker: (1) an invention of the mass media. (2) A computer user who takes pride in violating computer security systems designed to exclude unauthorized users, or to prevent unauthorized duplication of commercial software. (3) Originally, a self-taught programmer.

Handshaking signals: a set of electrical signals (and associated connector pins) used in communication applications to ensure that data are sent and received properly.

Hardcopy: physically palpable output, such as a printed page, as opposed to more transient types of output (i.e., data shown on a display screen). See also Softcopy.

Hard disk: a common type of secondary memory used with microcomputers, so called because the storage medium (the disk itself) is rigid. The disk is usually permanently mounted inside a disk drive. As with floppy disks, data can be recorded (written) and retrieved (read) under machine control and are organized via concentric tracks and radial sectors. Hard disk media and drives employ more precise mechanical tolerances than floppy systems, thus increasing memory capacity. Hard disks can store between 2 and 40 megabytes, depending upon design details. See also Disk and Disk drive.

Hardware: the physical part of a computer or other system, as opposed to the "logical" part. Computer hardware includes all of the functionally separate parts (central and peripheral) that make up the electronics and machinery of a computer system. See also Firmware and Software.

Hard-wired: a process implemented with hardware. Faster, more permanent, and less flexible than a process implemented with software.

Half-duplex: a serial asynchronous communication protocol which allows sending and receiving of information, but requires devices to "take turns." An example of a half-duplex system is citizens' band (CB) radio. In half-duplex data communication, a character is sent from a data source to a receiver. Thereafter, the receiver may become a source. There is no "echo-back" feature as found with full-duplex communication. Half-duplex is optional with most MODEMs and most time-shared computer systems. See also Full-duplex and Simplex.

Header: a sequence of characters appearing at the top of a page. Many word processing systems let the user define a header, then automatically place it at the beginning of each page.

Help screen: a feature of many computer programs by which the user is reminded of program options and commands. Help screens may be called up or invoked with little effort and are usually organized as menus. Help screens are characteristic of friendly programs.

Heuristic: a problem-solving method employing "rules of thumb" or empirical approximations to get answers. Many heuristic methods are designed and evaluated in consideration of human problem-solving performance. The emphasis is on useful solutions, rather than perfect solutions.

Hexadecimal: sixteen. Referring to the base-16 number system. The digits 0 through 9 and the letters A through F represent values in this system. Each digit in a hexadecimal number is a power of 16. The "hex" system is used extensively in 8-bit and 16-bit computers.

Hierarchical structures: a way of organizing data, processes, tasks or people in which elements are subsets or suprasets of each other. Organizational charts and outlines are examples of hierarchical structures. Many computer programs are organized in this manner (major tasks, divided into subtasks, divided into sub-subtasks). Hierarchical structures are strong in clarity and weak in flexibility. See also Networked structures.

High-level language: a category of computer language relatively similar to natural language and relatively independent of particular computer hardware. High-level languages are easier to learn and use than low-level languages. Programs written in people-friendly, high-level languages must be translated into machine-friendly, low-level languages. This is accomplished via interpreters or compilers. Examples of high-level languages include BASIC, FORTRAN, and Pascal. See also Computer language, Low-level language, and Translator.

Hollerith card: a binary storage medium consisting of a stiff paper card in which holes are punched in columns and rows to "remember" data. Sometimes called "IBM" cards, Hollerith cards were developed by Herman Hollerith to help tabulate the results of the

United States census of 1890. These cards are generated with a "keypunch" machine; information on them is converted into electronic signals via a card reader. Until the mid-1970s, punched cards were the major secondary memory media used with computers. They are rapidly being replaced by floppy disks, which are less bulky, cheaper, and correctable.

Housekeeping functions: a class of low-level computer operations of little or no interest to users, but which are necessary anyway. For example, floppy disks must be formatted (initialized) before they are used. This is done with help from a disk-operating system (DOS), a system program (software) which "writes" a blank "table of contents page" (technically, a volume control block) on the disk. Friendly systems manage housekeeping functions. Some systems even do windows.

HPIB: acronym for "Hewlett-Packard interface bus," a system originally developed by the Hewlett-Packard Corporation to expedite data communication among measurement instruments (e.g., signal analyzers) and computers. This parallel interface system allows each device connected to a daisy-chain bus to serve as a "talker," a "listener," or both. The HPIB protocol is now standardized (IEEE technical standard 488) and is used by many other firms. Also called GPIB ("general purpose interface bus").

IBM card: see Hollerith card.

Icon: a pictorial representation of an object or function. Some computer systems use icons (shown on a display screen and selected with a cursor) to let the user control the system. A very friendly feature.

IEEE-488: the technical standard for the proprietary HPIB interface for connecting microcomputers to laboratory control and measurement devices. See also HPIB.

IEEE-696: the technical standard for the S-100 bus, an internal interconnection scheme (nonproprietary) for microcomputers. See also S-100 bus.

Image processing: a category of computer application focusing on the generation or enhancement of images from (typically) nonoptical sensing systems in order to reveal static or dynamic features otherwise indiscernible. Examples include computerized axial tomography (the "CAT scan"), computerized holography, and geophysical resource management. Also called "imaging."

Impact printer: a type of printer employing an inked ribbon and a striker mechanism to place images on paper. Some impact printers use discrete character systems (see also Daisy-wheel printer); others use matrices of individual dots (see also Dot-matrix printer).

Index variable: a numeric (integer) variable used to designate a particular element of an array (i.e., a subscript), or to tally the number of iterations of a loop (i.e., a counter). See also Numeric variable and String variable.

Information: meaningful symbols, text, images, or other signals derived from originally unorganized data. More generally, data and the programs which process data.

Information processing: the acquisition, manipulation, and disposition of information by electronic means.

Information retrieval system: see Data management system.

Initialize: to prepare for use. In computer programs, variables must be initialized (set to zero values) before they are used. In computer systems, disks must be initialized (erased, then given a blank "table of contents") prior to use.

Ink-jet printer: a type of printer that places images on paper by means of a matrix of tiny pens, each fed by a separate ink supply, or by means of a single stream of ink directed by puffs of air. This nonimpact printer technology is relatively fast and produces excellent quality images and graphics.

Input: any information (data or programs) entered into a computer. Input may include characters, graphics, electrical signals—virtually anything. See also GIGO.

Institute of Electrical and Electronic Engineers (IEEE): ("eye triple-e") an association of engineers and scientists with professional interests in electronics. The IEEE promulgates technical standards and recommended practices for computers, communications, and related systems.

Instruction: a command issued to a computer system by a computer program. Groups of allowable instructions (instruction sets) differ across central processing units (hardware) and across computer languages (software). In the most general sense, instructions include verb-analogs (called operations) and noun-analogs (called operands—the things operated on). Also called "statement."

Integer: a positive or negative number consisting only of a whole-number part, without fractions. See also Floating point.

Integrated circuit (IC): a miniaturized electronic circuit containing the equivalent of dozens, hundreds (MSI—medium-scale integration), or even thousands (LSI—large-scale integration) of discrete components.

Integrated software: a relatively new development for microcomputers in which different categories of application software (e.g., word processing programs, data base management programs, and graphics preparation programs) share a common data file structure. Thus, a user must enter data only once. More advanced integrated software allows several different programs or tasks to be "active" at the same time in a multitask environment. Integrated software requires specialized hardware and a specialized operating system. See also Networked structures.

Interface: (1) a device (hardware) that makes it possible for a central processing unit (or computer system) to communicate with peripheral hardware. For example, a printer interface lets a computer direct output to a printer. "Interface" is usually reserved for hardware, but many practical interfaces include firmware to make the hardware work. Interface programs are called "driver routines." (2) More generally, the place and manner in which dissimilar things meet (e.g., the "man–machine" interface).

International Standards Organization (ISO): a nongovernmental organization of national standards groups (e.g., ANSI) which develops and distributes technical standards for applications that transcend national boundaries.

Interpreter-oriented language: a category of computer languages that accomplish translation of source code (written by a programmer) into object code (required by the computer) at the level of the program statement or line. In other words, each program statement is translated into machine language as it is encountered, one line at a time. The resulting object code cannot be stored, but is executed immediately. A program must be translated each time it is executed. Interpreter-oriented languages are slower than compiler-oriented languages, but they are also easier to learn, write, and edit. BASIC and LOGO are examples of languages of this type. See also Translator.

Interrupt: a signal or event which causes a computer to pass control to a special interrupt-handling routine. Interrupts are used to tell a computer that a particular peripheral device needs attention.

I/O: input and output.

I/O-limited (or bound): a process or task, the most demanding feature of which is the entry and display of information. For example, generating form letters with a word processor consists mostly of output operations and entails very little actual processing of data. See also Process-limited.

Iterative process: a process that is repeated, usually many times. Examples include clinical activities such as giving, recording, and interpreting "routine" screening tests of articulation, language, and hearing, as well as much therapy drill work. Iterative processes, especially those which are formatted and rule driven, are prime candidates for computerization. Most high-level computer languages include control structures to facilitate iteration. Examples include the "FOR–NEXT" structure in BASIC and the "DO loop" in FORTRAN.

Joystick: a control device (hardware) consisting of two potentiometers (variable resistors), each wired as a voltage divider and connected to an analog-to-digital converter. The two "pots" are aligned in an *X–Y* coordinate pattern and are manipulated by a lever similar to an aircraft control stick (joystick). Alternatively, lever position may be sensed by optical techniques. Joysticks are used to provide two-dimensional control information to computers for applications ranging from games to industrial robotics.

Junk: information (data or programs) of no value.

Keyboard: a matrix of buttons arranged like a typewriter keyboard, but with additional keys for "CONTROL," "ESCAPE," special functions, cursor position control, repeat, and some or all of the following special symbols: <>, [,], { ,}, ~ , ˇ , ı . Keyboards are a major input device for microcomputers. This may seem trivial, but is not: in most cases, data are entered by keyboard, not by magic. This requires time and a typist. Although ASCII standardizes character codes for computers, computer keyboards are not standardized in terms of numbers, layout, size, or shape of keys.

Keypad: a specialized keyboard consisting of the numbers 0 through 9, and (on some keypads) additional keys for mathematical operators, the "RETURN" key, and other keys. Used primarily for numerical data entry.

Keypunch: an electromechanical device (hardware) equipped with a keyboard and used to place holes in Hollerith (IBM) cards. Keypunch machines were developed in the 1930s. They are rapidly becoming extinct, except in university computer centers.

Kilo (K): (1) metric prefix for one thousand. (2) In computer parlance, two to the tenth power (1,024).

Kilobyte: 1,024 bytes, or approximately one thousand bytes.

Knowledge base: see Expert system.

Language: see Computer language and Natural language.

Laser disk: see Video disk.

Laser printer: a relatively expensive type of printer used in large word processing and mainframe computer installations which uses a directed beam of coherent light to burn images onto the surface of a page. Laser printers produce extremely high-quality text and graphics at extremely high speed.

LCD: acronym for "liquid crystal display," an image technology developed in the late 1960s and used in calculators, digital watches, computer display screens, and contemporary microminiature televisions. LCDs are light-weight, low-resolution, low-power systems suitable for use with portable computers and computer terminals which do not require large numbers of characters.

LED: acronym for "light emitting diode," a solid state display technology developed in the middle 1960s and still used in some calculators and digital watches.

LIFO: acronym for "last-in, first-out." Information stored in a stack is managed on a LIFO basis.

Light pen: a control device (hardware) used to point to locations on a video display screen. A light pen is a stylus (connected to a computer or computer terminal by a wire) which senses the presence of illumination, as well as the synchronization pulse of video display. This allows identification of specific places on the screen. Light pens can be used to select options from a menu, or to move a cursor around on the display screen.

Line: (1) a group of characters on a single horizontal plane of a display screen. (2) A single statement in a computer program. (3) An I/O port of a computer or computer terminal. (4) A single channel of a communication network. (5) A speech to persuade a member of the opposite sex.

Linear programming: a style of programming in which subtasks are organized and sequenced in a "straight-line" manner from beginning to end. Linear programming avoids use of unconditional branching and subroutines. It tends to be useful only for fairly simple problems. See also Modular programming and Structured programming.

LISP: acronym for "LISt Processing language," a high-level computer language developed in 1958 by John McCarthy. LISP is a non-numerical language designed to process data organized in hierarchical structures (lists). It has seen extensive use in artificial intelligence and in the development of compilers. Originally, LISP was an interpreter-oriented language; it is also available as a compiler-oriented language.

Load: to move information from a peripheral (such as a disk drive) to a computer. See also Download and Upload.

Local-area network (LAN): a communication system for computers and/or computer terminals which uses dedicated interconnecting cables and permits exchange of messages, data, and programs among users of the network. LANs are used primarily as "inhouse" systems. See also Long-haul network (LHN).

Logic: hardware and/or software that perform operations employing deductive logic.

Logical decision: the ability of computer languages and programs to use arithmetic and Boolean logic to compare things (variables) and to act differentially on the basis of the result of the comparison. Boolean operations include relations such as identity (*a* equals *b*, *a* does not equal *b*), ordinality (*a* is less than *b*, *a* is greater than *b*), conjunction (logical AND, implying "both"), and disjunction (logical OR, implying "either"). The ability to use such operations makes possible sorting, merging, sequencing, and organizing of numerical and non-numerical data. Practical applications include alphabetizing names, categorizing disease states, and matching verbal discriptors (e.g., "normal intelligence") to numerical data (e.g., "IQ score = 105). Most high-level computer languages include control structures to facilitate logical decisions (e.g., the "IF-THEN" structure in BASIC and FORTRAN).

Logical organization: the way the resources of a computer system are organized for the user, as distinct from how they are organized for the computer. For example, a user may invoke a variable named "MEAN" to represent the result of a computation. The computer deals with that variable as an equation, the result of which is stored in a particular location in memory.

LOGO: a high-level computer language developed at the Massachusetts Institute of Technology by Papert in 1969 to teach children logical reasoning. Based upon the theories of Piaget, LOGO lets the learner "teach" the computer to do things. This language features strong graphics capabilities (via robots or screen display cursors called "turtles") and the ability of routines to invoke themselves (recursion). LOGO is an interpreter-oriented language available on many microcomputers.

Long-haul network (LHN): a communication system for computers and/or computer terminals which uses existing telecommunication systems and permits exchange of messages, data, and programs among users of the network. LHNs are used in cases where users are separated by significant distances. See also Local-area network (LAN).

Loop: a group of instructions or statements in a computer program that may be executed more than once. The number of times a loop is executed may be tallied by an index variable known generally as a "trip-counter."

Low-level language: a category of computer language relatively unlike natural language and relatively dependent upon particular computer hardware. Low-level languages are harder to learn and use than high level languages. Examples of low-level languages include assembly language and machine language. See also Computer language, High-level language, and Translator.

LSI: acronym for "large-scale integration," a manufacturing technology which places the equivalent of 5,000–100,000 discrete transistors on a single integrated circuit.

Machine language: a class of low-level computer languages using only numbers to express commands (operation codes), variables, and memory locations. Machine language is device dependent, that is, different central processing units employ different repertoires of commands. These are not compatible across processors. Machine language is not at all user friendly, but it is the fastest class of computer language.

Macro command: a group of commands in a computer program (software) treated as a unit; a command made up of a set of more primitive commands.

Magnetic bubble memory: see Bubble memory.

Magnetic disk: see Disk, Floppy disk, and Hard disk.

Main memory: see Primary memory.

Mainframe computer: initially the only computer configuration, "mainframe" now designates the largest of computers—large in size, memory capacity, and function. Modern mainframe computers employ from 1 to 1,024 megabytes of primary (main) memory and can access disk systems with billions of bytes of secondary memory. Mainframes accommodate from dozens to thousands of users simultaneously, each communicating with the computer via time-sharing terminals. Mainframe systems typically support multiprocessing, multiprogramming, and multitasking, and can operate at speeds up to 1,000 mHz. The first commercial mainframe computer was the Univac 1, introduced in 1951. The largest mainframe system now available is the Cray S-2, announced in 1983. See also Microcomputer and Minicomputer.

Mark-sense: a data-entry system by which pencil marks on formatted paper are converted to a digital code for subsequent processing by computer. The pencil marks (present or absent) constitute a binary code.

Mass memory: secondary memory of significant capacity.

Master control unit (MCU): a functional component of a central processing unit which decodes machine language instructions into actions and which coordinates the actions of other components (e.g., the arithmetic logic unit).

Mega (M): (1) metric prefix for one million. (2) In computer parlance, two to the twentieth power (1,048,576).

Megabyte: 1,048,576 bytes, or approximately one million bytes.

Memory: the systems used by a computer to store and recall data and programs. Memory size is expressed in numbers of bytes: one byte is equal to one typed character. Primary (or main) memory is that which can be directly addressed and controlled by the central processing unit. Modern systems use RAM, ROM, PROM, and EPROM for primary memory; microcomputers are available with 4–1024 kilobytes of main memory. Secondary (mass) memory is that which can be indirectly accessed by the central processor through an interface. The most common form of secondary memory is the magnetic disk. Disk systems for microcomputers can store from 80 kilobytes to 40 megabytes. Technologies for primary and secondary memory differ widely. See also Primary memory and Secondary memory.

Memory dump: an output or listing of the contents of a computer's primary memory. These data are "raw" in the sense that they are expressed in the internal number base (octal or hexadecimal) of the computer.

Menu: a list of program options available to a user, typically shown on a display screen. An option is selected with a single keystroke. Menus are characteristic of friendly systems.

Menu-driven software: a type of computer program that lets the user communicate with the program through selection of options from one or more menus. Programs of this type are easy to learn, but limited in flexibility. See also Menu and Command-driven software.

Merge: a process or program by which data from two or more files are combined to form a new file on the basis of some common attribute. For example, name–address files for 50 states might be combined in a new file organized alphabetically by name, or by zip codes in ascending order.

Microcomputer: a relatively small, freestanding computer system based upon a microprocessor. Microcomputers tend to be used as dedicated systems, but some can support up to 16 simultaneous users. See also Mainframe computer, Microprocessor, and Minicomputer.

Microprocessor: a large-scale integrated (LSI) circuit containing most or all of the components of a central processing unit. Microprocessors are available in 4-, 8-, 16-, and 32-bit configurations. Most microcomputers employ 8- or 16-bit microprocessors operating at speeds ranging from 1 to 10 mHz. See also Central processing unit (CPU).

Minicomputer: a middle-sized computer, larger than a microcomputer and smaller than a mainframe computer. Minicomputers are heavily used in laboratory and manufacturing settings and can support from dozens to hundreds of time-sharing users. Many minicomputer systems support multitasking and multiprogramming. See also Mainframe computer and Microcomputer.

Minifloppy disk: a 5.25-inch floppy disk, also called a diskette. See also Floppy disk.

Mnemonic: an acronym or other symbol used in place of something else that is harder to remember.

Mode: a condition or situation in which a particular set of rules apply.

Modeling: a category of computer application focusing on the simulation of real or imaginary people, places, processes, events, or things. Modeling employs mathematical and logical relations to mimic behavior and to predict outcomes of future events and hypothetical situations. Heavily used in business, engineering, science, education, and recreational gaming.

MODEM: acronym for "MODulator–DEModulator," a device (hardware) used to let data terminal equipment (DTEs, such as computers and computer terminals) communicate with each other over communication networks. The most common application of MODEMs is conditioning digital signals for communication over telephone lines. This is accomplished by *modulation* (binary signals from DTEs are changed into analog signals of different frequencies for sending) and *demodulation* (tonal analog signals are converted back into digital signals to be sent to DTEs). Connection to the telephone system may be by means of a connector or an acoustic coupler. MODEMs operate at different speeds (from 100–9600 baud) and in different configurations (originate only, answer only, originate–answer). MODEMs are a type of data communication equipment (DCE) designed to "expect" standardized (RS-232) asynchronous serial signals. See also Acoustic coupler, Asynchronous, Baud, Data terminal equipment, Data communication equipment, and Serial transmission.

Modular programming: a style of programming in which subtasks are configured as separate entities, then joined together to form an entire program. Subtasks are usually organized as subroutines, accessed as needed by the program. Modular programming is well suited to complex tasks, and to subtasks that can be "reused" in different programs. See also Linear programming and Structured programming.

Monitor: (1) a closed-circuit television set, that is, one without a channel selector (tuner). Video monitors are available as monochrome and color units. Some color monitors employ composite video signals. Others require separate signals for each color "gun" of the CRT (red, blue, green). Monitors generally produce higher resolution images than receivers. See also Receiver. (2) A system software program written in machine language that services relatively primitive functions, such as viewing the contents of a particular cell or location in primary memory.

Motherboard: the primary printed-circuit board of a small computer, often equipped with connectors to accept daughterboards.

Mouse: a control device (hardware) used to position a cursor on a video display screen. A mouse is a small box (connected to a computer or computer terminal by a wire) that can be moved across a flat surface. A ball bearing on the bottom of the mouse controls two potentiometers wired as voltage dividers. The signals from the "pots" feed a pair of analog-to-digital converters to index X-Y coordinate positions on the display screen. This allows two-dimensional placement of the cursor for menu and icon selection. Alternatively, a mouse may use optical techniques to detect position on a surface enscribed with a gridwork of lines. A very friendly feature, but one requiring sophisticated software.

MS-DOS: acronym for "MicroSoft disk-operating system," an operating system developed by Microsoft Corporation for use with 8086 and 8088 microprocessors. Originally, MS-DOS was very similar to CP/M, but recent revisions are more like the UNIX operating system. The current version of MS-DOS incorporates provisions for software integration (multitasking) and windows (i.e., screen display of up to four processes at one time). See also CP/M, Integrated software, UNIX, and Windows.

MSI: acronym for "medium scale integration," a manufacturing technology which places the equivalent of 100–5,000 discrete transistors on a single integrated circuit.

MTBF: acronym for "mean time between failures," a statistical estimate of the minimum use-life of hardware.

Multiplexing: simultaneous transmission of several sets of signals over a single communication channel. Multiplexing is commonly used in satellite communication, cable television systems, and computer communication systems.

Multiprocessing: processing accomplished by two or more computers (or central processing units) working in tandem and sharing a common work load.

Multiprogramming: the ability of a computer system to simultaneously execute programs written in different programming languages.

Multitasking: the ability of a computer system to execute more than one program or process at one time. In most such systems, one task is a foreground program, while others are background programs. See also Background and Foreground.

Native code: the machine language code for any particular central processing unit. A program may be written in several machine languages (one for each of several central processors), then distributed in "native code." See also P-code.

Natural language: human languages such as English, French, and German. Natural languages are less structured and more flexible than computer languages, but both types of language share common features (syntax, semantics, pragmatics). See also Computer language.

Natural language processing: a category of computer application with the goal of "understanding" natural languages as used by people in written and oral communication. An experimental area, most attempts at natural languge processing use syntax parsing and relational logic to resolve semantic content (meaning). Some work in natural language processing is based upon neurological evidence; other work has stimulated neurologic and linguistic research. See also Artificial intelligence.

Nesting: placing one or more subroutines inside of another subroutine. For example, a program which sorts elements in a name and address file might contain a routine to alphabetize names within a routine to order zip codes within a routine to alphabetize states.

Network: an interconnection of computers, computer terminals, and/or other devices. See also Local-area network (LAN) and Long-haul network (LHN).

Networked structures: a way of organizing data, processes, tasks, or people in which elements are related to each other in functional ways, rather than hierarchical ways. "Unorganized" social groups, self-help groups, and natural river systems are examples of networked structures. Some application programs (which integrate word processing, graphics preparation, and data base management) employ this structure to allow users to work on several tasks more or less simultaneously. Networked structures offer many paths for moving data and program control from one element to another. Thus, they are strong in flexibility, but weak in clarity. See also Hierarchical structures.

Nibble: half a byte or 4 bits.

Noise: any unwanted signal, electrical, acoustical, or conceptual.

Number crunching: a class of computer application involving large quantities of numerical data and/or large quantities of mathematical operations on data.

Numeric variable: a variable whose value is a number, either integer or floating point (real). See also Index variable and String variable.

Nyquist limit: a rule of thumb for sampling rate in applications involving analog-to-digital conversion: sampling rate should be at least 2.5 times the highest frequency component of the analog signal.

Object code: the binary version of a program, directly executable by a central processing unit.

Octal: eight. Referring to the base-8 number system. The digits 0 through 7 represent values in this system. Each digit in an octal number is a power of eight.

Off-line: a resource, process, or device not under direct control of a computer because it is incompatible, not connected, or turned off. Some operations are off-line because they are too complex or too poorly understood to be managed by machines. Others are "service" operations performed by people, for example, putting a disk into a disk drive.

On-line: a resource, process, or device under direct control of a computer, such as a disk drive or printer.

Operand: the variable "operated on" by a machine language command, distinct from an operation code (the command itself). For example, if an operation code (op code) indicates "add x," the operand is the quantity x.

Operating system: see Disk-operating system.

Operation code (op code): a command in machine language or the mnemonic for such an instruction in assembly language.

Optical character reader (OCR): a device (hardware) that converts standardized character shapes printed on a page into digital code for subsequent processing by computer.

Optical disk: see Video disk.

Optical scanner: any device (hardware) that converts image information of any type into digital code for machine processing.

Output: anything produced by a process, program, or computer and shown on a display screen, printer, or other such device. See also GIGO.

Packaged: see Canned.

Pagination: to number pages in ascending order. More generally, the format of printed material produced by a word processor or text processor, including justification, margins, line spacing, paragraph indentation, page numbering, and the use of headers and footers.

Parallel transmission: one of two major ways of sending electrical signals between central processing units and peripherals, and between computers and other devices. Parallel transmission employs several wires (usually, eight), each of which carries information. Coded information is sent as an ensemble of bits (zeros and ones) deployed across the set of wires. Parallel transmission is very fast, but operates well only over relatively short distances. See also Serial transmission.

Parity checking: a way to determine the validity of transmitted binary information. For each digital "word" of information, the sum of bits (zeros and ones) will always sum to either an odd number or an even number. Part of the word is a parity bit, the value of which (odd or even) is "set" when information is sent. If, at the receiving point, the parity bit equals the sum of the other bits, then (presumably) no information has been lost in transmission.

Pascal: (1) a high-level computer language developed in 1971 at the University of California at San Diego and licensed for use on many microcomputers. A highly standardized language, Pascal forces the use of very explicit structures in designing and writing programs. Pascal is well suited to tasks involving graphics, numerical operations, and character manipulations. Although it employs a straightforward syntax, it is harder to learn than LOGO or BASIC. Programs written in Pascal execute very quickly, but require a large amount of primary memory. Pascal is a compiler-oriented language. Pascal object code is expressed in p-code, a highly "portable" language. See also P-code, P-system, and Portable. (2) A seventeenth century French scientist, noted for his contributions to physics and mathematics and developing an early mechanical calculator. (3) The metric unit for pressure.

Patch: a temporary, ad hoc repair to a program. By connotation, an action directed at symptoms, rather than causes. Too many patches produce bombs.

Pattern recognition: a category of computer application which focuses on the identification of patterns extracted from real-world events for the purpose of subsequent machine action. Examples include speech recognition, robotic "vision," and the recognition of disease states from descriptions of symptoms. Identification is usually accomplished through comparison of digitized samples (things to be recognized) to normalized templates of exemplars (targets). Originally an area of artificial intelligence, pattern recognition has become a practical engineering art.

PC-DOS: A proprietary version of MS-DOS developed for use with 8088-based microcomputers manufactured by IBM and other firms.

P-code: an intermediate-level computer language which is machine language for an idealized "pseudomachine" emulated on a large number of real microprocessors. Emulation is usually accomplished by an interpreter (written in native code) each time a p-code program is executed. See also P-system.

P-system: an operating system developed at the University of California at San Diego (UCSD) and commercially marketed by Softech Microsystems in 1979. The p-system is independent of hardware, meaning that it works with microcomputers based upon any of a large number of microprocessors (e.g., 6502, Z80, 8080, 8086, 8088, 68000, 9900). This is accomplished by the contrivance of a "pseudomachine" which is emulated on real microprocessors through p-code translators (a different translator for each microprocessor). The advantage of the p-system is that programs written in p-code (or translated into p-code from high-level languages such as BASIC, Pascal, Forth, or FORTRAN) can be executed without modification on a large number of different microcomputers. The p-system supports several utility programs and several high-level languages.

Peripheral: in a strict sense, any device (hardware) distinct from a central processing unit. More generally, any devices physically separate from a computer (e.g., graphic tablets, touch pads, printers, plotters, and disk drives).

PILOT: acronym for "programmed inquiry learning or teaching." PILOT is a high-level computer language designed for use in interactive computer-assisted instruction. It is available in several dialects which differ significantly in ease of use and efficiency. PILOT is one of several authoring languages developed for teaching purposes; it is available on several microcomputers.

Pixel: the smallest manipulable element of a graphic display.

Plotter: see Digital plotter.

Polling: one of several ways a computer checks peripherals to see if they have anything to communicate. When an interrupt signal occurs, peripherals are sampled until one is found that needs service (input or output). Polling is also used in communication networks to determine the status of terminals.

Port: a communication channel, or the connector (hardware) associated with that channel.

Portable: (1) the ability of computer hardware to be moved from one location to another. (2) The ability of computer software to be executed on more than one manufacturer's hardware.

Primary (main) memory: all the memory (of whatever technology—RAM, ROM, PROM, EPROM) that can be directly addressed and modified by the central processing unit of a computer. Distinct from secondary memory, which requires the intervention of an interface, primary memory usually requires less time to access than secondary memory, but has less information capacity. See also Memory.

Printed circuit board (PCB): see Circuit board.

Printer: a device (hardware) that places characters and/or graphics on paper. See also Character printer, Dot-matrix printer, Impact printer, Ink-jet printer, Laser printer, and Thermal printer.

Process: any action taken with data which modifies the value, form, format, location, or organization of data.

Process control: a category of computer application in which a computer manipulates external events by means of a predefined set of rules, modified as necessary by responses sampled from the real world. Examples include industrial robots used in manufacturing and the heating, ventilation, and energy systems of large buildings. An additional example is in laboratory research in the behavioral and physiological sciences, where events and signals can be controlled to stimulate a subject and where responses can be acquired and analyzed in real time.

Process limited (or bound): a process or task, the most demanding feature of which is the set of operations that intervene between the entry of data and the display of results. For example, computing Fourier transforms (spectra) of speech waveforms requires a great deal of processing and relatively little effort in data input and data output. See also I/O limited and Number crunching.

Program: (1) a sequence of instructions which tells a computer to do something. (2) The directions given to a computer by a person.

Program counter unit (PCU): a functional component of a central processing unit which contains the memory addresses of instructions in a program. The PCU keeps track of the last and the next step in the program. See also Central processing unit.

Program generator: a category of software (application or system, depending upon perspective) which writes programs. Program generators ask the user questions about form, format, and quantity of input data, the form, format, and quantity of output data, and the processes that intervene between input and output operations. Programs of this type differ in terms of the computer languages in which they generate programs, and in the efficiency of the resulting code. Program generators attempt to bridge the gap between natural language and computer languages, but they still require sophisticated users. They are most successful in data base management tasks and less successful in other application areas.

Program line editor (PLE): a category of utility software which helps a programmer enter and edit source code. PLEs are essentially specialized word processors optimized for particular computer languages to simplify typing of commands, moving to particular locations in the source code, and editing statements or variable names with minimal retyping. PLEs are found in some (not all) disk-operating systems, and are available as separate utility programs.

Programming: (1) the process of analyzing problems, defining algorithms, coding those algorithms in a particular computer language, entering and editing program code, testing and debugging the program, and documenting the finished product. Programming also entails maintaining the program over time and instructing end-users in the implementation of the program. (2) An art form involving computers.

Programming language: see Computer language.

PROM: acronym for "programmable read-only memory," an information storage technology used in microcomputers. PROMs are integrated circuit devices (hardware) which store binary information indefinitely. They are irrevocably programmed by applying relatively high voltages, thus burning away tiny traces inside an integrated circuit. PROM is nonvolatile, requiring no power to retain information.

Prompt: (1) a symbol or text issued by a computer, a computer terminal, or a computer program which signals the operator that a response is possible or required. System prompts include cursors of various shapes to tell the user the current mode of operation or computer language. (2) An explicit question (e.g., "WHAT IS TODAY'S DATE?") or instruction (e.g, "PRESS RETURN TO CONTINUE") issued by a computer program.

Punched-paper tape: an early secondary memory storage medium which used patterns of punched holes to represent alphanumeric, control, and other types of characters. Hole patterns followed either the 7-bit ASCII code or the 5-bit Baudot code. Paper tape was generated and read by specialized devices commonly associated with electromechanical teletypes (TTYs). Punched-paper tape was inexpensive and (with proper care) relatively nonvolatile; it was also slow and limited in capacity. See also ASCII, Baudot, and TTY.

Queue: an ordered, temporary sequence of data, processes, tasks, programs, or people. For example, a print queue might consist of a set of reports of client evaluations, each awaiting its "turn" at the printer. Also, what computer idiots and computer nerds stand in while waiting for unemployment checks.

QWERTY keyboard: the standard typewriter keyboard layout for English.

RAM: acronym for "random-access memory." RAMs are integrated circuit devices (hardware) which store binary information until electrical power is removed. RAMs differ in access speed (from 1–4 mHz), memory capacity per chip (1–256 kilobytes), and requirements for maintenance of stored information. Dynamic RAM must be continuously refreshed by the computer to retain information; static RAM does not require refreshing. Dynamic RAM can be accessed more rapidly than static RAM. RAM is preferred as primary (main) memory in modern computers.

Random access: a way of accessing a particular location in memory directly by its address. See also Sequential access.

Random data file: a collection of data stored in secondary memory and organized by records consisting of one or more fields. For a particular file, all records must have the same number of characters. Random data files are more economical of storage space and allow faster access to individual records than do sequential data files. Random data files also permit access to individual records and fields in any order. See also Sequential data files.

Raster graphics: a method for implementing graphics on a display screen which creates images with hundreds or thousands of pixels. Low-resolution raster graphics are characterized by "straight" lines that look like staircases. See also Character graphics and Vector graphics.

Read/write memory: a class of computer memory that allows the user to put information into memory (write) and recall information from memory (read).

Real-time process: a process or event that happens at rates independent of a computer.

Real-time clock: an electronic device (hardware) that keeps time in terms important to people, that is, year, month, day, hour, minute, second, millisecond. Distinct from the clock associated with the central processing unit of a computer.

Real number: see Floating point.

Receiver: (1) a television set equipped with a channel selector (tuner) to sense commercial broadcasts. Many small computers are able to use receivers as display devices, but with less resolution than can be obtained with a monitor. See also Monitor and RF modulator. (2) Any device which accepts signals from another device (source).

Record: a category of information consisting of several related fields. In a file of names and addresses, a record might be the name, street number, street name, city, state, and zip code for a particular individual. In this example, the "unit of record" is the person. See also Field and File.

Recursion: the ability of a process to invoke simpler versions of itself or parts of itself. A linguistic example of recursion is the sentence, "Nothing is absolute, including the statement 'nothing is absolute.'" Some computer languages allow recursion (e.g., Pascal), others do not (e.g, BASIC and FORTRAN).

Reflective video disk: see Video disk.

Register: a section of memory in a central processing unit set aside for temporary storage of data, results, and memory addresses. Most processors contain several registers.

Repeat key: a special key on a keyboard which, when pressed simultaneously with another key, causes the character produced by the other key to be repeated.

Reset key: a special key on a computer keyboard that causes the central processing unit to stop, then restart as if the computer had just been turned on. This voids the contents of primary memory, resulting in the loss of program and data.

Reserved word: a sequence of characters which may not be used as a variable name because that sequence has special meaning to a computer language or operating system. See also Variable.

Resolution: the detail and clarity of an image (graphics or characters) on a display screen or printed page. In video monitors and receivers, resolution is largely a function of the bandwidth of the device: the higher the bandwidth, the better the resolution.

Return: to exit a subroutine and go back to the program that called it.

Return key: a standard key on a computer or computer terminal keyboard that causes the current line of characters to be sent to the central processing unit for action. The return key usually also causes the cursor to drop down a line and return to the left margin of the display screen.

RF modulator: "Radio-frequency" modulator, a device (hardware) that converts the video output of a computer (or video game) into a signal detectable by the tuning section of a television receiver.

RGB monitor: see Monitor.

RJE: acronym for "remote job-entry terminal," a workstation from which data and programs may be directed to a minicomputer or mainframe computer located some distance away. Many RJEs consist of computer terminals, card readers, high-speed line printers, data concentrators, multiplexers, and MODEMs.

Robot: a programmable, electromechanical device (hardware) capable of limited sensing and manipulation, independent of other machines. The word "robot" was coined in 1922 by Karel Capek, a Czechoslovakian dramatist.

ROM: acronym for "read-only memory." ROMs are integrated circuit devices (hardware) which store binary information indefinitely. The information in ROM is recorded when the chip is manufactured and cannot be erased. ROM is used to store low-level system software that must always be available to the central processing unit (e.g., the programs that service the keyboard and boots the system).

RS-232: a standard for serial communication between data terminal equipment (DTE) and data communication equipment (DCE). The standard specifies electrical signal levels, connector size and shape, and signal functions. RS-232 designates several configurations ranging from a simple three-wire system to a more complex system with multiple handshaking lines. The most common of these is RS-232C.

Rubout key: a special key on a keyboard which causes the cursor to backspace and erase a character.

Rule-driven process: a task which can be completed through application of a set of rules for making decisions. Examples include interpretation of tympanograms and methods for administering standardized receptive vocabulary tests. When the rules for a process are both explicit and unambiguous, that process may be well suited to automation.

S-100 bus: an internal interconnection scheme by which certain 8-bit microprocessors communicate with computer subsystems located on separate printed circuit boards. Subsystems include primary memory and a variety of interfaces for peripheral equipment (disk drives, printers, MODEMs, etc.). Developed in the mid-1970s for microcomputers based upon 8080, 8085, and Z-80 microprocessors, the S-100 bus is the most common nonproprietary computer bus now available. See also IEEE-699.

Search-and-replace: a feature of some word processors, text editors, and program line editors by which a user can find one, some, or all occurrences of a specified set of characters and replace that set with a new sequence of characters.

Secondary memory: memory electronically addressed and modified by a central processing unit working through an interface (i.e., indirectly). Secondary memory is used to store relatively large programs and bodies of data, and is generally nonvolatile (persists when electrical power is removed). Examples include magnetic and video disk systems. See also Memory.

Semiconductor: a substance (e.g., silicon treated with trace elements) which behaves as an insulator or as a conductor of electrons, depending upon how energy is applied to it. Semiconductor materials are used extensively in transistors, integrated circuits, microprocessors, and other solid state devices.

Sequential access: a way of accessing a particular location in memory indirectly through reference to relative position. See also Random access.

Sequential data file: a collection of data stored in secondary memory and organized in serial order. For a particular file, individual records and fields may contain different numbers of characters. Sequential data files are less economical of storage space and more time consuming to access than random data files, but they are simpler to understand and use. To access a particular element in a sequential file, it is necessary to first access all of the preceding elements. See also Random data file.

Serial transmission: one of two major ways of sending electrical signals between central processing units and peripherals, and between computers and other devices. Serial transmission employs a minimum of three wires (one to send, one to receive, and one electrical ground). Additional wires may be used to control information flow (i.e., handshaking lines). Coded information is sent as a sequence of bits (zeros and ones), one after another. The sequence for a coded character includes seven or eight data bits. Additional bits may be included to signal the start and stop of a character, and/or to check the validity of transmission (a parity checking bit). Serial transmission rates are generally slower than parallel transmission rates, but serial transmission can be used over much greater distances. The RS-232 standard specifies the most common serial transmission protocol. See also Handshaking signals, Parallel transmission, Parity checking, and RS-232.

Scrolling: the horizontal or vertical movement of characters across the face of an electronic display device (e.g., a video monitor).

Sheet feed: a mechanism found on some printers by which single sheets of paper can be automatically positioned for printing. Also called "cut-sheet feed." See also Tractor feed.

Simplex: a serial asynchronous communication protocol which allows sending of information in only one direction. An example of a simplex system is transmission of information from a computer to a printer. Other examples include classroom lectures, sermons, and similar one-way conversations. See also Half-duplex and Full-duplex.

Simulation: see Modeling.

SLSI: acronym for "super large scale integration," a manufacturing technology which places the equivalent of more than 1,000,000 discrete transistors on a single integrated circuit.

Softcopy: transient, physically insubstantial output, such as that shown on a video monitor, as opposed to more permanent output (i.e., a printed page). See also Hardcopy.

Softkey: a programmable or user-defined function key on the keyboard of a computer or computer terminal. See also Function key.

Software: the "logical" part of a computer or other system, as opposed to the physical part. Computer software includes programs written to serve the application needs of users, the utilitarian needs of users and programmers, and the system needs of the computer itself. See also Hardware and Firmware.

Solid state: electronic components which use solid materials, such as transistors, LCDs, LEDs, and integrated circuits. Solid state devices differ from vacuum tubes, incandescent lamps, coils, condensers, and other components which use gas or liquids.

Sort: a process or program by which data in a file are placed in an ordered sequence on the basis of values of a common attribute. For example, elements of a name-income file of speech-language pathologists might be placed in order of ascending salary. Sorting often involves counting the number of elements in a file which share identical values of a common attribute (e.g., all certified speech-language pathologists whose income exceeds the average income of programmers). See also Merge.

Source code: a computer program as written by a programmer. Source code must be translated into object code before it can be executed.

Special characters: printing and nonprinting characters other than numbers and letters. For example: !, #, ð $, %, ^, &, *, (,), <,>, ?, ", ', :, ;, { ,}, [,], - , _, and ~ . Nonprinting characters include control characters and escape sequences.

Special purpose computer: a computer of any class (micro-, mini-, or mainframe) which is used for only one purpose, or for a very small number of specialized tasks. Special purpose computers usually support only one or two computer languages. Examples include computers used for cryptography, medical image processing, industrial process control, and evoked-response audiometry. See also General purpose computer.

Speech recognition: a category of computer application with the goal of "understanding" human speech. This is accomplished by "training" the recognition system with repetitions of words or phrases. A "template" is generated from these exemplars. An utterance to be recognized is compared to each template. The comparison yielding the smallest discrepancy index designates the "recognized" utterance. Small systems are capable of recognizing up to 64 words spoken by one talker; larger systems are capable of recognizing thousands of words spoken by any of several talkers. All such systems require limited "vocabularies." Speech recognition systems are used in inventory and process control, as well as security work.

Speech synthesis: a category of computer application intended to generate speech by one of several methods: digital recording and playback of speech waveforms, dynamic mathematical modeling of the vocal tract, or dynamic mathematical modeling of the acoustical parameters of speech. Current synthesizers differ considerably in intelligibility and quality. Some systems employ text-to-speech translation software capable of reasonable prosody. Speech synthesis systems are used in toys, vending machines, watches, unattended banking services, and voice-output communication aids (VOCAs).

Spooler: a hardware or software buffer which allows information to be output without the "attention" of the central processing unit (CPU), thus making the CPU available for other tasks. Spooling is often used in word processing to permit simultaneous printing and editing. See also Buffer.

Spreadsheet: a category of computer application in which a user can enter, modify, and manipulate data organized in rectangular arrays of rows and columns (tables). A given cell in the array may contain numerical data, a mathematical equation, or a logical relation that uses data placed elsewhere in the table. This computational ability makes it possible to answer "what if" questions about data. Spreadsheet programs are used in financial planning, business record keeping, and clinical applications based upon single subject designs.

Sprite: a graphic figure treated as a unit and capable of being moved about on a display screen. Some microcomputer systems allow use of several sprites simultaneously, reserving a "plane" for each one. Sprites are used in recreational games and computer animation.

Stack: a reserved area in memory used to temporarily store information in a one-dimensional array. A stack (analogous to a pile of dishes) is referenced by order, rather than by address. Data are entered and retrieved from a stack on a LIFO (last-in, first-out) basis: the last datum "pushed" onto the top of a stack will be the first datum "popped" off the stack.

Statement: a line of code in a computer program, analogous to a sentence in natural language. See also Instruction.

Statistical processing: a category of computer application which summarizes the characteristics of samples (descriptive statistics), or which tests hypotheses about the characteristics of samples or populations (inferential statistics). Previously in the domain of mainframe computers, statistical processing is now common on microcomputers.

Status line: (1) an electrical connection (hardware) which conveys information about the state of a process or device. (2) A line of characters (software) shown at the top or bottom of a display screen which conveys information about the state of a program, or about the options currently available to the user.

Stringy floppy: a device (hardware) employing magnetic tape as a memory storage medium. Stringy floppies can store vast amounts of information, but are too slow to use as secondary memory. They are used primarily to backup hard disk systems. See also Backup and Hard disk.

String variable: a variable, the value of which is a sequence of alphanumeric characters treated as a unit. For example, a BASIC string variable named Day$ might have a value equal to the characters "March 30." String variables may include letters, numbers, punctuation marks, and some special characters. Where numbers are used as strings, they are treated as literal symbols, rather than numerical quantities. Most computer languages that support string varibles permit concatenation and limited logical operations on strings. See also Index variable and Numeric variable.

Structured programming: a style of programming which places special emphasis on creating explicitly organized, formatted, and annotated source code. Structured programming employs modules (subroutines) organized in a top-down pattern and avoids unconditional branching. It was developed to manage teams of programmers so as to simplify program construction, debugging, and maintenance. Some computer languages are inherently structured (e.g., Pascal); others are not (e.g., BASIC). See also Linear programming, Modular programming, and Top-down design.

Synchronous: timed. Synchronous communication protocols require that both ends of a communication channel share a common pacemaker (clock signal). Synchronous systems can operate at higher speeds than asynchronous systems.

System: a collection of interactive and interdependent elements, such as a school system, the human nervous system, or a computer system. The elements of a system may include goals, people, hardware, processes, inputs, outputs, and feedback signals, any of which may vary in time. In computer parlance, "system" denotes integration of hardware and software. See also Hardware and Software.

System analysis: a profession which focuses on the interaction (sequential, hierarchical, networked, or otherwise) of functionally related elements, usually for the purpose of improving the effectiveness, efficiency, or clarity of the system. Systems analysis is based on a more fundamental discipline variously referred to as "system science," or "system theory," the goal of which is understanding and predicting the behavior of complex assemblages of interdependent parts. See also System.

System software: a class of computer programs designed to solve low-level problems directly associated with the functioning of a particular computer system. Examples include disk-operating systems, computer programming languages, and I/O device drivers. See also Application software and Utility software.

Subroutine: a self-contained segment of a larger program or process. Subroutines are modules designed to accomplish a particular task, constituent to the overall purpose of a larger program. They can be accessed (called) by the larger program as often as necessary. For example, a program that computes means and standard deviations might contain one subroutine to input data from a keyboard, another to trap typing errors (e.g., the letter O instead of the number 0), another to show results on a display screen, and another to list results on a printer. In most computer languages, subroutines can be nested inside of other subroutines.

Table: any organization of information in a rectangular array of rows and columns.

Table look-up: a programming technique which circumvents long or difficult computations by storing results in a table (array) that can be accessed by a program or subroutine. Particular cells in the table are retrieved through the use of subscripts. See also Variable.

TDD: acronym for "telecommunications device for the deaf." Originally called "teletypewriters" (TTYs) because they transmit text over distances, the first TDDs were surplus devices rented or given to deaf persons by firms engaged in commercial telegraph and telephone communication. Because they are relatively old, proprietary systems, TDDs use communication protocols which differ from those used with modern computers. See also TTY.

Telecommunication: generally, communication over distance. More specifically, electronic communication involving machines (or people and machines) which uses existing telephone, radio, and television systems. Voice, text, photographs and other images, and handwriting are among the signals that can be sent and received via telecommunication.

Terminal: generally, an input or output device (hardware) at one end of a communication network. More specifically, "terminal" refers to a computer console. See also Console.

Text: Any alphanumeric information.

Text editor: a computer program or system which does text editing. See also Text editing.

Text editing: a category of computer application which allows electronic entry, editing, manipulation, and printing of textual information, usually in the context of programming. Although "text editing" is often used as a synonym for "word processing," the two differ. Text editors were originally used to enter and edit source code computer programs. Hence, they employ automatic line-numbering and variable name cross-referencing functions not present in word processors. Text editing systems are often line oriented (i.e., the line is the smallest accessible unit of text), whereas word processing systems are character oriented. The two applications are otherwise very similar. See also Program line editor (PLE) and Word processing.

Text file: a data file coded in the form of ASCII character codes, as opposed to binary codes.

Text processing: a category of computer application which accepts print format commands, then processes a file of textual material in the manner specified by those format commands. "Text processing" is often used synonymously with "word processing," although the text processing function is only one of those associated with word processing. See also Word processing.

Text processor: a computer program or system which does text processing. See also Text processing.

Thermal printer: a type of dot-matrix printer employing thermally sensitive paper and a print mechanism consisting of a matrix of electronic wires. When current passes through individual wires, heat is generated and a pattern of dots is placed on the paper. Thermal printers are fast, quiet, and inexpensive, but they require relatively expensive paper.

Throughput: the ability of a computer or other system to do work, expressed in terms of speed. Throughput is a "bottom line" concept influenced by all the hardware and software components of a given system. See also Input and Output.

Time sharing: a style of computer use in which several users (from a handful to hundreds) can simultaneously access programs available to a computer, as well as enter and execute their own programs. In this mode, the computer interacts with users, sharing time with each as necessary. Access to time-sharing computers is usually via MODEMs and telephone lines. See also Batch processing and Multitasking.

Top-down design: a way of developing computer programs in a modularized hierarchy which proceeds from general (at the top) to specific (at the bottom). The top-down approach involves the design, coding, and testing of high-level modules before low-level modules. Top-down design is the opposite of bottom-up design, in which low-level (detailed) tasks are approached first. See also Hierarchical structures and Modular programming.

Touch pad: a control device (hardware) which senses the position of a stylus or finger on a flat rectangular surface. Touch pads offer less resolution than graphics tablets, but can be used to effectively control the position of a cursor in graphics, gaming, or program control operations. See also Graphics tablet.

Touch screen: a control device (hardware) which senses the position of a finger on a display screen. Touch screens are used to select menu options from graphic or alphanumeric lists of alternatives. They typically use arrays of light-emitting diodes (LEDs) and light-sensing diodes placed around the perimeter of a video screen. When a finger interrupts a pair of invisible infrared light beams, the X-Y coordinate position of the interruption is sent to a computer via an interface. Touch screens offer low resolution (16-by-16 LED arrays are typical), but are very friendly.

Trackball: a control device (hardware) similar in purpose and operation to a joystick, but which uses a movable sphere instead of a lever. Trackballs can be designed to sense velocity as well as direction. They are used in real and simulated weapons systems. See also Joystick.

Tractor feed: a mechanism found on some printers by which edge-perforated, continuous-sheet paper can be automatically positioned for printing. See also Sheet feed.

Transceiver: a communication device (hardware) capable of transmitting and receiving information.

Transistor: a semiconductor device that can control electron flow discretely (gating) or continuously (valving). Transistors are the building blocks of integrated circuits used in digital applications.

Translator: a system program (software) which converts source code (written by a programmer) into object code (required by computers). Translators may accomplish conversion one line at a time as a program is entered (interpreters), or at the level of the entire program (compilers). Written in machine language, translators are (or should be) transparent to the user. See also Compiler-oriented language, Interpreter-oriented language, Object code, and Source code.

Tree structures: a way of organizing data, processes, tasks, or people in a strict heirarchy somewhat like a family tree. In a binary tree structure, for example, each node (junction point) gives rise to a pair of branches, each of which ends in a subsidiary node. Tree structures are used in studies of deterministic decision making. See also Hierarchical structures and Networked structures.

TTL: acronym for "transistor–transistor logic," a category of semiconductor technology used for digital logic and control. The TTL family is fast and enjoys wide use, but requires more electrical power than the CMOS family. See also CMOS.

TTY: acronym for "TeleType," an electromechanical computer terminal device (hardware) consisting of a keyboard, printer, paper tape reader-punch, and interface circuits. TTYs were developed in the late 1940s and for 25 years served as the major means by which people communicated with computers. TTYs also were used for electronic written communication between people over distance. Relatively slow (100–300 baud), noisy, serial asynchronous systems, TTYs have been all but replaced by CRT terminals. The term "TTY"

is sometimes used to refer to any device which uses the RS-232 communication protocol. Although "TTY" has been used to refer to telecommunication devices for the deaf (TDDs), the two systems do not share compatible protocols. See also TDD.
Turing test: a criterion for machine "intelligence" posed by Alan Turing, British mathematician and contributor to the development of modern computers. If an intelligent human interacts with a computer by means of a terminal and cannot distinguish the behavior of the computer from that of a person, then the computer is "intelligent."
Turn-around time: the time elapsing between the beginning and completion of a program, process, or task.
Turnkey system: a self-contained, integrated system of hardware and software delivered as a "plug-it-in-and-turn-it-on" product.
Turtle: a special cursor used with the LOGO computer language to generate graphics (turtle tracks). Originally, turtles were limited to display screens. Later, hardware turtles were developed (small, wheeled robots capable of holding pens). In LOGO parlance, turtles can be "taught" to make pictures, graphic designs, and geometric shapes. Thus, the "teachers" (young programmers) learn to use coordinate systems.
UART: acronym for "universal asynchronous receiver transmitter," an integrated circuit device (hardware) which converts external serial signals into parallel signals for use by a computer, and vice versa. UARTs are used to facilitate communication among computers and peripherals. See also Serial transmission and Parallel transmission.
Unbundled: see Bundling.
UNIX: an operating system developed at Bell Laboratories in the late 1960s. UNIX is a multiuser, multitasking system based on a "toolbox" concept of utility programs to allow "piping" results from one program to another through "filters" that sort, count, and tag data. UNIX also uses tree structures to organize large numbers of disk files into smaller groups of files. UNIX requires more primary memory than other 16-bit operating systems (too much for 8-bit computers), but is extremely powerful. See also Xenix.
Upload: the process of directing data files or program files from a small computer, computer terminal, or other device to a large computer via a communication network.
Up time: an interval during which a system functions properly. See also Down time.
Upward compatible: a feature of computer systems by which early versions of hardware and software remain compatible with newer versions. Upward compatibility is sometimes more hope than fact.
User friendly: see Friendliness.
Utility software: a class of computer programs designed to handle more-or-less routine tasks. Utility programs may be dependent or independent of particular microprocessors. Very often, they are distributed as enhancements to operating systems (system software). Examples include debuggers, program line editors, and sort–merge programs. See also Application software and System software.
Variable: a named quantity whose value can be changed. For example, a quantity named "SRT" might be set equal to 25. In most computer languages, variables can be subscripted in one or two dimensions. A one-dimensional variable is called a "scalar array" and a two-dimensional variable is called a "vector array" or "table." A variable named "AGE (7)" might equal 30, the age in years of the seventh person in a group. "IQ (2,5)" might refer to the intelligence quotient of the fifth child in a second-grade class. In the last example, grade might be symbolized by "G" and child by "K." Thus the expression "IQ (G,K)" refers generally to a two-dimensional array, of which "G" and "K" are subscripts or index variables. Variables may refer to numeric values or simply to strings of symbols (numbers or letters). See also Index variable, Numeric variable, and String variable.
Vector graphics: a method for implementing graphics on a display screen which plots lines between points specified in terms of X-Y coordinates. See also Bit-mapped graphics, Character graphics, and Raster graphics.

Video disk: a type of secondary memory which stores information on a rigid, removable platter capable of digitally storing video images, audio signals, data, and computer programs. Information is recorded by a device that produces an intense beam of coherent light (a laser) that burns pits onto the surface of the disk. Because recording permanently alters the disk, video disks are read-only memory. Information is retrieved by a low-intensity laser reflected from the surface of the disk. Video disks require specialized disk drives, hardware interfaces, and file management software. They are true mass-storage systems because they can store billions of bytes of information. Also called "reflective" or "optical" video disks to distinguish them from capacitive video recording methods (which use disks, but employ an incompatible recording principle). Video disks are currently used in advertising and computer-assisted instruction. See also Disk and Disk drive.

Video monitor: See Monitor.

Videotex: a commercial telecommunication subscription service by which individuals using telephone lines, a MODEM, and a computer terminal can view electronic newspapers, magazines, and advertising, as well as access shopping and banking services. Videotex also supports electronic mail and computer time-sharing services.

Virtual machine: a computer capable of simulating several different computer systems simultaneously in real time. Virtual machine simulation is accomplished logically, rather than physically.

Virtual memory: a way of managing primary memory that effectively expands capacity beyond what is physically available. This is accomplished by an operating system that "swaps" parts of data or program files between primary and secondary memory. This is done transparently (i.e., rapidly and without demands on the attention of the user).

Voice-output communication aid (VOCA): a category of computer application which combines speech synthesis with a variety of specialized input control devices and microcomputers or microprocessors to facilitate communication. VOCA systems may be based upon general purpose or special purpose computers and are most often used by persons with cerebral palsy, dysarthria, or other neuromotor difficulties that preclude normal speech production. VOCAs have also been used by laryngectomy patients and (experimentally) by stroke victims.

Voice processing: a category of computer application which treats speech signals as data to be recorded, transmitted, and reproduced in a manner analogous to electronic mail. Used primarily in business communication. See also Electronic mail.

Voice recognition: see Speech recognition.

Voice response: see Speech synthesis.

Volatile memory: a category of computer memory which requires the presence of electrical power to maintain information. When power is lost, so is information. RAM is volatile; ROM, magnetic disks, and video disks are not.

VLSI: acronym for "very large scale integration," a manufacturing technology which places the equivalent of 100,000 to 1,000,000 discrete transistors on a single integrated circuit.

Wand: a hand-held device (hardware) equipped with an optical scanner to read universal product code (bar code) information. Wands contain a solid state device which senses the width and number of blank vertical bars printed on a white background. The wand is connected to a computer or terminal by means of a cable and an interface. Wands are used in retail applications to electronically read product codes, manage inventory, and generate customer invoices.

Warm start: the process of starting a computer by stopping, then restarting the central processor, or by rebooting the computer system. Electrical power is not interrupted, but information in primary memory is lost. See also Cold start.

Wild card: a special character used (literally) in the place of other characters in a command to a program. Wild cards (an asterisk in some programs) are inserted in formatted commands to indicate "any string of characters is acceptable."

Window: a viewing area on a display screen. More generally, a mode of information display in which several different tasks can be shown simultaneously on a high-resolution video monitor. Windows make it possible for a user to access, control, and see the status of several application programs (e.g., word processing, spreadsheets, graphics preparation) at one time. Thus, a user can use the display screen as if it were the top of a desk. "Windowing" is new to microcomputers and requires special hardware, special application software, and special system software (all of which are proprietary at present). Windowed systems require integrated software; they typically use virtual memory, icons (to indicate control options), and a mouse (to select icons). An extremely friendly feature. See also Icons, Integrated software, Mouse, and Virtual memory.

Winchester disk: see Hard disk.

Word: the smallest unit of information that can be addressed by a computer. Most microcomputers use 8-bit (1-byte) or 16-bit (2-byte) words; some mainframe computers use 32- or 64-bit words. "Longer" words usually permit faster, more precise processing.

Word processing: a category of computer application which allows electronic entry, modification, editing, and printing of textual information. Word processing can facilitate production of formatted correspondence (e.g., clinical reports), material subject to revision (e.g., research reports), and lengthy documents (e.g., books). Word processing systems require (at least) a computer, a keyboard, a display screen, a printer, disk memory, and software. Most such systems let the user electronically duplicate, delete, and move blocks of text (words, sentences, and paragraphs) in a document. A major strength of word processors is that the printed format of a document can be manipulated independently of the text itself; paragraph indentation, justification, vertical spacing, page width and length, and other format features can be changed by simple commands, rather than by retyping text. Various auxiliary programs exist to support word processing (spelling checkers, thesauruses, grammar aids). See also Header, Footer, Pagination, and Search-and-replace.

Word processor: a computer program or system which does word processing. See also Word processing.

Write enable: a hardware or software method to allow placement of new information in secondary memory. For example, when the notch on a 5.25-inch floppy disk is uncovered, information can be placed on the disk. A write-enabled system works as read–write memory. See also Write protect.

Write protect: a hardware or software method to ensure against unintended loss of information in secondary memory by "overwriting" old information with new information. Floppy disks contain notches (hardware) which, when covered, prevent recording of information. (Audio cassette tapes use an opposite technique: when the plastic tab on the edge of the cassette is removed, sound cannot be recorded.) Most disk-operating systems include commands (software) which write protect specified files of information on a disk. A write-protected system works as read-only memory. See also Write enable.

Xenix: a commercial version of the UNIX disk operating system marketed by Microsoft Corporation. See also UNIX.

X-Y plotter: see Digital plotter.

Author Index

A

Abbs, J., 190
Adams, P., 211
Adams, R., 150
Adams, S., 244
Adams, T., 211
Ahl, D., 27
Allard, K., 157
Allen, D., 149
Allen, J., 117
Anderson, J., 248
Anthony, A., 152
Archambault, P., 150
Artwick, B., 88, 90, 91, 92, 109, 111, 114
Atal, B., 117

B

Bailey, D., 85
Bar, A., 22
Baughman, S., 272
Becker, S., 255, 256
Bejar, I., 98
Bennett, R., 26, 27
Berger, K., 161
Berryman, J., 166
Berst, J., 60, 67, 68, 75
Beukelman, D., 27, 161
Billingham, K., 85, 190
Bird, R., 177
Birnbaum, M., 67, 68, 69
Bishop, J., 235
Blache, S., 159
Blodgett, A., 85
Blumenthal, H., 56, 57, 58, 73
Bogle, D., 152
Bolton, B., 28
Bonner, P., 75
Boothroyd, A., 150
Borko, H., 86, 93
Bowers, J., 60
Bruman, J., 66
Budoff, M., 254
Bull, G., 85, 191

C

Cahill, B., 83
Carlson, F., 30
Carrick, R., 255
Carter, J., 116
Carterette, E., 85, 114
Casbon, S., 65
Castelewitz, D., 57
Chapman, R., 160
Chin, K., 257
Ciarcia, S., 110, 111
Cohen, C. G., 127
Cohen, V. B., 126, 127
Collopy, D., 69, 70, 250
Consumer Reports, 5, 244
Cook, S., 127, 142
Cox, L., 200
Craik, F., 10
Cross, T., 27
Cush, 11, 244

D

Data Sources, 85, 120
Datapro, 22, 23
Datapro Research Corp., 127, 128, 129, 130, 131
Daynes, R., 98
Deloche, G., 153
Demartino, M., 72
Dence, M., 194
Deruyter, F., 30
Dickerson, L., 149
Dillon, R., 84
Dirks, D., 85, 114
Durrett, H., 85

E

Eckerman, D., 85, 112
Edwards, W., 148, 153, 156
Eggebrecht, L., 93
Elliott, L., 149

Elovitz, H., 117
Enderby, P., 161
Engebretson, A., 85

F

Faucett, R., 148, 168
Fawcette, J., 75
Feldman, H., 85
Feldman, W., 190
Fields, T., 149, 151
Fitch, J., 27, 29, 149, 152, 244
Flanagan, J. L., 176, 179
Flannagan, J., 113, 116
Flavey, N., 149
Flowers, J., 85, 177
Foltz, G., 85, 98, 112
Fons, K., 118
Fontana, D., 10
Foree, D., 85, 112
Fox, A., 57
Fox, B., 147, 149, 152, 157, 162, 163
Frankel, P., 127, 131, 133
Frillman, L. W., 176
Fritz, B., 212
Fuchs, V., 73

G

Gabel, D., 156
Gagne, R., 194
Galland, F., 56
Gans, D., 161
Garetz, M., 92
Gargagliano, T., 118
Garrett, E., 150
Gibbs, L., 66
Glatzer, H., 130, 244
Gleason, G., 135, 149, 252, 269
Golas, K., 216
Gold, J., 238
Goldband, S., 108
Goldes, H., 212
Goldsbrough, P., 114
Gordon, W., 85, 112
Graham, N., 126, 127, 142
Gras, A., 127, 131, 133
Grossnichle, D., 197
Grosswirth, M., 66
Gruschow, J., 235
Gupta, A., 85, 143

H

Hanauer, H., 117
Hannaford, A., 127, 131, 250, 252
Hannan, J., 58
Hansen, J., 116
Harden, R. J., 149
Harden, R. W., 149
Harlan, D., 7
Hartmann, J., 238
Hartnell, T., 56, 57
Hazen, M., 211
Hedberg, G., 27
Heidt, M., 19
Heilborn, J., 57
Helms, H., 56
Herschler, M., 205
Hertz, S., 117
Heyer, J., 10
Heywood, S., 91
Hight, R., 149, 152
Hirsh, A., 181
Hixson, J., 7
Hoffberg, A., 70, 71
Hoffman, R., 250
Hoffmeister, A., 27, 247
Holland, A., 150
Holmes, G., 215
Hon, D., 98, 214
Houston, J., 92
Humphrey, M., 214
Hutten, L., 254

I

Ingram, T., 152

J

Jacoby, L., 10
Janke, R., 65
Jarrett, T., 97
Jay, T., 215
Johnson, R., 117, 166
Jones, B., 147, 161

K

Kafatou, T., 57, 75
Kalikow, C., 149, 150, 151
Kamm, C., 85, 114
Katz, K., 7, 153, 161

Katz, R., 7, 153
Kehberg, K., 162
Keller, E., 178
Kieras, D., 85
Kihneman, K., 152
King, T., 90, 91
Kirchner, G., 214
Kleinman, G., 214
Knight, B., 90, 91
Kolotkin, R., 85, 190
Kramer, J., 148, 168
Kruglinski, D., 238
Kursan, B., 196
Kusak, J., 60

L

Laefsky, I., 98
LaPointe, L., 165
Larkins, P., 7
Larson, D., 93
Lasky, E., 10
Lathrop, A., 128, 135, 136
Leger, D., 177, 85
Leibson, S., 100, 110, 111
Lemmons, P., 86
Levin, W., 214
Levine, S., 18, 24
Levinson, S., 113
Liberman, M., 113
Lieff, J., 71, 72
Lombardino, L., 157
Lowe, D., 85
Lund, T., 114
Lutman, M. E., 178, 179
Lutus, P., 244

M

Macurik, K., 149, 153, 156
Mager, R., 20
Malinconico, M., 70
Marchionini, G., 61, 70
Margolis, A., 83
Martin, J., 238
Mason, M., 73
Matthews, J., 151
Mau, E., 83
Mayer, R., 85
McCarr, J., 162
McCorkell, W., 9
McCullough, L., 149
McDonald, E., 152
McDougal, A., 211

McHugh, A., 117
McIsaac, M., 152
McNiff, M., 127, 142
McWilliams, P., 84
Meilach, D., 72, 77
Messial, S., 149
Metzger, E., 70, 71
Milich, M., 116
Miller, J., 160, 244
Miller, M., 85
Mills, R., 147, 149, 157, 158, 165
Minifie, F., 266
Mitchener, J., 133
Moberg, D., 98
Montague, C., 83
Moore, M., 97
Moran, T., 97
Mordecai, D., 155, 159, 160, 177
Morgan, C., 255, 256, 257
Morgan, D., 85, 114
Moulard, J., 153
Moursund, D., 11, 29
Munro, A., 116

N

Nagy, V., 153
Naiman, A., 18, 20, 23
Naisbitt, J., 263
Nakatani, L., 117
Nash, K., 66
Newton, M., 159
Nickerson, R., 8, 10, 12, 13
Norris, M., 149
Norwood, D., 23, 61, 75

O

O'Shea, T., 193, 209, 214
Ojala, M., 65
Okada, M., 173, 178
Onosko, T., 214
Oratio, A., 178
Orwig, G., 194
Ozley, C., 148, 168

P

Page, J., 238
Palin, M., 159, 160, 177
Palmer, C., 159, 160, 177
Papert, S., 9, 11, 210, 271
Park, O., 209, 214

Perera, T., 83
Peterson, H., 149
Pierrehumbert, J., 117
Plum, T., 212
Plummer, H., 17
Poirot, J., 19
Poltrock, S., 85, 112
Poole, L., 57, 127, 142
Popelka, G., 85, 161
Power, D., 147, 161
Price, D., 211
Pritchard, W., 149
Purnelle, J., 176, 181, 190

Q

Quigley, S., 147, 161

R

Rabiner, L., 116, 117
Raleigh, C., 10
Raskin, J., 84
Rayner, J., 114
Reed, A., 85
Reid, B., 157
Remer, D., 255, 256
Renshaw, S., 149, 151
Rienhoff, E., 57
Roberts, D., 238
Roberts, F., 209, 214
Roberts, S., 64
Roblyer, M., 127, 131, 216
Rochowansky, W., 244
Rockman, I., 63
Rodwell, P., 126, 244
Rogers, E., 23
Rojas, A., 194
Roose, T., 59
Rosen, A., 244
Rothchild, E., 98
Rothfeder, J., 75, 248
Rouselle, M., 153
Roworth, M., 161
Rubin, C., 67, 72
Rudow, R., 190
Rushakoff, G., 27, 29, 131, 135, 147, 148, 149, 150, 153, 157, 165, 169, 196
Russell, S., 9, 11
Ryder, A., 200

S

Salathiel, R., 152
Sarisky, L., 97
Saxon, J., 212
Scanland, W., 193, 197
Schafer, R., 116, 117
Schmeltz, L., 244
Schneider, W., 83
Schwejda, P., 95, 112
Sclater, N., 116
Sebestyn, L., 214
Segal, H., 60, 75
Self, J., 193, 209, 214
Seron, X., 153
Shaffer, R., 255
Shaffert, T., 18, 24
Shane, H., 12
Shea, R., 250
Shea, T., 250
Shoemaker, F., 23
Shore, J., 117
Silverman, F., 174, 175
Simpson, D., 235
Sims, D., 214
Sippl, C., 56
Slattery, D., 193, 197
Sloane, E., 250
Smith, A., 66
Sohr, D., 135, 136
Somers, R., 149, 150, 152
Sonies, B. C., 7
Spindler, L., 235
Stallard, C., 25
Stanton, J., 244
Steffin, S., 201
Steinberg, E., 201
Steinkamp, M., 147, 161
Stephens, J., 251
Stephenson, J., 83
Stevens, K., 149, 150, 151
Stiefel, M., 235
Stilwell, T., 84
Stolker, B., 3
Sturdivant, P., 139
Sutton, D., 98
Swallow, L., 71

T

Taber, F., 11, 23, 57, 75, 127, 131, 133, 252
Telage, K., 150, 152, 178
Terrio, L., 149, 152
The, L., 97
Thomas, A., 85

Thomas, R., 147, 149, 157, 158, 165
Thorkildsen, R., 157
Tidwell, A., 148, 168
Tilley, B., 200
Titus, C., 93
Titus, J., 93
Tompkins, W., 190
Toong, H., 85, 143
Tossi, M., 147, 149, 150
Trachman, P., 196, 200
Traynor, C., 161
Troutner, J., 214

V

Valente, J., 9, 11
Vanderheiden, G., 12, 31, 85, 112
Vaughn, G., 12, 148, 168
Vegley, A., 149
Veit, S., 101
Vinson, B., 149
Voiers, W., 118

W

Wagner, W., 194
Wainer, H., 8
Walk, R., 10
Wasserman, P., 69
Watts, N., 149
Weiner, F., 159, 163, 165, 166
Weir, S., 9, 11
Welch, M., 83
Wells, R., 244
Wertz, F., 162
Wertz, J., 162
Whitacker, L., 83
Whitney, T., 84
Wilber, L., 147
Williams, A., 61
Willis, J., 85
Wilson, M., 147, 148, 152, 157, 162, 163
Witten, I., 109, 110, 116, 174, 184
Wolf, C., 95, 106
Woznak, D., 10

Y

Yorkston, R., 27, 161
Yutzy, M., 10

Z

Zicker, J., 190
Zinagle, T., 91
Zweiner, C., 85

Subject Index

A

Ada, 212
   see also languages
Adaptive testing, 8
   see also applications software
   see also clinical applications
ADC
   see analog to digital conversion
Administrative applications, 5-7, 149-150, 165-166, 233-244
   custom software applications, 222-233
   data base management, 6, 165-166, 190-191, 235-240
   private practice, 28-29, 233-245
      see administrative functions
   school settings, 26-27, 166
      see administrative functions
   spread sheets 190-191, 233-235
   word processing, 166, 190-191, 240-244
Administrative applications in research, 190-191
Administrative functions, 5-7, 219-221
   custom programs, 221-223
      see applications software
   microcomputer functions, 219-220
   packaged programs, 220
      see vertical applications software
Agencies and associations, 60-62
   clearinghouses, 61
   consortiums, 60-61
   funding agencies and associations, 61-62
   professional associations, 60
   state education agencies, 61
Algorithms, 80
Analog data, 80
Analog to digital conversion, 114-115, 174, 175, 183-188
Apple Education Foundation, 46-47
   see also funding sources
Applications
   administrative, 209-215
   clinical, 147-171
   instructional, 193-218
   research, 173-191
Applications software, 127, 142, 219-221
   general purpose software, 127, 142, 219-221

      see general purpose software
   vertical applications software, 127, 220
      see also software types
Applying microcomputer instruction, 197-201
   advantages of CAI, 8-10, 197-198
Artificial intelligence, 177, 181
Assessment programs, 27, 147-148, 159-161
Attitudes, 22-23, 27, 260-262
   see also selection criteria
Authoring programs, 213-214

B

Backup policies, 137-138
   see software selection criteria
Basic, 209-210
   see languages
Baud rate, 107
Benchmark testing, 82, 130
   see evaluating software
Billing, 224
   see custom software
Bit, 88
Bit width, 88
Byte, 82

C

C, 212
   see Languages
CAI, 8-11, 193-217
   see computer assisted instruction
CAI for anatomy of the ear, 204-206
Central Institute for the Deaf, 149
Central processing unit, 2, 86-92
   design, 88-91
   selection, 91-92
   variations in CPU design, 88-91
Checklists/rating scales, 133
   see software selection criteria
Chronicle of Higher Education, 39-40
   see funding opportunities
Client assessment, 7-8, 27
   see clinical applications

Subject Index

Client census information, 224
  see custom software
Client processing, 149-150, 224
  see custom software
Clinical applications, 7-11, 147-171, 222-240
  aphasia, 153
  articulation assessment, 152
  articulation therapy, 153-155
  augmentative communication, 30
  blissymbols, 162
  child language, 152-153
  client assessment, 7-8
  clinician microcomputer education, 29, 168
  clinics & hospitals, 30-31
  data base management, 165, 235-240
  existing applications, 7-11, 158-165
  generating clinical reports, 165-166, 221-223
  hardware needs, 155-158
  historical developments, 149-155
  limitations, 167-168
  private practice, 28-29
  rationale, 147-149
  remedial/instruction, 8-11
    see CAI
  school settings, 25-28
  software availability, 166
  speech recognition, 156-157
  spread sheets, 233-235
  word processing, 166, 240-244
Clinical software, 3-4, 7-8, 158-165
  analysis software, 7, 27, 159-161
  therapy software, 8, 161-165
Committee on Personal Computers and the Handicapped, 14
Communication aids, 31
  see input devices
  see output devices
Communication buses, 92-93
Communication devices, 3, 106-108
  MODEMs, 3, 106-108
Communication packages, 107
Compatibility
  functional, 83-84
  hardware compatibility, 83-84, 98-99 100-101, 105, 107, 108, 115, 116, 118
  operator compatibility, 84
  physical, 83-84
  software compatibility, 4, 84, 98-99, 100-101
Compiler programs, 142
  see languages
Component costs, 6, 12
  see trends in microcomputer technology
Component size, 12
  see trends in microcomputer technology
Computer assisted instruction, 8-11, 193-202
  advantages of CAI, 195-196
  CAI characteristics, 193-194
  costs, 200-201
  drill and practice, 11
  instructional applications in speech hearing, 196-197
  interactive video, 214-215
  microcomputer teacher function, 194
  outline of the CAI program, 194
  simulation, 11
  tutorial, 10
  uses for CAIs, 195-196
Computer literacy
  levels of computer knowledge, 2, 247-248
  cyperphobia, 271-272
Computer Users in Speech and Hearing (CUSH), 244
  see users groups
  see informational resources
Computers and other information processors 79-81
  characteristics of information processing systems, 80
  computers as information processors, 81
Conduit, 61
  see informational resources
Considerations
  compatability, 83-85
  costs, 6, 264-265, 272
  funding, 37-38
  improvement, 269-270
  limitations, 270-272
  misapplications, 270
  parallel systems, 24
  rate of adoption, 23
Consortium and network proposals, 37
  see proposal types
Consultants, 5, 22, 37, 67-70, 129
  determining needs, 68, 127
  locating consultants, 69-70
  selecting a consultant, 68-69
  services provided, 67-68
  systems investigation, 22, 128-131
  see informational resources
Controllers, 98
COPH-2, 14
  see Committee on Personal Computers and the Handicapped
Coprocessor, 92
Copyright Act (1980), 255
Copyrights, 255-256
Costs of microcomputer systems, 6, 94, 96, 107, 108, 114, 115, 116, 264-265, 270, 272
Costs, software
  computer assisted instruction, 200-201
  direct costs, 140
  see software selection criteria

indirect costs, 140
   see software selection criteria
Costs: Hardware
   analog to digital converters, 114-115
   memory, 94, 96
   MODEMs, 107
   output devices, 6, 101-108, 115-119
   real time clocks, 108
   speech recognition, 30, 114
CPU
   components, 86-88
   selection, 91-92
      see central processing unit
   special applications, 91
Curriculum proposal, 36
   see proposal types
Custom software, 221-233
   see applications software
   billing, 224
   client processing, 5-7, 149-150, 165-166, 223
      see administrative applications
   clinic census, 224
      see administrative applications
   student processing, 222-233
      see administrative applications
Cyberphobia, 248-250
   see issues and controversies

D

DAC, 80
   see digital to analog conversion
Data
   analog data, 80
   digital data, 80
Data base management, 235-240
   ASHA clock hour requirements, 222-224
   limitations, 236, 237
   retrieval of information, 236, 237
   types of, 236-238
      see packaged software
Data base searches, 59
Data sampling rate, 184-188
Dealers, 72-75
   services provided, 72-73
      see microcomputer dealers
Dedicated function keys, 135
   see ease of use, software
Demonstrations, software, 129-130
   see software selection criteria
Department of Education, 48-49
   see funding sources
Detectors
   event detectors, 182
   level detectors, 182

Determining software requirements, 127
   see software evaluation steps
Digital data, 80
Digital to analog converters, 119, 188-189
Digitized speech
   see speech synthesis
Direct memory access, 91
Disk operating system, 126, 141, 143
   see systems software
Documentation, 135-137
   feature organization, 136
      see software selection criteria
   reference manuals, 135-137
      see software selection criteria
   task organization, 136
      see software selection criteria
   tutorials, 136
   types, 136
      see software selection criteria
DOS
   see disk operating system

E

Earnet, 66
   see online databases
Ease of use, software, 4, 133-135
   menu driven, 3
Electronic mail, 66
   see teleconferencing
ENIAC, 12, 86
Equipment proposal, 36, 37
   see proposal types
Error trapping, 134-135
   see usability
Evaluating hardware systems, 81-86
   general evaluation parameters, 81-84
   the evaluation process, 81-84
Evaluating software, 127-131
   benchmark testing, 130
   demonstration, 129, 130
      see software evaluation steps
Expanded CAI features, 202-205

F

Fatal error, 134
   see ease of use
Features, programming languages, 142-143
Federal Grants and Contracts Weekly, 38
   see funding opportunities
Fipse, 49
   see funding sources
Firmware, 81

Floppy disks, 96-97
FORTH, 4, 211-212
   see instructional languages
Framework for research, 176-180
   thinking clinically, 179
   thinking numerically, 177-178
   thinking patterns and symbols, 178-179
Functions of information processing systems, 81
Funding considerations, 37-38
Funding opportunities, 38-40, 61-62, 63
   Chronicle of Higher Education, 39-40
   Medical Research and Funding Bulletin, 38
   National Institutes of Health Bulletin, 39
   National Science Foundation Bulletin, 39
   News Notes—The Grant Advisor, 39
   Research Monitor, 38-39
Funding Sources, 45-50
   Apple Education Foundation, 46-47
   Department of Education, 48-49
   FIPSE, 49
   National Science Foundation, 49
   NINCDS, 47-48
   state agencies, 49-50
   Tandy TRS-80 Program, 45-46

G

General applications software
   word processing, 190-191, 240-244
General architecture for microcomputers, 86
General purpose peripherals, 99-108
   communication devices, 106-108
   input devices, 99-101
   output devices, 101-106
   real time clocks, 108
General purpose software
   data base management, 165-166, 235-240
   electronic spread sheets, 190-191, 233-235
   see administrative applications
Generating clinical reports, 165-166
Generations of computer technology, 86
Graphics displays, 189
Graphics, 102

H

Hard disks, 97-98
   see secondary memory
Hardware
   decision making parameters, 85-86
   documentation, 84
   selection guides, 81-84
Hardware evaluation, 81-86
   benchmark testing, 35-36, 82
   parameters, 81-84
   process, 85-86
   strategy, 81
Hardware implications
   interfaces, 88-89
Hardware operating requirements, 82
Hardware systems
   architecture for microcomputers, 86
   central processing units (CPUs), 2, 86-92
   communication buses, 92-93
   computers and information processors, 79-81
   evaluating hardware systems, 81-86
   general purpose peripherals, 99-108
   implications for communication disorders, 119-120
   interfaces, 108-111
   memory systems, 82, 86, 93-99
   special purpose devices, 111-119
   the marketplace and costs of progress, 120
High level languages, 3-4, 141-142
   see programming languages
Hollerith cards, 93

I

I/O channels, 181-182
IEEE-488 (HPIB) interface standard, 110-111
IEP programs, 8, 166
   see applications software
Impact of microcomputers, 266-272
   awareness of limitations, 270-272
   present status of utilization, 267-268
   professional reactions, 268-269
   utilization of microcomputers, 267-270
Impacts on research directions, 176-180
   answering research questions, 180
   interactive research, 179
Implementing microcomputers, 25-31
   academic settings, 29-30, 171-191, 222-223, 232-240
   see instructional applications
   applications in schools, 25-28, 235-244
   see clinical applications
   clinical & hospital, 30-31, 233-245
   private practice, 28-29, 221-244
   see clinical applications
Implications: hardware
   input devices, 2, 100-101
   output devices, 105-106, 107-108
   primary memory, 82, 86, 94-95
   secondary memory, 82, 86, 95-99
Increasing reliability, 13
   see trends in microcomputer technology

Information processing systems
  characteristics, 53-78
Informational resources
  agencies and associations, 5, 14, 60-62
  books and journals, 57-58, 84-85
  Committee on Personal Computers and the Handicapped, 14
  consultants, 5, 67-70
  dealers, 72-75
  libraries, 53-60
  outline data bases, 62-67
  users groups, 14, 70-72, 76
Input devices
  cursor, 100
  functions, 99
  general purpose, 99-101
  keyboards and keypads, 9-100
  light pen, 100, 157
  mouse, 100
  special purpose, 112-115
  touch sensor, 100, 157
Installation, software, 130-131, 139
  see software selection criteria
Instructional applications, 3-4, 8-11, 193-218
  advantages of CAI, 195-196
  disadvantages of CAI, 198
  instruction for young children, 198-200
  kinds of CAI programs, 10-11
    see CAI
  meeting instructional demands, 200-201
  needs for instructional applications, 196-197
  what CAI can offer, 8-10
    see CAI
Instructional languages, 3-4, 208-212
  see languages
Interactive video instruction, 214-215
Interfaces
  classes of interfaces, 108-109
  digital interfacing, 181-182
  standards for interfaces, 109-111
Interfacing analog signals, 183-190
  analog to digital converters, 114-115, 183-188
  digital to analog converters, 188-189
  precision, 183-184
  sampling rate, 184-188
  schmitt triggers, 183
Interfacing responses, 181-182
  simple switches, 182
Internal proposals, 44-45
Interpreter programs, 142
  see languages
Issues and controversies, 14, 247-258
  computer literacy, 2, 247-248, 271-272
  cost effectiveness, 264-265, 270
  cyberphobia, 248-250
  piracy, 14, 254-257

privacy, 14, 98-99
qwerty phenomenon, 271
software development, 252-254
software selection, 250-252
software validation, 265-266
trends, 12-14
Issues in selecting software, 3-4, 250-252
Issues in software development, 252-254

J

Joysticks and other devices, 189

K

Keyboards, 145
  see input devices

L

Lamps and relays, 115
Languages, 3-4, 141-143, 208-212
  Ada, 21
  Basic, 4, 200-201, 209-210
    see high level languages
  C, 212
    see high level languages
  computer language, 3-4, 208-220
  features, 208
    see programming languages
  FORTH, 4, 211-212
    see high level languages
  high level, 3-4, 199-200, 208, 210
    see programming languages
  Logo, 4, 11, 199-200, 208, 210
    see high level languages
  low level languages, 142-143
  Pascal, 211
    see high level languages
  Pilot/Superpilot, 211
    see high level languages
Large scale integration, 81
Leasing
  software, 138
Library services, 54-60
  data base search services, 59
  dictionaries & encyclopedias, 56
  directories, 56-57
  indexes and abstracts, 57-58
  journals, 57-58, 84-85
  microcomputer books, 57
  reference books, 56-57
Logo, 9-10, 11, 199-200, 210-211

see instruction languages
Low level languages, 142-143, 208
   assembly language, 142-143, 208
      see programming languages
   machine language, 142, 208
      see programming languages
LSI, 81
   see large scale integration

M

Magic cymbals, 30
   see therapy programs
Making a CAI program, 202-207
Medical Research and Funding Bulletin, 38
   see funding opportunities
Memory, 82, 86, 93-99, 143
   requirements, 143-144
Memory access, 91, 94-96
Memory capacity, 82
   byte, 82
Memory systems, 82, 83-99
   primary memory, 82, 86, 94-95
   secondary memory, 82, 86, 96-99
   system implications, 98-99
Microcomputer assisted assessment, 8-11, 27, 147-148
Microcomputer dealers, 72-75
   see dealers
Microcomputers
   considerations for adoption, 25
   constraints, 31
   functions, 220
   reasons for adoption, 17-18
Microsift, 61
   see information resources
MODEM, 3, 106
   types, 106-108
      see communication devices
Monitors
   RGB, 102
   monochrome, 103
   LCD, 103
MTBF (mean time between failures), 83
   see hardware evaluation

N

National Institutes of Health Bulletin, 39
   see funding opportunities
National Science Foundation Bulletin, 39
   see funding opportunities
Needs analysis, 20-21, 127
   see phases of implementation

News Notes — The Grant Advisor, 39
   see funding opportunities
NINCDS, 47-48
   see funding sources

O

Online databases, 62-76
   electronic mail, 66
   funding information from databases, 63
   hardware and software, 66
   merits of use, 63
   microcomputer databases, 62
   speech & hearing databases, 62
   using data bases on microcomputers, 65
   using online data bases, 65
Operating systems, 141
   see systems software
Operations evaluation, 24, 81, 129-130, 133-135
   see phases of implementation
Oregon, 11
   see computer assisted instruction
Outline of the CAI program, 194-195
Output devices, 101-108
   communication devices, 106-108
   functions, 101
   general purpose, 101-106
   monitors, 101, 103, 156-157
   printers, 3, 103-106, 156
   print spoolers, 116
   real time clocks, 108
   special purpose, 115-119
   video terminals, 101

P

Packaged software programs, 233-244
   see applications software
   data base management, 235-240
      see administrative applications
   word processing, 190-191, 240-244
      see administrative applications
   spread sheets, 233-235
      see administrative applications
Parallel interfaces, 108-109, 111
Pascal, 211
   see instructional languages
Performance, software, 132-133
   see software selection criteria
Peripherals, 144
Perspectives, 249-273
   historical point of view, 262-263
   impact on the profession, 267-272

microcomputers as technological achievements, 266-267
microcomputers in perspective, 263-267
reflections of trends in society, 263-264
state of the art, 259-262
Phases of implementation, 17-25
   Phase I: Planning and Preparation, 18-20 67-68
   Phase II: Task Analysis, 20
   Phase III: Needs Analysis, 21-22, 220, 233-244
   Phase IV: Systems Investigation, 21-22, 67-68, 81-86, 272
   Phase V: Staff Preparation, 22-23, 70-72, 75-77
   Phase VI: System Installation, 23-24, 130-131, 139-140
   Phase VII: Operations Evaluation, 24, 131-137
Pilot/Superpilot, 211
Piracy, 14, 254-257
   copyright protection, 255-256
   Legal protection methods, 255-256
Planning and preparation, 18-20
   see phases of implementation
Portability
   hardware, 83
   software, 83
Primary memory, 94-95
   characteristics, 86, 94
   EEPROM, 95
   EPROM, 95
   PROM, 95
   RAM, 94
   ROM, 94
   types, 86, 94-95
Print spoolers and buffers, 116
Processing data
   batched processing, 177
   real time processing, 177
Professional impacts, 263-264, 266-267
Programming languages
   see languages
Project special, 6, 7
   see database management
Proposal contents, 40-43
Proposal generation, 40-44
   contents, 40-43
   strategy, 40
Proposal strategy, 40
Proposal types, 35-40
   consortium or network proposals, 37
   curriculum proposal, 36
   equipment proposal, 36-37
   requests for proposals, 37
   research proposal, 35-36

   special projects, 37
Protection
   hardware, 98-99
   software, 137-138, 256-257

R

RAM, 44
   see random access memory
Random access memory types, 94-95
   dynamic ram, 94
   static ram, 94
Rate of adoption, 23
   see considerations
Read only memory, 94-95
Real time clocks, 108
Recommendations, CAI, 216
Register types, 90-91
Remate, 12, 168
Requests for proposals, 37
   see proposal types
Research applications, 173-191
   a research framework, 174-176
   impacts of microcomputers on research, 176-180
   objective measurements, 175-176
   reliability and validity, 175
   strategies for research applications, 180-190
Research monitor, 38-39
   see funding opportunities
Research proposal, 35-36
   see proposal types
RF modulator, 102
RGb, 101-102
   see output devices
Rollover, 100
   see keyboards
ROM, 94-95
   see read only memory
RS-232C interface, 109-110, 185

S

Schmitt triggers, 183
Schneier Communication Unit, 30
   see clinical applications
Screening software information, 128-129
   see software evaluation
Secondary memory
   characteristics, 95-96
   floppy disks, 96-97
   functions, 95
   hard disks, 97-98
   random access, 95-96

Subject Index

sequential access, 96
Security
    hardware, 98-99
    piracy, 255-257
    privacy, 14, 98-99
    software, 137-138, 256-257
        see protection
Sercc, 5
Serial interfaces, 109
Servicing, 83
Simulation problems: CAI, 205
Single entry function, 224, 226, 231
Software
    reasons for considering, 132
    turnkey programs, 139
Software command types
    command driven software, 134
        see usability
    menu driven software, 3, 134
        see usability
Software evaluation, 127-131
    determining requirements, 127, 233-234
    feature specification, 133
    installation, 130-131
    rating forms, 133
    screening information, 128-129
    software selection, 4-5, 130
    standards, 133
    steps, 127-131
Software features
    user friendliness, 4, 133-134
Software in audiology, 7
    see applications software
    hearing aid fitting, 7
Software installation, 131
    see software evaluation steps
Software rating forms
    see software evaluation steps
Software selection, 131-141
    see software evaluation steps
Software selection criteria, 131-141
    checklists/rating scales, 5, 133
    costs, 140
    documentation, 135-137, 250-252
    ease of use, 3, 133-135
    software performance, 132-133
    support, 137-139
Software standards
    see software evaluation
Software system considerations
    memory, 127, 222-233
Software types, 3-4, 126
    applications software, 127, 222-233
        see custom software
        see packaged software
    systems software, 4, 126, 141, 143

    see systems software
Special net, 66
    see online databases
Special project proposals, 537
    see proposal types
Special purpose devices, 111-119
    input devices, 112-115
    output devices, 115-119
    special tasks, data and users, 111-112
Special purpose input devices, 112-115
    analog to digital converters, 114-115, 183-188
    graphic tablets, 113
    paddles and joysticks, 113-114
    speech recognition systems, 30, 113-114
    switch closures, 112
Special purpose output devices, 115-119
    digital to analog converters, 119, 188-189
    lamps and relays, 115-116
    printers and spoolers, 3, 116
    sound effects and music, 118-119
    speech synthesis systems, 3, 30, 117-118
Speech recognition, 3, 30, 113-114, 156-157
    clinical applications, 156-157
    direct speech recognition, 113-114
    dynamic speech recognition, 113-114
Speech synthesis
    linear coding, 117-118
    linear predictive coding, 117-118
    pulse coding modulation, 117-118
    systems, 3, 30, 116-118, 153, 155, 157-158
Spread sheets, 190-191, 233-235
    see packaged software
Staff preparation, 22-23, 75-76, 139-140
    see phases of implementation
State and local agencies, 49-50
    see funding sources
Strategies for research applications, 190-191
    graphic displays, 189-190
    interfacing analog signals, 183-190
    interfacing responses, 181-182
    joysticks and other devices, 189
Student practicum, 222, 224
    see custom software
Student processing, 222, 224
    see student practicum
Support services, 137-138
    dealer support 73-75, 138
        see software selection criteria
    manufacturer support, 137-138
        see software selection criteria
Switch closures, 112
System installation, 23-24, 130-131
    see phases of microcomputer implementation
Systems investigation, 21-22, 81, 86, 127-131, 271-272
    see phases of microcomputer analysis

Systems software, 4, 81, 141, 143
see types, software

T

Talking Blissapple, 30
see therapy programs
Tandy TRS-80 Educational Grants Program, 45-46
see funding sources
Task analysis, 20
see phases of microcomputer implementation
Teleconferencing, 14, 27
Template matching, 113
see speech recognition
The computer teaching program, 201-208
diagram of the CAI, 208
expanded CAI features, 201-208
making a CAI program, 201-208
outline of CAI teaching program, 205-208
simulation problems: CAI, 205
The microcomputer teacher concept, 193-197
see computer assisted instruction
Therapy programs, 162-165
Throughput, 82
Trace Center, 12, 30
Training sources, 75
Trends in instructional use and developments for CAI, 14-16, 213-215
Trends in microcomputer technology
decreasing component cost, 12, 264-265, 270
see costs
decreasing component size, 12
increasing reliability, 13
professional implications, 13-14
see issues
Turnkey software, 139
see ease of use
Types of secondary memory, 82, 86, 96-98
see core memory

U

Usability, 133-135
command structure, software, 3, 135
see software selection criteria
error trapping, 134-135
see software selection criteria
User friendly, 134, 212-213
see usability
User friendly instruction, 212-213
User's groups, 14, 70-72
locating user's groups, 70-72, 76
Utilities software, 81, 126

see systems software

V

Vertical applications software, 222-223
see custom applications
Video disks, 98
see secondary memory
Views of microcomputers, 260-263

W

Word processing, 166, 190-191, 240-244
administrative applications, 243-244
clinical applications, 244
see packaged software
functions, 240-244
Write enabled disks, 97
Write protected disks, 97